Epilepsy in Children and Adolescents

Epilepsy in Children and Adolescents

Edited by
James W. Wheless, MD
Department of Pediatric Neurology
University of Tennessee Health Science Center
Le Bonheur Comprehensive Epilepsy
Program and Neuroscience Institute
Le Bonheur Children's Hospital
Memphis, TN, USA

WILEY-BLACKWELL
A John Wiley & Sons, Ltd., Publication

This edition first published 2013 © 2013 by John Wiley & Sons, Ltd

Wiley-Blackwell is an imprint of John Wiley & Sons, formed by the merger of Wiley's global Scientific, Technical and Medical business with Blackwell Publishing.

Registered office: John Wiley & Sons, Ltd, The Atrium, Southern Gate, Chichester, West Sussex, PO19 8SQ, UK

Editorial offices: 9600 Garsington Road, Oxford, OX4 2DQ, UK
The Atrium, Southern Gate, Chichester, West Sussex, PO19 8SQ, UK
111 River Street, Hoboken, NJ 07030-5774, USA

For details of our global editorial offices, for customer services and for information about how to apply for permission to reuse the copyright material in this book please see our website at www.wiley.com/wiley-blackwell.

Library of Congress Cataloging-in-Publication Data

Epilepsy in children and adolescents / [edited by] James W. Wheless.
p. ; cm.
Includes bibliographical references and index.
ISBN 978-0-470-74123-8 (cloth)
I. Wheless, James.
[DNLM: 1. Epilepsy. 2. Adolescent. 3. Anticonvulsants–therapeutic use. 4. Child.
5. Epilepsy–therapy. WL 385]
616.85′300835–dc23

2012024368

A catalogue record for this book is available from the British Library.

Wiley also publishes its books in a variety of electronic formats. Some content that appears in print may not be available in electronic books.

Cover image: 4 year old with Lennox-Gastaut Syndrome, slow spike and wave complexes in sleep, courtesy of Dr James W. Wheless.

Set in 10/12pt Times by Aptara Inc., New Delhi, India
Printed and bound in Singapore by Markono Print Media Pte Ltd

First Impression 2013

Contents

List of contributors

Matthew Byrne, BA
Uniformed Services
University of the Health Sciences
Bethesda, MD
USA

Asim F. Choudhri, MD
Departments of Radiology and Neurosurgery
University of Tennessee Health Science Center
Le Bonheur Children's Hospital
Memphis, TN
USA

David F. Clarke, MBBS, ABPN (Child Neurology and Sleep), ABCN
Dell Children's Comprehensive Epilepsy Program
Dell Children's Medical Center of Central Texas
Austin, TX
USA

Susan E. Combs, MD
Department of Neurology
Children's National Medical Center
The George Washington University School of Medicine
Washington, DC
USA

Dewi Frances T. Depositario-Cabacar, MD
Neurology and Pediatrics
George Washington University Medical Center
Children's National Medical Center
Washington, DC
USA

Georgann Ferrone, MD
Center for Neuroscience and Behavioral Medicine
Children's National Medical Center
Washington, DC
USA

Stephen Fulton, MD
Department of Neurology and Pediatrics
University of Tennessee Health Science Center
LeBonheur Comprehensive Epilepsy Program
Le Bonheur Children's Hospital
Memphis, TN
USA

Marie Francisca Grill, MD
Department of Neurology
University of California San Francisco
San Francisco General Hospital
San Francisco, CA
USA

Eric V. Hastriter, MD
Mayo Clinic Hospital
Phoenix, AZ
USA

David T. Hsieh, MD
San Antonio Military Medical Center
Division of Child Neurology
Wilford Hall Medical Center
Lackland AFB, TX
USA

Sucheta M. Joshi, MD, MS
Pediatrics and Communicable Diseases
Division of Pediatric Neurology
University of Michigan
Ann Arbor, MI
USA

Karen Keough, MD
'Specially For Children'
Austin, TX
USA

Susan Koh, MD
Children's Hospital Colorado
Aurora, CO
USA

Rama Maganti, MD
Department of Neurology
Barrow Neurological Institute
St Joseph's
Hospital and Medical Center
Phoenix, AZ
USA

William McClintock, MD
Neurology and Pediatrics
George Washington University Medical Center
Children's National Medical Center
Washington, DC
USA

Amy L. McGregor, MD
Department of Pediatrics
Division of Child Neurology
Le Bonheur Comprehensive Epilepsy Program
University of Tennessee Health Science Center
Memphis, TN
USA

Bhagwan Indur Moorjani, MD, FAAP, FAAN
Hope Neurologic Center, La Quinta
JFK Memorial Hospital
Indio, CA
USA

Yu-Tze Ng, MD, FRACP
University of Oklahoma
Health Science Center and The Children's Hospital
Pediatric Neurology
Oklahoma city, OK
USA

Kristen Park, MD
Children's Hospital Colorado
Aurora, CO
USA

Phillip L. Pearl, MD
Department of Neurology
Children's National Medical Center
The George Washington University School of Medicine
Washington, DC
USA

Freedom F. Perkins Jr, MD
Seton Healthcare and Dell Children's Hospital
Austin, TX
USA

Tom Reehal, BA
University of Sheffield School of Medicine Dentistry and Health
Sheffield
UK

Jay Salpekar, MD
Center for Neuroscience and Behavioral Medicine
Children's National Medical Center
Washington, DC
USA

Kate Van Poppel, MD
Department of Pediatric Neurology
University of Tennessee Health Science Center
Le Bonheur Comprehensive Epilepsy Program and Neuroscience Institute
Le Bonheur Children's Hospital
Memphis, TN
USA

James W. Wheless, MD, FAAP, FACP, FAAN
Department of Pediatric Neurology
University of Tennessee Health Science Center
Le Bonheur Comprehensive Epilepsy Program and Neuroscience Institute
Le Bonheur Children's Hospital
Memphis, TN
USA

Preface

Of all the neurological disorders that affect infants, children, and adolescents, epilepsy is a profound challenge for the patients, caregivers, and physicians and demands expertise to evaluate and treat. As with every illness, gathering a clinical history is an important first step in helping define the problem. However, remarkable improvements in our ability to image brain structures, define physiological patterns, and select medications has made the task of caring for the child with epilepsy more effective than in past years. I envision this book to be a resource for all physicians and other professionals taking care of children with seizures or epilepsy. The goal was for each chapter to be succint, so a physician confronted with a child who has seizures would have an efficient resource for answering questions and designing treatment. I thank the authors for their focus and persistence. I am ever mindful of the patients and their families who bear the challenge of epilepsy with courage. I have learned from them and am keenly aware of our responsibility to do the very best for their care.

James W. Wheless
Memphis, TN, USA
June, 2012

Preface

[illegible]

Section 1

Epidemiology and classification of childhood epilepsies

Phillip L. Pearl

1 Epidemiology and common comorbidities of epilepsy in childhood

Jay Salpekar[1], Matthew Byrne[2], and Georgann Ferrone[1]

[1]Center for Neuroscience and Behavioral Medicine, Children's National Medical Center, Washington, DC, USA
[2]Uniformed Services University of the Health Sciences, Bethesda, MD, USA

Epilepsy is a common illness in childhood, and the epidemiology has been well described. However, epilepsy is also complex and controversial in terms of optimal methods for diagnosis and treatment. Classification schemes for seizures have been refined over the years and improved treatment options have allowed better outcomes for children with epilepsy. Understanding of comorbidity, particularly psychiatric comorbidity, has also improved over recent years, yet in many cases it is difficult to resolve whether psychiatric illness is coincidental or associated with the underlying seizure disorder. This chapter addresses the incidence and prevalence of childhood epilepsy and strategies for identifying and managing common psychiatric comorbidities.

1.1 Epidemiology

An epileptic seizure is defined as the clinical manifestation of abnormal or excessive discharge of neurons in the brain [1]. Epilepsy is defined as recurrent seizures, specifically two or more seizures separated by 24 hours but within 18 months of one another [1,2]. This common consensus is based on observations that children who experience one seizure have

Epilepsy in Children and Adolescents, First Edition. Edited by James W. Wheless.

an approximately 50% chance of recurrence within 2 years [3,4]. It is important to note that febrile seizures are not included in most epidemiological studies of epilepsy.

Population-based studies concerning seizures and epilepsy have been done in numerous communities around the world. Although many international studies of prevalence are based on small communities, the results can be extrapolated to reflect wider regions of the world. In the United States, there are approximately 2.3 million people diagnosed with epilepsy, which reflects an incidence of approximately 1% of the population [5]. The pediatric population, however, has a higher prevalence of epilepsy; 4–10% of children will experience a seizure before the age of 16. Thus, a working knowledge of epilepsy is very important for primary and specialty clinicians in pediatrics, as well as for pediatric neurologists [6].

Terminology review

Incidence: The rate at which new cases of disease occur in a population during a given period of time.

Prevalence: The proportion of a population who have a disease during a given time period.

1.2 Incidence and prevalence

In the general population, the incidence of epilepsy is reported at between 40 and 70 cases per 100 000 [7]. The incidence of childhood epilepsy has been reported to be 82.2 per 100 000 children, markedly higher than that of the overall population [8]. A meta-analysis of over 40 epidemiological studies found that the highest incidence of epilepsy occurs in childhood and in the geriatric population. Interestingly, the incidence of epilepsy has been decreasing over the past 50 years. This decrease in incidence could be explained by more stringent and/or universally followed diagnostic criteria or perhaps from a decrease in exposure to epilepsy risk factors [8].

The overall number of children affected by epilepsy, or the prevalence of the disease, is higher than the incidence because of the chronic nature of epilepsy. A significant variation in prevalence is found in international epidemiology studies [9–12]. In the United States, epilepsy prevalence averages 3.83 per 1000 children, while in northern Tanzania, it is 7.39 per 1000 [13,14]. This discrepancy may result from a variety of factors including possible misclassification of a single seizure as epilepsy. Environmental factors, access to healthcare, and different methods of reporting may also account for some of the variability. The prevalence of epilepsy in varying regions across the world is described in Table 1.1.

1.3 Gender and age

Studies have consistently found that males are diagnosed with epilepsy more often than females [18]. While the difference between the genders is slight, this trend holds true for most populations [13]. Although there are exceptions to this trend, they are rarely statistically significant in children [10,11]. Analysis of prevalence among children of varying ages found that epilepsy was most common in children under the age of 5, with a gradual decline

Table 1.1 International epidemiology studies.

Location	Years of study	Epilepsy prevalence	Age range	Limits/comments
Okayama Prefecture, Japan [9]	1999	5.3 per 1000	0–12 years	Removed data resulting from only one seizure
Kayenta, Shiprock, and Crowpoint Reservations, Navajo Nation, USA [10]	1999–2002	6.46 per 1000	0–19 years	Only those who went to hospital; excluded those who used tribal medicine
Hordaland count, western Norway [12]	1995	5.13 per 1000	6–12 years	Small sample area, limited age range
Northern Tanzania (14)	2003–2004	7.39 per 1000	0–19 years	Only villages polled around centralized hospital location
Rochester, Minnesota [13]	1950–1980	3.83 per 1000	0–14 years	Very comprehensive
Estonia [15,16]	1995–1997	3.7 per 1000	0–19 years	Much of data came from one hospital, University of Tartu
Canada [17]	1994–2001	2.5 per 1000	0–11 years	Utilized national census data
		4.4 per 1000	12–14 years	

in occurrence in older age groups [15]. Figure 1.1 demonstrates the peak of prevalence at a young age and a gradual decrease in children as they age.

1.4 Classification

When studying the epidemiology of epilepsy, means of classification must be clarified to ensure uniformity in standards. Since 1909, the International League Against Epilepsy

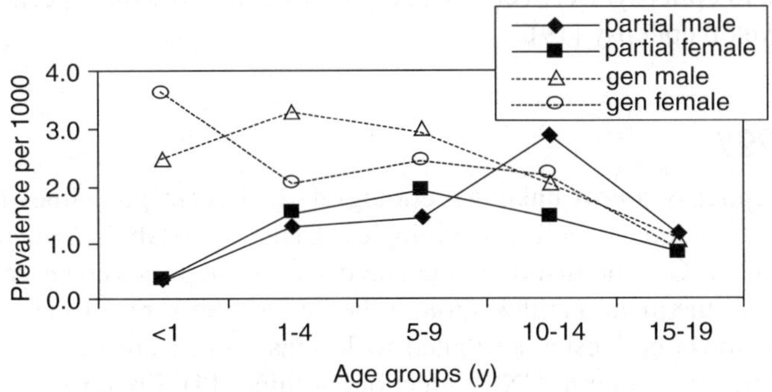

Figure 1.1 Graph showing prevalence of epilepsy (per 1000) in children by year from age 1 to 19 [16].

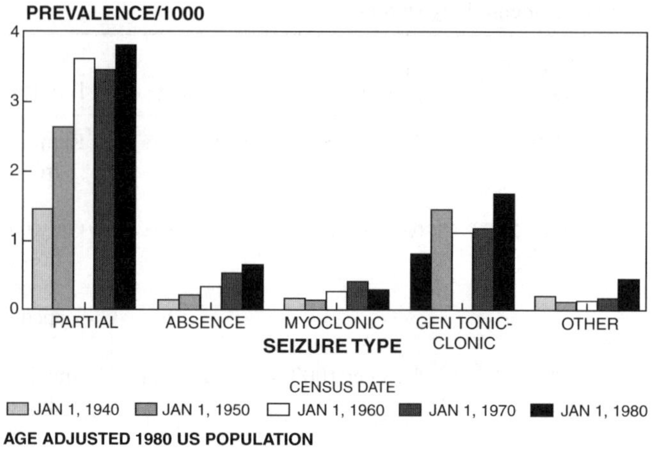

Figure 1.2 Bar graph of relative prevalence of adolescent seizure etiologies (per 1000) [13].

(ILAE) has worked toward identifying, studying, and classifying all variations of seizure disorders. Epilepsy syndromes can be classified as localization-related or generalized. The syndromes are determined by multiple criteria, with particular emphasis on seizure type as well as associated patient characteristics such as age of onset, comorbidities including neurodevelopmental status, presence of associated family history, and identification of an underlying etiology [1]. Distinguishing characteristics of seizure types can range from loss or modification of consciousness and responsiveness, along with total or partial motor control impairment [2].

A 40-year detailed study done in Rochester, Minnesota, found that partial seizures are the most prevalent, followed by generalized tonic-clonic, absence, and then myoclonic. Details for prevalence are represented in Figure 1.2 [13].

1.5 Febrile seizures

Febrile seizures are a common seizure disorder for children under the age of 3 years. Between 2% and 4% of children will suffer from one febrile seizure, and only one-third of these children will have a second seizure [18]. Most importantly, a febrile seizure will not always lead to epilepsy. Between 2% and 10% of children who experience one febrile seizure will develop epilepsy [19].

1.6 Etiology

Most cases of epilepsy are of unknown etiology [12]. Recent guidelines have identified three main classifications of epilepsy etiologies: Genetic, metabolic/structural, and idiopathic/unknown [2]. Genetic disorders include diseases due to a known genetic defect in which seizures are the main manifestation of the disease. Seizures of metabolic/structural etiology can be those epilepsies attributed to lesions, which are often a result of head trauma, central nervous system (CNS) infection, or tumor [4]. Epilepsy of unknown etiology represents the most common designation for epilepsy in childhood.

1.7 Psychiatric comorbidity

Psychiatric and psychological complications are commonly associated with pediatric epilepsy [20–23]. In pediatrics, the classic Isle of Wight epidemiology study reports psychiatric illness present in 16% of patients with chronic medical illness; however, if that illness happened to be epilepsy, the psychiatric comorbidity was 29% [24]. Subsequent studies have confirmed an overrepresentation of psychiatric illness associated with epilepsy as compared to many other chronic medical illnesses. Some studies report a two- or three-fold greater prevalence of psychiatric illness associated with epilepsy as compared to diabetes or asthma [25,26]. Of particular concern is evidence showing an overrepresentation of epilepsy among children and adolescents hospitalized for suicide attempts [27]. Despite numerous reports confirming high levels of comorbidity, many children and adolescents with epilepsy do not receive treatment for psychiatric illness [28]. In many cases, the psychiatric comorbidity may be more impairing to quality of life for children and families than the seizures themselves [29].

This consistently high level of psychiatric comorbidity suggests that epilepsy is a complicated illness that may have neuropsychiatric symptoms well beyond discrete seizures. However, the etiology of psychiatric comorbidity in children and adolescents with epilepsy is still controversial. Psychiatric illness may be difficult to isolate as an independent disorder in the context of seizure events. Some symptoms may be clearly related to ictal or postictal phenomena, but more often, psychiatric symptoms occur during interictal time periods and may be viewed as only indirectly related to epilepsy pathophysiology [30]. Classic views of forced normalization, in which psychiatric symptoms increase when the epilepsy stabilizes (the EEG "normalizes"), complicate conceptualization of comorbidity in relation to epilepsy pathophysiology [31]. Nevertheless, the frequent occurrence of psychiatric disorder has raised awareness of the need for an interdisciplinary approach to management of epilepsy [32,33]. The existing literature tends to focus upon one of three potential explanations for psychiatric comorbidity: symptoms related to psychosocial stress of chronic disease; symptoms related to medication side effects; and symptoms directly related to epilepsy pathophysiology.

1.8 Psychological and psychosocial stress related to chronic disease

Studies of health-related quality of life consistently report marked psychosocial stress for children and families [34]. Because seizures may involve sudden loss of consciousness and social embarrassment, epilepsy may be expected to carry a higher level of psychosocial sequelae. The disruption to the quality of life may be significant, as is the potential stigmatization of the child suffering publicly witnessed seizures [35]. Social difficulties are commonly reported among children with epilepsy, and lifestyle changes may occur among families, including limitations on activities and hindered development of social independence for the child facing the risk of spontaneous seizures [36]. Classroom teachers have reported discomfort in having a child with epilepsy in the classroom and favored increased restrictions upon the child's activity [37]. Children with epilepsy have been noted to have lower self-esteem, often associated with a negative attitude toward illness and a lack of a sense of control [38].

Although social stigma and stress related to chronic epilepsy are significant, many groups do not consider that these issues sufficiently account for the marked overrepresentation of psychiatric illness associated with epilepsy. One body of literature that is well developed is the study of "new-onset" epilepsy. By assessing patients early in their treatment course, the impact of psychosocial stress or treatment side effects leading to psychiatric dysfunction would be minimized. Psychiatric illness identified at "baseline" may be plausibly considered to result from underlying neurological disease rather than from the stress or stigma of chronic epilepsy. Well-designed studies with sibling controls identify high levels of anxiety and depression very early in the course of epilepsy [39]. Such anxiety and mood disorder cannot be attributed to a reactive depression resulting from the stress of chronic disease.

1.9 Psychiatric symptoms related to medication side effects

Studies of psychiatric side effects resulting from antiepileptic medication treatment are common, although few focus upon the pediatric population [40]. Although psychiatric and behavioral problems may potentially be associated with any medicine, the risk with some medicines has been more commonly reported. Phenobarbital has been well known to increase the possibility of depression, irritability, and disinhibition [41–43]. Irritability has also been associated with levetiracetam [44]. Impairments in short-term memory, verbal fluency, and cognitive processing speed have been reported with topiramate [45]. However, it should be noted that antiepileptic drugs are commonly used as primary treatments for psychiatric illness; many psychiatric symptoms may be improved by judicious selection of antiepileptic drugs. In some cases, psychiatric symptoms and seizures may be improved simultaneously by the same anticonvulsant medicine [46]. Behavioral symptoms may be misattributed as a side effect instead of representing a comorbid psychiatric illness that would be an appropriate target of anticonvulsant medicine.

Despite the association of some anticonvulsants with psychiatric symptoms, medication side effects may not account for the broad spectrum of psychiatric comorbidity present in children and adolescents with epilepsy. Recent studies in the new-onset population confirm that internalizing behavior problems such as depression or anxiety are commonly found prior to the start of antiepileptic treatment [47].

1.10 Psychiatric comorbidity related to epilepsy pathophysiology

Over the past decade, a paradigm shift has occurred such that epilepsy pathophysiology is considered to play a direct role in comorbid psychiatric illness. Many researchers and clinicians now consider that the impaired neural function related to epilepsy pathophysiology may directly cause behavioral and cognitive difficulties. In this sense, a structural lesion or seizure focus may concurrently cause epilepsy and psychiatric symptoms. It is possible that a transactional process occurs between psychiatric illness and epilepsy, in that one condition may aggravate or even precede exacerbations of the other [48]. Improved characterization of seizures has fueled speculation that specific seizure types or localizations in the brain may present higher risks of psychological or psychiatric complications. Although psychiatric comorbidity is understudied and conclusions are difficult to make given varying

Table 1.2 Common psychiatric comorbidities with epilepsy and their associated prevalence.

Psychiatric comorbidity	Prevalence
Attention-deficit/hyperactivity disorder (ADHD)	20–38% [50,51]
Anxiety	20–33% [59,60]
Depression	26–33% [60,61]
Intellectual and developmental disability (IDD)	10–33% [70,71]

methodology, some specific childhood psychiatric disorders have emerged as particularly associated with epilepsy (Table 1.2).

1.11 Attention-deficit/hyperactivity disorder (ADHD)

Attention-deficit/hyperactivity disorder is the most common psychiatric comorbidity associated with pediatric epilepsy; the prevalence ranges from 20% to 38% depending upon assessment methods and samples [49,50]. ADHD is described in terms of subtypes: primarily inattentive, primarily hyperactive or impulsive, and combined type. Symptoms of absence epilepsy may appear similar to ADHD-primarily inattentive subtype, and the latter is a common differential diagnosis for pediatric epileptologists [51]. One recent report suggests a bidirectional relationship such that ADHD increases risk for seizures and that more patients with epilepsy have ADHD [52]. A sizeable literature suggests that EEG spikes are found in children with ADHD though it is unclear whether they go on to develop frank epilepsy [53,54].

Case 1

M is an 8-year-old female who presents to her pediatrician after a referral from school. Despite seeming to be bright and capable, teachers note that she is frequently "off task" and inattentive. She occasionally has trouble organizing material and remembering to turn in completed worksheets. Several times a day, she does not respond when teachers call her name and ask her a question, though with prompting she will acknowledge the teacher. She is below grade level on academics despite coming from a highly educated family. She is described as a quiet child who is well-behaved and friendly, but at times seems distant and even confused. One incident was noted by a playground attendant when M stood motionless, almost "frozen" for about 10 seconds when it was time to line up to go back into the classroom. She is successful with many outside activities, including soccer, and she enjoys playing complex, strategy-based computer games. Physical exam was unremarkable.

Comment

The case of M illustrates the sometimes difficult differential diagnosis of absence epilepsy and ADHD-inattentive subtype. Sometimes absence seizures may appear as periods of inattention and are considered to be symptomatic of ADHD. ADHD is characterized by the presence of impairing symptoms in multiple settings, which often having academic and social sequelae. Careful history-taking will correctly place more emphasis upon the playground incident as evidence of disruption of consciousness. M also has interests and periods of intact functioning not characteristic of a child who is chronically inattentive. The astute pediatrician consulted a pediatric neurologist, who ordered an EEG that revealed generalized spike and wave discharges at a rate of 3 per second, consistent with absence epilepsy.

Case 2

J is a 7-year-old male with a 2-year history of partial complex seizures who presents to his pediatric neurologist with a chief complaint of disruptive behavior. He has been seizure free for 8 months on a stable dose of lamotrigine. J is described as always "on the go" from preschool age, and is unable to stay in any one place, including the dinner table, for more than 5 minutes. He will often get up out of his seat in school, and will disturb other students by talking to them or going to their desks while they are trying to complete their assignments. He has performed poorly in school because of not finishing assignments and losing textbooks and materials necessary for class. He is below grade level despite his teachers believing that he is very smart when he is focused. Two separate teachers completed an ADHD rating scale, which was overwhelmingly positive for hyperactivity, impulsivity, and inattention. He is forgetful and does not seem to listen when spoken to directly. His parents report that he is very hyperactive – much more than his two older brothers were at his age. They report trying behavioral strategies and counseling to no avail. Now they are exhausted and need help. Physical and neurological examination is unremarkable.

Comment

The case of J illustrates a typical case of comorbid epilepsy and ADHD. Confidence in the diagnosis of ADHD is paramount to treatment planning, and clinicians should seek corroborating information from several sources. Historically, clinicians have been hesitant to use stimulant medication in children with epilepsy for fear of exacerbating seizures. However, several recent studies report that stimulants are well tolerated and effective for patients with stable epilepsy, defined as less than one seizure per month [55–57]. Given that alternative management strategies have been attempted without success, J was given sustained-release methylphenidate, and within 2 weeks showed marked improvement in attention span and impulse control. The parents are grateful.

1.12 Anxiety

Anxiety is a common feature in pediatric epilepsy. Anticipatory anxiety regarding possible seizure events is often present to some extent though it may not rise to the level of a formal psychiatric illness. Social anxiety symptoms such as isolation and fear of being in public places are often noted. Anxiety is also notable as an experiential phenomenon in patients with temporal lobe seizure foci, especially amygdalar foci. Sensations of fear or anxiety may occur in the context of a seizure aura or throughout the ictal period. Several studies note anxiety disorder prevalence ranging from 20% to 33% by using either structured psychiatric interviews or validated rating scales [58,59].

Case 3

D is 13-year-old female with a history of complex partial seizures and secondary generalization. She has a 5-year history of epilepsy, and has had three seizures over the past 6 months, usually in the context of a viral illness. She has been stable with levetiracetam. She had a generalized seizure in school approximately 6 weeks ago in Physical Education class, and was brought to the emergency room. Her parents have brought her to the pediatric neurologist because since that time she complains of feeling dizzy. She had to come home from school twice last week because of the dizzy feeling. The dizziness does not occur at home or when she visits her grandmother's house. Physical examination is unremarkable, as is the MRI scan, EKG, and chemical and hematological studies. The parents are worried that this is a medication side effect, and want to switch medications.

Comment

After the neurologist is satisfied that the medical and neurological status is at baseline, consideration of a psychiatric or psychological stressor should occur. Publicly witnessed seizures are stressful for adolescents and may have long-lasting impact upon social function. The neurologist referred D to a clinical social worker for psychotherapy. Within several weeks, the social worker helped her process her anxiety regarding having recurrent seizures, and the dizziness resolved. Treatment focus included helping her discuss epilepsy with close friends. The neurologist provided educational materials to the school nurse, who provides periodic check-ins with the patient during the school day.

1.13 Depression

Depression is a particularly worrisome comorbidity of pediatric epilepsy. Pediatric studies are uncommon, but recent reports found a prevalence of depression ranging from 26% to 33% [58,60]. Suicidal ideation has been reported to be several-fold higher than in patients without epilepsy [61]. Suicide has been reported as responsible for 10% of deaths in adults with epilepsy as compared to 1% in the general population [62]. A recent report suggests that seizures with a temporal lobe focus may lead to a higher risk for depression [63]. Recent precautions from the US Food and Drug Administration (FDA) have raised concern about antiepileptic drugs as a class leading to increased risk of suicidal thoughts and behaviors. However, this risk has not been isolated independent of comorbidity of depression [64,65]. Clinicians are well advised to screen for depression in children and adolescents with epilepsy.

Case 4

R is a 15-year-old male with a history of complex partial seizures with a left temporal lobe focus since age 9. He presents to his pediatric neurologist for a routine follow-up visit. He has been taking topiramate for 3 years with fair result, although he has seizures approximately every 3 months. Over the past 6 months, his parents have noted a significant departure from his usual function. He has lost interest in seeing his friends or participating in organized youth group activities. He often skips meals, and says he just does not feel hungry. His academic performance has worsened and he often skips assignments. He has an unhappy expression on his face, and usually goes to his room and sleeps, often going to bed at 7 pm. A week ago, he told his parents that he had no reason to live. The parents are concerned that this is a medication side effect.

Comment

Depression may have an insidious onset, and often builds very gradually. Some reports state that seizure focus in the temporal lobe yields a higher risk for depression, but results are inconsistent, and pediatric studies are uncommon [66–68]. R demonstrates worrisome symptoms, particularly given his hopelessness and thoughts of death. He is promptly referred to a pediatric psychiatrist, who initiates treatment with fluoxetine. After a few weeks he has more energy and is more engaged socially and academically.

1.14 Intellectual and developmental disabilities (IDD)

The presence of epilepsy in children with IDD ranges from 10% to 30% depending on how the diagnosis of autism is made. Some groups report that complex partial seizures and temporal lobe EEG abnormalities may be particularly common with autism [69,70]. There are some cases of improved behavior and cognition in autistic children treated with antiepileptic drugs [71,72].

1.15 Conclusion

Epilepsy is a complex medical condition that has a high prevalence in pediatrics. Psychiatric comorbidity is very common and in some cases may be more debilitating than the seizure disorder itself. The etiology of psychiatric comorbidity is still difficult to resolve, but interdisciplinary management from both neurology and psychiatry is well indicated for many patients with epilepsy and psychiatric comorbidity. Although the evidence base is limited regarding treatment for the most common comorbidities of ADHD, depression, anxiety, and IDD, strategies are similar to those utilized for patients without epilepsy. Future studies will improve understanding of the relationship between psychiatric illness and specific epilepsy types. Ultimately, treatment outcome studies are needed in order to minimize morbidity related to psychiatric illness and to maximize quality of life for children and adolescents with epilepsy.

References

[1] ILAE Commission Report. The epidemiology of the epilepsies: future directions. International League Against Epilepsy. *Epilepsia* 1997;**38**:614–618.
[2] Berg AT, Samuel F, Berkovic M, *et al. Revised Terminology and Concepts for Organization of the Epilepsies: Report of the Commission on Classification and Terminology*. International League Against Epilepsy, 2009.
[3] Various. Proceedings and abstracts of the Canadian League Against Epilepsy 2007 Conference. *Can J Neurol Sci* 2009;**36**(Suppl. 2):S1–106.
[4] Berg AT. Risk of recurrence after a first unprovoked seizure. *Epilepsia* 2008;**49**(Suppl. 1):13–18.
[5] Hirtz D, Thurman DJ, Gwinn-Hardy K, Mohamed M, Chaudhuri AR, Zalutsky R. How common are the "common" neurologic disorders? *Neurology* 2007;**68**:326–337.
[6] McAbee GN, Wark JE. A practical approach to uncomplicated seizures in children. *Am Fam Physician* 2000;**62**:1109–1116.
[7] Sander JW, Shorvon SD. Epidemiology of the epilepsies. *J Neurol Neurosurg Psychiatry* 1996;**61**:433–443.
[8] Kotsopoulos IA, van Merode T, Kessels FG, de Krom MC, Knottnerus JA. Systematic review and meta-analysis of incidence studies of epilepsy and unprovoked seizures. *Epilepsia* 2002;**43**:1402–1409.
[9] Oka E, Ohtsuka Y, Yoshinaga H, Murakami N, Kobayashi K, Ogino T. Prevalence of childhood epilepsy and distribution of epileptic syndromes: a population-based survey in Okayama, Japan. *Epilepsia* 2006;**47**:626–630.
[10] Parko K, Thurman DJ. Prevalence of epilepsy and seizures in the Navajo Nation 1998–2002. *Epilepsia* 2009;**50**:2180–2185.
[11] Jones JE, Watson R, Sheth R, *et al.* Psychiatric comorbidity in children with new onset epilepsy. *Dev Med Child Neurol* 2007;**49**:493–497.
[12] Hoie B, Sommerfelt K, Waaler PE, Alsaker FD, Skeidsvoll H, Mykletun A. The combined burden of cognitive, executive function, and psychosocial problems in children with epilepsy: a population-based study. *Dev Med Child Neurol* 2008;**50**:530–536.
[13] Hauser WA, Annegers JF, Kurland LT. Prevalence of epilepsy in Rochester, Minnesota: 1940–1980. *Epilepsia* 1991;**32**:429–445.
[14] Winkler AS, Kerschbaumsteiner K, Stelzhammer B, Meindl M, Kaaya J, Schmutzhard E. Prevalence, incidence, and clinical characteristics of epilepsy: A community-based door-to-door study in northern Tanzania. *Epilepsia* 2009;**50**:2310–2313.
[15] Kolk A, Beilmann A, Tomberg T, Napa A, Talvik T. Neurocognitive development of children with congenital unilateral brain lesion and epilepsy. *Brain Dev* 2001;**23**:88–96.
[16] Beilmann A, Napa A, Soot A, Talvik I, Talvik T. Prevalence of childhood epilepsy in Estonia. *Epilepsia* 1999;**40**:1011–1019.
[17] Tellez-Zenteno JF, Pondal-Sordo M, Matijevic S, Wiebe S. National and regional prevalence of self-reported epilepsy in Canada. *Epilepsia* 2004;**45**:1623–1629.
[18] Hauser WA. The prevalence and incidence of convulsive disorders in children. *Epilepsia* 1994;**35**(Suppl. 2):S1–6.
[19] Shinnar S, Pellock JM. Update on the epidemiology and prognosis of pediatric epilepsy. *J Child Neurol* 2002;**17**(Suppl. 1):S4–17.
[20] Pellock JM. Understanding co-morbidities affecting children with epilepsy. *Neurology* 2004;**62**(5 Suppl. 2):S17–23.
[21] Dunn DW. Neuropsychiatric aspects of epilepsy in children. *Epilepsy Behav* 2003;**4**:101–106.
[22] Salpekar JA, Dunn DW. Psychiatric and psychosocial consequences of pediatric epilepsy. *Semin Pediatr Neurol* 2007;**14**:181–188.
[23] Plioplys S, Dunn DW, Caplan R. 10-year research update review: psychiatric problems in children with epilepsy. *J Am Acad Child Adolesc Psychiatry* 2007;**46**:1389–1402.

[24] Rutter M, Graham P, Yule WA. *A Neuropsychiatric Study in Childhood.* Philadelphia: JP Lippincott, 1970.

[25] Austin JK, Huster GA, Dunn DW, Risinger MW. Adolescents with active or inactive epilepsy or asthma: a comparison of quality of life. *Epilepsia* 1996;**37**:1228–1238.

[26] Hoare P. The development of psychiatric disorder among schoolchildren with epilepsy. *Dev Med Child Neurol* 1984;**26**:3–13.

[27] Brent DA. Overrepresentation of epileptics in a consecutive series of suicide attempters seen at a children's hospital, 1978–1983. *J Am Acad Child Psychiatry* 1986;**25**:242–246.

[28] Ott D, Siddarth P, Gurbani S, *et al.* Behavioral disorders in pediatric epilepsy: unmet psychiatric need. *Epilepsia* 2003;**44**:591–597.

[29] Cushner-Weinstein S, Dassoulas K, Salpekar JA, *et al.* Parenting stress and childhood epilepsy: the impact of depression, learning, and seizure-related factors. *Epilepsy Behav* 2008;**13**:109–114.

[30] Austin JK, Dunn DW. Progressive behavioral changes in children with epilepsy. *Prog Brain Res* 2002;**135**:419–427.

[31] Krishnamoorthy ES, Trimble MR, Sander JW, Kanner AM. Forced normalization at the interface between epilepsy and psychiatry. *Epilepsy Behav* 2002;**3**:303–308.

[32] Kanner AM, Palac S. Neuropsychiatric complications of epilepsy. *Curr Neurol Neurosci Rep* 2002;**2**:365–372.

[33] Goldstein J, Plioplys S, Zelko F, *et al.* Multidisciplinary approach to childhood epilepsy: exploring the scientific rationale and practical aspects of implementation. *J Child Neurol* 2004;**19**:362–378.

[34] Ronen GM, Streiner DL, Rosenbaum P. Health-related quality of life in childhood epilepsy: Moving beyond 'seizure control with minimal adverse effects'. *Health Qual Life Outcomes* 2003;**1**:36.

[35] MacLeod JS, Austin JK. Stigma in the lives of adolescents with epilepsy: a review of the literature. *Epilepsy Behav* 2003;**4**:112–117.

[36] Williams J, Steel C, Sharp GB, *et al.* Parental anxiety and quality of life in children with epilepsy. *Epilepsy Behav* 2003;**4**:483–486.

[37] Baumann RJ, Wilson JF, Wiese HJ. Kentuckians' attitudes toward children with epilepsy. *Epilepsia* 1995;**36**:1003–1008.

[38] Dunn DW, Austin JK, Huster GA. Symptoms of depression in adolescents with epilepsy. *J Am Acad Child Adolesc Psychiatry* 1999;**38**:1132–1138.

[39] Austin JK, Dunn DW, Caffrey HM, Perkins SM, Harezlak J, Rose DF. Recurrent seizures and behavior problems in children with first recognized seizures: a prospective study. *Epilepsia* 2002;**43**:1564–1573.

[40] Loring DW, Marino S, Meador KJ. Neuropsychological and behavioral effects of antiepilepsy drugs. *Neuropsychol Rev* 2007;**17**:413–425.

[41] Devinsky O. Cognitive and behavioral effects of antiepileptic drugs. *Epilepsia* 1995;**36**(Suppl. 2):S46–65.

[42] Robertson MM, Trimble MR, Townsend HR. Phenomenology of depression in epilepsy. *Epilepsia* 1987;**28**:364–372.

[43] Brent DA, Crumrine PK, Varma R, Brown RV, Allan MJ. Phenobarbital treatment and major depressive disorder in children with epilepsy: a naturalistic follow-up. *Pediatrics* 1990;**85**:1086–1091.

[44] Dinkelacker V, Dietl T, Widman G, Lengler U, Elger CE. Aggressive behavior of epilepsy patients in the course of levetiracetam add-on therapy: report of 33 mild to severe cases. *Epilepsy Behav* 2003;**4**:537–547.

[45] de Araujo Filho GM, Pascalicchio TF, Lin K, Sousa PS, Yacubian EM. Neuropsychiatric profiles of patients with juvenile myoclonic epilepsy treated with valproate or topiramate. *Epilepsy Behav* 2006;**8**:606–609.

[46] Salpekar JA, Conry JA, Doss W, *et al.* Clinical experience with anticonvulsant medication in pediatric epilepsy and comorbid bipolar spectrum disorder. *Epilepsy Behav* 2006;**9**: 327–334.

[47] Dunn DW, Austin JK, Caffrey HM, Perkins SM. A prospective study of teachers' ratings of behavior problems in children with new-onset seizures. *Epilepsy Behav* 2003;**4**:26–35.

[48] Kanner AM. The behavioral aspects of epilepsy: an overview of controversial issues. *Epilepsy Behav* 2001;**2**:8–12.

[49] Hermann B, Jones J, Dabbs K, *et al.* The frequency, complications and aetiology of ADHD in new onset paediatric epilepsy. *Brain* 2007;**130**:3135–3148.

[50] Dunn DW, Austin JK, Harezlak J, Ambrosius WT. ADHD and epilepsy in childhood. *Dev Med Child Neurol* 2003;**45**:50–54.

[51] Williams J, Griebel ML, Sharp GB, *et al.* Differentiating between seizures and attention deficit hyperactivity disorder (ADHD) in a pediatric population. *Clin Pediatr (Phila)* 2002;**41**:565–568.

[52] Hamoda HM, Guild DJ, Gumlak S, Travers BH, Gonzalez-Heydrich J. Association between attention-deficit/hyperactivity disorder and epilepsy in pediatric populations. *Expert Rev Neurother* 2009;**9**:1747–1754.

[53] Hughes JR, DeLeo AJ, Melyn MA. The electroencephalogram in attention deficit-hyperactivity disorder: emphasis on epileptiform discharges. *Epilepsy Behav* 2000;**1**:271–277.

[54] Holtmann M, Becker K, Kentner-Figura B, Schmidt MH. Increased frequency of rolandic spikes in ADHD children. *Epilepsia* 2003;**44**:1241–1244.

[55] Gross-Tsur V, Manor O, van der Meere J, Joseph A, Shalev RS. Epilepsy and attention deficit hyperactivity disorder: is methylphenidate safe and effective? *J Pediatr* 1997;**130**:670–674.

[56] Gucuyener K, Erdemoglu AK, Senol S, Serdaroglu A, Soysal S, Kockar AI. Use of methylphenidate for attention-deficit hyperactivity disorder in patients with epilepsy or electroencephalographic abnormalities. *J Child Neurol* 2003;**18**:109–112.

[57] Baptista-Neto L, Dodds A, Rao S, Whitney J, Torres A, Gonzalez-Heydrich J. An expert opinion on methylphenidate treatment for attention deficit hyperactivity disorder in pediatric patients with epilepsy. *Expert Opin Investig Drugs* 2008;**17**:77–84.

[58] Caplan R, Siddarth P, Gurbani S, Hanson R, Sankar R, Shields WD. Depression and anxiety disorders in pediatric epilepsy. *Epilepsia* 2005;**46**:720–730.

[59] Williams J, Steel C, Sharp GB, *et al.* Anxiety in children with epilepsy. *Epilepsy Behav* 2003;**4**:729–732.

[60] Ettinger AB, Weisbrot DM, Nolan EE, *et al.* Symptoms of depression and anxiety in pediatric epilepsy patients. *Epilepsia* 1998;**39**:595–599.

[61] Plioplys S. Depression in children and adolescents with epilepsy. *Epilepsy Behav* 2003; **4**(Suppl. 3):S39–45.

[62] Jones JE, Hermann BP, Barry JJ, Gilliam FG, Kanner AM, Meador KJ. Rates and risk factors for suicide, suicidal ideation, and suicide attempts in chronic epilepsy. *Epilepsy Behav* 2003;**4**(Suppl. 3):S31–8.

[63] Verrotti A, Cicconetti A, Scorrano B, *et al.* Epilepsy and suicide: pathogenesis, risk factors, and prevention. *Neuropsychiatr Dis Treat* 2008;**4**:365–370.

[64] Gangwisch JE, Jacobson CM. New perspectives on assessment of suicide risk. *Curr Treat Options Neurol* 2009;**11**:371–376.

[65] Hesdorffer DC, Kanner AM. The FDA alert on suicidality and antiepileptic drugs: Fire or false alarm? *Epilepsia* 2009;**50**:978–986.

[66] Sanchez-Gistau V, Pintor L, Sugranyes G, *et al.* Prevalence of interictal psychiatric disorders in patients with refractory temporal and extratemporal lobe epilepsy in Spain. A comparative study. *Epilepsia* 2010;**51**:1309–1313.

[67] Schmitz B. Depression and mania in patients with epilepsy. *Epilepsia* 2005;**46**(Suppl. 4):45–49.

[68] Richardson EJ, Griffith HR, Martin RC, *et al.* Structural and functional neuroimaging correlates of depression in temporal lobe epilepsy. *Epilepsy Behav* 2007;**10**:242–249.

[69] Tharp BR. Epileptic encephalopathies and their relationship to developmental disorders: do spikes cause autism? *Ment Retard Dev Disabil Res Rev* 2004;**10**:132–134.
[70] Ballaban-Gil K, Tuchman R. Epilepsy and epileptiform EEG: association with autism and language disorders. *Ment Retard Dev Disabil Res Rev* 2000;**6**:300–308.
[71] Hollander E, Dolgoff-Kaspar R, Cartwright C, Rawitt R, Novotny S. An open trial of divalproex sodium in autism spectrum disorders. *J Clin Psychiatry* 2001;**62**:530–534.
[72] Di Martino A, Tuchman RF. Antiepileptic drugs: affective use in autism spectrum disorders. *Pediatr Neurol* 2001;**25**:199–207.

2 Classification and definition of seizures and epilepsy syndromes in childhood

Susan E. Combs and Phillip L. Pearl

Department of Neurology, Children's National Medical Center, The George Washington University School of Medicine, Washington, DC, USA

2.1 Introduction

Seizures and epilepsy syndromes each require their own classification system, as seizures represent the cardinal clinical manifestation of epilepsy, while the epilepsies represent clinical conditions that are recognizable by a pattern of seizure characteristics in addition to a panoply of clinical features, ranging from neurodevelopmental status to age of onset, inheritance pattern, and prognosis. Hence, a working knowledge of the definitions and classification of both seizures and epilepsy is essential for the practicing physician.

2.2 Purpose and goals of definitions and classification

Rigorous diagnostic criteria and precision based on current evidence-based data allow accurate and objective distinction between different forms of seizures and epileptic syndromes, and are thus important for making informed decisions about management and therapy. Furthermore, using a defined and shared vocabulary facilitates communication and collaboration among clinicians, researchers, and patients. A classification scheme that elucidates

Epilepsy in Children and Adolescents, First Edition. Edited by James W. Wheless.

the common and unique characteristics of these diagnostic entities provides an organizational framework for seizures and syndromes. Criteria need to be explicit, objective, and specific enough to reproducibly distinguish one diagnostic entity from another.

Recent debate on the classification of seizures and epilepsy has recognized that a dynamic system must exist for ongoing clinical and research usefulness [1]. Classification systems may need to be customized for the purpose of presurgical evaluations or clinical trials. Epileptologists have argued for the creation of two separate entities – an empirically-based "diagnostic scheme" to guide traditional clinical management, and a "taxonomic system" based on known and developing pathophysiological mechanisms that defines distinct natural classes [1–3].

2.3 Systems of classification and definitions

The International League Against Epilepsy (ILAE) first published the International Classification of Epileptic Seizures (ICES) in 1981 [4] and a Classification of Epilepsies and Epileptic Syndromes in 1985 [5], followed by a revised classification of syndromes in 1989 [6]. Both the classification and descriptive terminology were primarily based on the localization of seizure activity and observed semiology. The 1981 seizure classification reflected data from the recently proliferated video-electroencephalography (EEG) technique, allowing simultaneous observation and thus description of both electrophysiological and semiological aspects of an ictal period [4].

The ILAE's 1981 seizure classification and the 1989 syndrome classification remained unchanged until 2010, when the organization published a revised terminology and concepts for organization of both seizures and epilepsies (Box 2.1) [7]. The revisions did not drastically alter the original classifications, but did change or remove some outdated and misleading terms, and included some new syndromes. The ongoing debate of specific classes and terms makes it difficult to significantly rework the accepted and widely used language and organization established in 1981 and 1989, but a general agreement exists that any modifications should reflect more evidence-based information. Rapid updates in the molecular biology of the epilepsies and advanced neuroimaging will mandate ongoing alterations to any existing classification system.

2.4 Seizures

An epileptic seizure is defined as "a transient occurrence of signs and/or symptoms due to abnormal excessive or synchronous neuronal activity in the brain." The three elements of this definition are the mode of seizure onset and termination, ictal clinical manifestations, and abnormal enhanced neuronal synchrony [8]. The mode of seizure onset refers to the area or areas of the brain that initiate the seizure activity. Clinical manifestations can include motor, sensory, or autonomic processes, as well as changes in consciousness, memory, emotional state, or behavior [8]. The 2010 ILAE Classification implemented a few major revisions to the prior system, but the original criteria remain useful.

Self-limited epileptic seizures can be separated into two distinct categories: generalized and focal (partial), based on the mode of seizure onset. The 1981 ILAE classification of epileptic seizures differentiated seizure types based on observed physical characteristics as well as electrographic data to determine whether seizure activity was initiated in one part of the brain or whether it involved multiple parts and/or both hemispheres [4]. Recent

Box 2.1 ILAE classification of seizures (2010) [7]

GENERALIZED SEIZURES

- Tonic-clonic
- Clonic
- Tonic
- Absence:
  - Typical
  - Atypical
  - With special features
- Myoclonic:
  - Myoclonic
  - Myoclonic atonic
  - Myoclonic tonic
- Atonic

FOCAL SEIZURES

UNKNOWN

- Epileptic spasms

discussions have emphasized that the terms generalized and partial/focal may be misleading, as generalized seizures may not involve the entire cortex, and focal seizures are not likely limited to a distinct neuronal focus, as the name suggests. In the 2010 report, the ILAE Commission updated and clarified the meaning of "generalized" and "focal" with reference to seizures, stating:

- *Generalized* epileptic seizures originate at some point within, and rapidly engage, bilaterally distributed networks [7].
- *Focal* epileptic seizures originate within networks limited to one hemisphere, which may be discretely localized or more widely distributed [7].

In addition, the ILAE 2010 report recognizes that both generalized and focal seizures may originate in subcortical structures.

Unclassified epileptic seizures have been redefined as seizures with an unclear mode of onset, a category that contains epileptic spasms (including infantile spasms). In contrast, neonatal seizures formerly comprised an entity separate from generalized and focal seizures, but they are now classified as having generalized, focal, or unknown onset.

2.5 Generalized seizures

Generalized seizures demonstrate bilateral ictal encephalographic patterns, but discharges can be asymmetric and the location or hemisphere of seizure onset is not consistent from seizure to seizure [7]. Different types of generalized seizures are characterized by the signs and movements observed. These types of movement include tonic, clonic, and myoclonic, and also atonia (Box 2.2).

Box 2.2 Definitions of ictal motor events used to describe seizures [9]

- **Myoclonic**: Sudden, brief (<100 ms) involuntary single or multiple contractions(s) of muscle(s) or muscle groups of variable topography (axial, proximal limb, distal).
- **Clonic**: Myoclonus that is regularly repetitive, involves the same muscle groups, at a frequency of ~2–3 cycles/s, and is prolonged.
- **Tonic**: A sustained increase in muscle contraction lasting a few seconds to minutes.
- **Atonic**: Sudden loss or diminution of muscle tome without apparent preceding myoclonic or tonic event lasting ≥1–2 s, involving head, trunk, jaw, or limb musculature.

Tonic-clonic seizures

Tonic-clonic seizures include both types of motor elements in some combination, frequently tonic-clonic or clonic-tonic-clonic. This class includes *generalized tonic-clonic seizures* (GTCS), commonly referred to as *grand mal*. GTCS are characterized by a bilateral symmetric tonic contraction followed by bilateral clonic contractions of somatic muscles [9]. GTCS are usually associated with autonomic phenomena including loss of consciousness or apnea.

Tonic seizures

Tonic seizures, often resembling the "ballet posture" with extension of the arms above the head, have a predilection to occur during sleep but, in wakefulness, may result in a fall. EEG characteristically shows a low-voltage, fast pattern (≥9–10 Hz) or simply diffuse attenuation of the EEG activity [4].

Clonic seizures

Clonic seizures involve repetitive muscle jerks, usually involving both sides of the body. They may resemble myoclonic seizures, but patients with clonic seizures often lose consciousness and the repetition rate is less rapid. The typical EEG profile of a clonic seizure is fast activity (≥10 Hz) and slow waves (e.g., polyspike and slow wave complexes) [4].

Myoclonic seizures

Myoclonic seizures consist of a single or series of muscle contractions that occur unilaterally or bilaterally in any muscle group. Negative myoclonus is the interruption of a sustained contraction (tonic activity) for <500 ms without evidence of preceding myoclonias [9]. EEG typically shows polyspike and wave complexes or, less frequently, spike and wave or sharp and slow wave complexes [4].

Myoclonic atonic seizures include a myoclonic jerk of axial muscles preceding atonia. This motor pattern typically causes a sudden fall, causing so-called falling seizures or drop attacks. EEG recordings show a spike and slow wave complex, where the spike occurs with the myoclonic jerk and the slow wave with the loss of tone [10]. Myoclonic atonic seizures were previously called myoclonic-astatic seizures, but were only recognized as a distinct natural class of seizure by the ILAE in 2010 [7].

Absence seizures

Transient impairment of consciousness is a hallmark characteristic of absence seizures. The subclasses of absence seizures include typical, atypical, and absence with special features.

Typical absence seizures

These have two primary features:

- transient period of impaired consciousness;
- 2.5–4.5 Hz spike-and-slow wave or polyspike and slow wave complexes [11,12].

Typical absence seizures have abrupt onset and recovery, wherein the patient suddenly becomes unresponsive, appears to have a blank gaze, and then snaps back to consciousness. Though some children present without any additional semiology, in "typical absence" seizures, most patients demonstrate additional motor manifestations [13], including:

- *Clonic components* – typically mild twitching of eyelids, eyebrows, and mouth.
- *Atonic components* – decrease in muscle tone causing head drop, torso slump, loss of grip, but rarely falls.
- *Tonic components* – eyes and head roll back, truncal arching.
- *Automatisms* – repetitive, seemingly intentional movements, e.g. lip-smacking, swallowing, walking.

Patients may exhibit more than one of these components in a seizure or from seizure to seizure. Though the 1981 ILAE classification included these different presentations as independent seizure types, they are better used as descriptors of seizures rather than distinct taxonomic classes. This idea is reflected in the simplified, revised ILAE classification [7] (Table 2.1).

Atypical absence seizures

The two most common divergences from typical absence seizures that are labeled atypical are:

- more profound change in muscle tone (either tonic or atonic);
- more gradual or progressive initiation and conclusion of the seizure episode.

Atypical absence seizures frequently include the same motor events as typical absence, but these movements are more pronounced; for example, severe atonia may cause the patient to fall from a standing position. Patients with atypical absence seizures frequently have altered mental function, and their loss and gain of consciousness is not as abrupt as patients with typical absence seizures. The EEG of atypical absence seizures shows slow spike and slow wave complexes at less than 2.5 Hz (e.g., slow spike and wave).

Table 2.1 Comparison of classification/description of focal seizures.

1981 ILAE classification of partial seizures [4]	2010 ILAE descriptors of focal seizures [7]
Simple partial (consciousness not impaired) • With motor signs • With somatosensory or special-sensory symptoms • With autonomic signs • With psychic symptoms	**Without impairment of consciousness/awareness** • With observable motor or autonomic components • Involving subjective sensory or psychic phenomena only (aura)
Complex partial (with impairment of consciousness) • Simple partial onset followed by impairment of consciousness • With impairment of consciousness at onset	**With impairment of consciousness/responsiveness**
Partial seizures evolving to generalized tonic-clonic (GTC) seizures ("secondarily generalized")	**Evolving to a bilateral, convulsive seizure** (involving tonic, clonic, or tonic and clonic components)

Absence seizures with special features

The 2010 ILAE revisions add this new category, which includes:

- *Myoclonic absence* (absence episode with prominent myoclonus, as in Tassinari syndrome).
- *Eyelid myoclonia* (marked eye blinking with paroxysmal EEG including photosensitivity, as in Jeavon syndrome).

2.6 Focal seizures

Focal seizures, formerly also termed partial seizures, originate in cortical or subcortical structures of one hemisphere, but can propagate to other areas of the ipsilateral or contralateral hemisphere. The ILAE has simplified the classification of focal seizures and no longer recognizes the subclasses of simple, complex, and secondarily generalized. The rationale includes concern regarding imprecise definitions, and the terms used to define these classes have been abandoned all together. The ILAE recommends the continued use of impairment of consciousness or responsiveness and evolution into a bilateral convulsive seizure as descriptors of focal seizures rather than distinct natural classes [7]. Table 2.1 compares the former and current classification systems.

No simple taxonomy has been agreed upon to organize this varied and dynamic seizure type, though the further understanding of anatomical substrates, pathophysiological mechanisms, and patterns of propagation will facilitate the elucidation of distinct natural classes. Classification schemes for focal seizures in discussion emphasize anatomical correlations with onset and propagation patterns. Considerations include lobe of onset and neocortical versus limbic (hippocampal and parahippocampal) involvement [14].

Box 2.3 Definitions

- **Epilepsies**: neurological conditions involving chronic recurrent epileptic seizures [8].
- **Epilepsy syndrome:** a clinical entity that is reliably defined by a cluster of electroclinical characteristics and associated manifestations [6].

2.7 Syndromes

Epilepsy and epilepsy syndromes

Epilepsy describes a diverse group of disorders whose commonality is an abnormal predisposition to unprovoked seizures. The diagnosis of epilepsy requires at least a single seizure and a condition leading to a persistently decreased seizure threshold [8]. It is possible to identify a set of hallmark characteristics, beyond seizure type, that occur together as a recognizable syndrome (Box 2.3).

Not all epileptic disorders can be described by a syndrome. The 2010 ILAE revisions redefine syndrome to limit its use to entities reliably identified by a cluster of electroclinical characteristics [7]. These include age at seizure onset, EEG abnormalities, seizure types, associated neurodevelopmental features, inheritance, response to therapy, and prognosis. These electroclinical syndromes are precisely defined diagnostic entities, and are different from epilepsies secondary to a structural or metabolic abnormality without a defined electroclinical pattern. With advances in epilepsy genetics and further understanding of the neurobiology of epilepsy, more recognized syndromes are likely to evolve and existing classifications will be amended. The currently accepted electroclinical syndromes are listed in Box 2.4, and defined in this chapter according to age of onset.

Organization and classification of epileptic syndromes

The 2010 ILAE report has changed the system of syndrome classification, which previously relied on the terms localization-related versus generalized epilepsy, and was based on underlying etiology as idiopathic (and presumably genetic), symptomatic, or cryptogenic. The new system replaces the latter three categories with Genetic, Structural/Metabolic, and Unknown Cause.

Genetic epilepsy syndromes are meant to imply that the epilepsy is the direct result of a known or presumed genetic defect(s) in which seizures are the core manifestation. The genetic contributions may derive from specific molecular studies or information from the family history.

Structural-metabolic syndromes represent distinct conditions associated with a significantly increased risk of developing epilepsy, for example, acquired epilepsies following stroke, trauma, or infection, or genetically determined conditions such as tuberous sclerosis where there is a distinct disorder interposed between the genetic defect and the epilepsy.

Syndromes of "unknown cause" are viewed neutrally where the nature of the underlying cause is as yet unknown.

Box 2.4 Electroclinical syndromes arranged by age at onset [7]

Neonatal period

Benign familial neonatal epilepsy (BFNE)
Early myoclonic encephalopathy (EME)
Ohtahara syndrome

Infancy

Epilepsy of infancy with migrating focal seizures
West syndrome
Myoclonic epilepsy in infancy (MEI)
Benign infantile epilepsy
Benign familial infantile epilepsy
Dravet syndrome
Myoclonic encephalopathy in non-progressive disorders

Childhood

Febrile seizures plus (FS+) (can start in infancy)
Panayiotopoulos syndrome
Epilepsy with myoclonic atonic (previously astatic) seizures
Benign epilepsy with centrotemporal spikes (BECTS)
Autosomal dominant nocturnal frontal lobe epilepsy (ADNFLE)
Late-onset childhood occipital epilepsy (Gastaut type)
Epilepsy with myoclonic absences
Lennox–Gastaut syndrome
Epileptic encephalopathy with continuous spike-and-wave during sleep (CSWS)*
Landau–Kleffner syndrome (LKS)
Childhood absence epilepsy (CAE)

Adolescence–adult

Juvenile absence epilepsy (JAE)
Juvenile myoclonic epilepsy (JME)
Epilepsy with generalized tonic-clonic seizures alone
Progressive myoclonus epilepsies (PME)
Autosomal dominant epilepsy with auditory features (ADEAF)
Other familial temporal lobe epilepsies

Less specific age relationship

Familial focal epilepsy with variable foci (childhood to adult)
Reflex epilepsies

*CSWS is sometimes referred to as electrical status epilepticus during slow sleep (ESES).

The goal in the reclassification of epilepsy syndromes is to create a system that is flexible yet emphasizes proven and useful characteristics such as cause, age at onset, ictal and interictal EEG, structural imaging, prognosis, etc. Ongoing discussions propose incorporating natural evolution information into the syndrome classification schema, using *benign encephalopathy* (i.e., self-limited with spontaneous remission) or *epileptic encephalopathy* (wherein the epileptic activity itself – rather than the underlying pathology – causes neurological impairment) [7].

2.8 Specific age-related epilepsy syndromes

Neonatal period

Benign familial neonatal epilepsy (BFNE)

Defining features:

- Onset during days 2–15, commonly clustered in first week.
- Family history, autosomal dominant inheritance.
- Cluster of focal clonic seizures, often secondarily generalized or apneic.
- No specific EEG pattern, interictal background may be normal.
- Spontaneous recovery with favorable outcome.

This was the first epilepsy syndrome linked to a specific gene. More recently mutations of potassium channel genes *KCNQ2* and *KCNQ3*, and a nicotinic cholinergic receptor channel gene have been linked to this syndrome [15]. Seizures can occur as late as 3.5 months and occur later in premature infants.

Classification: familial (autosomal dominant) focal epilepsy [2].

Early myoclonic encephalopathy (EME)

Defining features:

- Onset of erratic myoclonus before 3 months (usually first 30 days).
- Massive myoclonus, focal seizures and late-onset tonic spasms also occur.
- Developmental arrest.
- Suppression-burst EEG pattern.
- Refractory to antiepileptic therapies.
- Poor outcome; 50% mortality in first year.

EME is frequently associated with inborn errors of metabolism, especially glycine encephalopathy, but no consistent gene association has been identified.

Classification: epileptic encephalopathy [2].

Ohtahara syndrome

Defining features:

- Onset of tonic spasms before 3 months (usually first 10 days).
- Developmental arrest.

Table 2.2 Myoclonic epilepsy syndromes of infancy.

Clinical features	Early myoclonic encephalopathy (EME)	Myoclonic epilepsy in infancy (MEI)	Dravet syndrome (severe MEI)
Age of onset	<3 months	First 2 years	<12 months
Seizure type	Myoclonic	Myoclonic	Clonic, myoclonic
EEG	Suppression-burst	Spike-wave with normal background	Spike-wave with focal abnormalities
Outcome	Poor	Favorable	Poor

- Suppression-burst EEG pattern.
- Refractory to antiepileptic therapies.
- Frequent progression West syndrome.
- Poor outcome; severe neurological impairment, death.

Also known as early infantile epileptic encephalopathy with suppression bursts, Ohtahara syndrome is the earliest onset of the epileptic encephalopathies. It is distinguished from EME by the absence of erratic myoclonus and the presence of tonic spasms at onset (Table 2.2). Ohtahara syndrome is frequently accompanied by structural lesions, whereas EME is typically associated with metabolic disorders.

Classification: epileptic encephalopathy [2].

Infancy

Epilepsy of infancy with migrating focal seizures

Defining features:

- Onset <6 months.
- Clusters of severe, polymorphous focal seizures, frequently evolving into generalized.
- EEG with epileptiform activity appears to migrate to neighboring areas.
- Progressive decline in psychomotor development.

Also known as malignant migrating partial epilepsy in infancy, this syndrome is characterized by early onset of severe focal seizures and also apneic seizures in early infancy. Within weeks to months, patients enter a "stormy phase" with frequent polymorphous focal seizures that become virtually continuous. EEG shows multifocal discharges, typically rhythmic theta activity, that progressively expand to adjacent cortical areas [16]. The ictal and interictal EEGs become indistinguishable, and the prognosis is poor.

Classification: symptomatic focal epilepsy [2], epilepsy of unknown cause [7].

West syndrome

Defining features:

- Onset before 1 year, peak 4–7 months.
- Clusters of spasms.

- Developmental arrest and psychomotor deterioration.
- Hypsarrhythmia interictal EEG pattern.
- Often refractory to antiepileptic therapies.
- Often poor outcome.

The spasms are myoclonic-tonic contractions and can be either flexor, extensor, head nods, or a combination that cluster upon drowsiness or arousal. *Hypsarrhythmia* is defined as a continuously abnormal background of high-voltage slow waves with irregular, shifting spikes and sharp waves. Various forms of modified hypsarrhythmia have been described, the most frequent of which is hypsarrhythmia with increased interhemispheric synchronization.

Classification: epileptic encephalopathy [2].

Myoclonic epilepsy in infancy (MEI)

Defining features:

- Onset of myolonic seizures at 4–36 months.
- Normal development before onset.
- Generalized, fast spike-wave and polyspike-wave discharges on EEG associated with myoclonic events, normal interictal background.
- Responsive to antiepileptic therapies.

MEI (formerly known as benign myoclonic epilepsy in infancy) is a rare disorder that affects previously healthy infants who frequently have a family history of epilepsy or febrile seizures. Occasionally MEI includes simple febrile seizures or a reflex seizure component [17], especially in response to visual patterns, but other seizure types do not occur. Seizures progressively increase in frequency and intensity, and some patients with MEI develop GTCS in adolescence. MEI is responsive to antiepileptic drugs and usually has a favorable outcome. However, some infants suffer from mild neurodevelopmental delays, which led to the removal of "benign" from the syndrome name [14].

Classification: idiopathic generalized epilepsy [2], epilepsy of unknown cause [7].

Benign infantile epilepsy and benign familial infantile epilepsy

Defining features:

- Onset 3–20 months.
- Clusters of brief partial seizures.
- Normal development before onset.
- Responsive to antiepileptic therapies.
- Favorable outcome.

The familial form is based on a family history of infantile convulsions without later development of other forms of epilepsy and is inherited in an autosomal dominant pattern. The peak age of seizure onset in the familial form is 4–7 months.

Classification: idiopathic focal epilepsy; *familial form*: familial (autosomal dominant) focal epilepsy [2].

Dravet syndrome

Defining features:

- Onset of febrile clonic or tonic-clonic seizures before 12 months.
- Normal development before onset.
- Secondary onset of myoclonic, atypical absence, and/or focal seizures (1–4 years of age).
- Refractory to antiepileptic therapies.
- Poor outcome with psychomotor retardation and other neurological deficits.

Formerly known as severe myoclonic epilepsy of infancy (SMEI), Dravet syndrome follows a characteristic pattern of febrile or hemiclonic seizures in the first year of life, with a later appearance of other focal and generalized seizure types (Table 2.2) [18]. Interictal EEG may be normal early in the course. Dravet syndrome is most commonly caused by a channelopathy, typically affecting *SCN1A* and other sodium channel genes [19]. As many patients never experience myoclonias, the name Dravet syndrome has replaced SMEI [14,18]. Dravet syndrome was originally classified as undetermined focal or generalized epilepsy, and shares characteristics of both classical idiopathic and symptomatic epilepsies. In the new classification, Dravet syndrome is labeled an epileptic encephalopathy and a genetic epilepsy.

Classification: epileptic encephalopathy [2], genetic epilepsy [7].

Myoclonic encephalopathy in non-progressive disorders

Defining features:

- Prolonged myoclonic status.
- Neurological impairment in infant prior to status.
- Interictal EEG: continuous, rhythmic, diffuse, slow spike-wave with asynchronous myoclonias.
- Neuropsychological impairment with onset of status.
- Poor prognosis.

This pattern is associated with Angelman syndrome.

Classification: epileptic encephalopathy [2].

Childhood

Febrile seizures plus (FS+)

Defining features:

- Onset 3 months to 6 years.
- Generalized tonic-clonic seizures (GCTS) occurring with fever.
- Continuation of febrile GCTS after 6 years of age *or* occurrence of afebrile GCTS.
- Family history of childhood febrile seizures.
- Normal interictal EEG.
- Favorable outcome.

FS+ is a phenotype of familial generalized epilepsy with febrile seizures plus (GEFS+) and is distinguished from non-syndromic febrile seizures by the persistence of febrile GCTS after 5 or 6 years of age or the presence of GCTS without fever. Many patients also experience febrile myoclonus [20]. The syndrome is associated with mutations of the *SCN1A* sodium channel gene.

Classification: idiopathic generalized epilepsy [2].

Panayiotopoulos syndrome

Defining features:

- Childhood onset (peak 5 years).
- Focal autonomic seizures or autonomic status epilepticus, frequently with emesis.
- Interictal EEG with shifting or multifocal high-amplitude spikes, often with occipital predominance.
- Favorable outcome with remission in 1–2 years and normal development.

The definition of Panayiotopoulos syndrome, previously called early-benign childhood seizures with occipital spikes, has been refined and renamed in recent years. Episodes are characterized by pronounced autonomic features, primarily vomiting, followed by more common ictal manifestations including loss of responsiveness, eye and head deviation, and atonia [21]. EEG spikes occur most commonly in the posterior areas of the brain including the occipital lobe, though 30% of patients show only extraoccipital discharges or normal EEGs; thus, the use of "occipital" in the name of this syndrome is now discouraged.

Classification: idiopathic focal epilepsy [2].

Epilepsy with myoclonic atonic seizures

Defining features:

- Onset between 18 months and 5 years (peak 3 years).
- Myoclonic atonic seizures are primary seizure type, but heterogeneous presentation.
- Interictal EEG with 4–7 Hz spike and slow-wave or polyspike and slow-wave complexes.
- Variable course and outcome.

This syndrome was formerly known as myoclonic astatic epilepsy of Doose [22]. The hallmark myoclonic atonic seizure, previously called myoclonic astatic, is an initial massive myoclonic jerk followed immediately by severe loss of muscle tone, often causing a fall and referred to as a drop attack. Most patients, however, experience heterogeneous seizure presentations, including myoclonic, atonic, absence, tonic, clonic, and generalized tonic-clonic seizures. About half of patients have positive outcomes with spontaneous remission, while the other half experience encephalopathic effects and suffer from persistent GTCS, myoclonic-atonic status, and dementia.

Classification: idiopathic generalized epilepsy [2].

Benign childhood epilepsy with centrotemporal spikes (BECTS or BCECTS)

Defining features:

- Onset between 2 and 13 years (peak 9–10 years).
- Normal development before onset and during course of epilepsy.
- Autosomal dominant inheritance.
- Focal seizures with motor signs without impairment of consciousness ("simple partial").
- Interictal EEG with high-voltage centrotemporal spikes on a normal background.
- Favorable outcome with recovery in adolescence.

BECTS, also known as benign rolandic epilepsy or sylvian epilepsy, is a syndrome characterized by focal seizures in childhood. Seizures are primarily hemifacial motor contractions, are frequently associated with oropharyngeal or somatosensory symptoms, and may evolve into GTCS [23]. The EEG trait of centrotemporal spikes follows an autosomal dominant inheritance pattern, but not all people with these centrotemporal spikes experience seizures.

Classification: idiopathic focal epilepsy [2].

Autosomal dominant nocturnal frontal lobe epilepsy (ADNFLE)

Defining features:

- Childhood/adolescent onset (mean 11 years).
- Autosomal dominant inheritance.
- Focal sensory-motor seizures occurring in NREM sleep.
- Ictal EEG with frontally dominant slow discharges.

ADNFLE is a recently defined epilepsy syndrome defined by nocturnal seizures of heterogeneous presentation. The defect has been identified as a nicotinic acetylcholine receptor (AChR) channelopathy that is inherited in an autosomal dominant manner with incomplete penetrance [24]. Seizures typically occur in NREM sleep with variable manifestations including prominent motor features such as jerking, dystonia, and automatisms, as well as vocalizations, and non-specific auras. Prognosis is typically favorable, without significant neurological impairment.

Classification: familial (autosomal dominant) epilepsy [2], genetic epilepsy [7].

Late-onset childhood occipital epilepsy (Gastaut type)

Defining features:

- Childhood onset (mean 8–9 years).
- Occipital seizures, primarily visual manifestations including hallucinations and temporary blindness.
- Interictal EEG with occipital spike-waves upon eye closure and with attenuation upon eye opening.
- Responsive to antiepileptic therapies.
- Favorable prognosis with remission in adolescence.

Formerly grouped with Panayiotopoulos syndrome as childhood occipital epilepsy, late-onset Gastaut type is now recognized as a separate diagnostic entity, with relatively later onset and without the prominence of autonomic symptoms. Focal seizures are frequent, brief, and variable, but frequently begin with a visual phenomenon that is followed by a hemiclonic seizure or automatisms [25].

Classification: idiopathic focal epilepsy [2].

Epilepsy with myoclonic absences

Defining features:

- Childhood onset (mean 7 years).
- Myoclonic absence seizures: loss of consciousness with severe, rhythmic myoclonic jerks.
- Ictal EEG showing bilateral, synchronous spike and slow-wave complexes at 3 Hz associated with myoclonus.
- Variable course and outcome.

This syndrome as recognized by Tassinari and colleagues consists of typical absence seizures accompanied by severe, violent myoclonic jerks [26]. The myoclonias are bilateral and rhythmic, maximally involving proximal limb muscles, and may be associated with a tonic contraction associated with raising the arms. Interictal EEG is variable and ranges from normal to background slowing and generalized spike and slow-wave activity. Many patients are resistant to drug therapy and have less favorable outcomes associated with poor seizure control.

Classification: idiopathic generalized epilepsy [2].

Eyelid myoclonias with absence as described by Jeavons [27] is defined by childhood onset of brief episodes of eyelid jerking and upward gaze with photosensitivity. Though eyelid myoclonia was recognized as a distinct type of absence seizure with special features, the syndrome is not categorized as an electroclinical syndrome in the 2010 ILAE report [7].

Lennox–Gastaut syndrome (LGS)

Defining features:

- Onset from 3 to 10 years (peak 3–5 years).
- Generalized seizures of multiple types, including tonic axial, atypical absence, and drop attacks.
- In wakefulness: diffuse slow spike and slow-wave ($\leq$2.5 Hz) complexes on EEG.
- In sleep: generalized fast paroxysms ($\sim$10 Hz) on EEG.
- Developmental delay and mental retardation.

LGS is classified as an epileptic encephalopathy. Up to 75% of Lennox–Gastaut patients are characterized as symptomatic, as they have an established etiology in the form of a previous encephalopathy [28].

Classification: epileptic encephalopathy [2].

Epileptic encephalopathy with continuous spike-and-wave during sleep (CSWS)

Defining features:

- Childhood onset (peak 4–7 years).
- Various generalized and focal seizures.
- Cognitive deterioration and behavioral disturbances.
- EEG with continuous spike and slow wave seen in at least 85% of slow-wave sleep.

This syndrome is characterized by a hallmark EEG presentation, called continuous spike-and-wave during sleep (CSWS), or electrical status epilepticus of slow-wave sleep (ESES), accompanied by seizure activity and neuropsychological deficits. Following seizure onset, often 2–5 years later, the CSWS pattern emerges, and is temporally associated with the emergence of neuropsychological and behavioral disturbances [29], as well as the onset of atypical absence seizures in wakefulness. There is no associated brain pathology, and patients typically see some improvement in neurological status once epileptiform activity has resolved.

Classification: epileptic encephalopathy [2].

Landau–Kleffner syndrome (LKS)

Defining features:

- Onset between 3 and 8 years (peak 5–7 years).
- Acquired aphasia (verbal auditory agnosia).
- Continuous spike and wave discharges on EEG, activated in sleep.
- Resolution of EEG abnormalities in adolescence.

Acquired auditory agnosia is the classic presentation; patients may present with expressive aphasia. Deterioration or significant fluctuation in language are indications to evaluate for LKS. Generalized or focal seizures occur in up to 80% of children and may precede or follow the onset of aphasia [30]. Seizures commonly resolve before age 15 years, although neuropsychological deficits tend to persist. Though the ILAE classifies LKS and epilepsy with CSWS as separate syndromes [7], many epileptologists consider the two presentations on a common syndromic spectrum and consider LKS a specific presentation of epilepsy with CSWS [14,30].

Classification: epileptic encephalopathy [2].

Childhood absence epilepsy (CAE)

Defining features:

- Onset between 4 and 10 years in a previously healthy child.
- Frequent typical absence seizures.
- Maintenance of neurological status and development during course of epilepsy.
- Ictal EEG: generalized, high-amplitude 3 Hz spike and slow-wave complexes, typically lasting 4–20 s.

Childhood absence epilepsy, also called "pyknolepsy" to recognize the "clustering" effect, is characterized by typical absence seizures. Seizures are generally responsive to antiepileptic drug (AED) intervention, usually with ethosuximide or valproate. About one-half of patients develop convulsive seizures, which are associated with a worse prognosis if the latter occur at onset.

Classification: idiopathic generalized epilepsy [2], genetic epilepsy [7].

Adolescence–adult

Juvenile absence epilepsy (JAE)

Defining features:

- Onset 7–17 years (peak 10–12 years) in a previously healthy child.
- Typical absence seizures.
- Secondary seizure type: GTCS.
- Ictal EEG: generalized, high-amplitude spike and slow-wave complexes ≥3.5 Hz, typically >4 s duration.

In contrast to children with younger onset, as in CAE, absence seizures in JAE are more sporadic. The majority of patients with JAE also experience GTCS. The EEG in untreated patients is similar to that in CAE but may be slightly faster, with generalized spike wave paroxysms of 3.5–4 Hz. Seizures are usually controlled with AEDs and the prognosis is favorable, though less so for patients with uncontrolled GTCS.

Classification: idiopathic generalized epilepsy [2].

Juvenile myoclonic epilepsy (JME)

Defining features:

- Onset 8 to 26 years (peak 12–18, mean 14 years).
- Bilateral myoclonic jerks, most frequently upon awakening.
- Secondary seizure types including GTCS and typical absence seizures.
- Ictal EEG with generalized high-amplitude polyspike-and-wave.

Patients with JME usually demonstrate a life-long predisposition to generalized seizures. The 2006 ILAE Task Force report discusses the need for further investigation into the distinction between CAE, JAE, and JME, given their similar and sometimes overlapping presentations [14].

Classification: idiopathic generalized epilepsy [2].

Progressive myoclonus epilepsies (PME)

Defining features:

- Severe myoclonias.
- Epilepsy with generalized seizures, especially tonic-clonic, clonic-tonic-clonic, and clonic.

- Progressive course including dementia and cerebellar manifestations.

Progressive myoclonus epilepsies are a group of rare genetic diseases that feature severe myoclonias, epilepsy, and a progressive course. EEG typically shows progressive background slowing, generalized and multifocal abnormalities, and photosensitivity [31]. The most prevalent PMEs are Unverricht–Lundborg disease (ULD) and Lafora disease. Onset of ULD occurs between 7 and 16 years of age (peak 9–13 years) and is characterized by severe myoclonias, generalized clonic-tonic-clonic seizures, and cerebellar ataxia. ULD has a slow progression, with little to no cognitive impairment, and is caused by a mutation in the cystatin B gene [32]. Lafora disease presents at a similar age, but has a severe prognosis including rapid progression to dementia and nearly constant myoclonus, with death in 2–10 years. Lafora disease has autosomal recessive inheritance and is caused by mutations in the enzyme laforin [33]. Other PMEs include the neuronal ceroid lipofuscinoses, sialidosis, and myoclonic epilepsy with ragged-red fibers (MERRF).

Classification: progressive myoclonus epilepsies [2].

2.9 Future directions

Definitions of seizure types will incorporate more objective and physiologically based characteristics. In the 2006 report of the ILAE Classification Core Group, Engel describes six new criteria for distinguishing seizure types, including pathophysiological mechanisms, neuronal substrates, response to antiepileptic drugs, ictal EEG patterns (with distinct anatomical and physiological correlates), propagation patterns and postictal features, and epilepsy syndromes associated with the seizure type [14].

Acknowledgements

Niki R. Delis BA and Mandira Mehra MD assisted with research toward preparation of the manuscript for this chapter.

References

[1] Wolf P. Of cabbages and kings: some considerations on classifications, diagnostic schemes, semiology, and concepts. *Epilepsia* 2003;**44**:1–4; discussion 4–13.

[2] Engel J Jr. A proposed diagnostic scheme for people with epileptic seizures and with epilepsy: report of the ILAE Task Force on Classification and Terminology. *Epilepsia* 2001;**42**:796–803.

[3] Berg AT, Blackstone NW. Concepts in classification and their relevance to epilepsy. *Epilepsy Res* 2006;**70**(Suppl. 1):S11–19.

[4] International League Against Epilepsy. Proposal for revised clinical and electroencephalographic classification of epileptic seizures. From the Commission on Classification and Terminology of the International League Against Epilepsy. *Epilepsia* 1981;**22**:489–501.

[5] Proposal for classification of epilepsies and epileptic syndromes. Commission on Classification and Terminology of the International League Against Epilepsy. *Epilepsia* 1985;**26**:268–278.

[6] Proposal for revised classification of epilepsies and epileptic syndromes. Commission on Classification and Terminology of the International League Against Epilepsy. *Epilepsia* 1989;**30**:389–399.

[7] Berg AT, Berkovic SF, Brodie MJ, *et al.* Revised terminology and concepts for organization of seizures and epilepsies: report of the ILAE Commission on Classification and Terminology, 2005–2009. *Epilepsia* 2010;**51**:676–685.

[8] Fisher RS, van Emde Boas W, Blume W, *et al.* Epileptic seizures and epilepsy: definitions proposed by the International League Against Epilepsy (ILAE) and the International Bureau for Epilepsy (IBE). *Epilepsia* 2005;**46**:470–472.

[9] Blume WT, Luders HO, Mizrahi E, *et al.* Glossary of descriptive terminology for ictal semiology: report of the ILAE task force on classification and terminology. *Epilepsia* 2001;**42**:1212–1218.

[10] Oguni H, Fukuyama Y, Tanaka T, *et al.* Myoclonic-astatic epilepsy of early childhood – clinical and EEG analysis of myoclonic-astatic seizures, and discussions on the nosology of the syndrome. *Brain Dev* 2001;**23**:757–764.

[11] Panayiotopoulos CP. Typical absence seizures and related epileptic syndromes: assessment of current state and directions for future research. *Epilepsia* 2008;**49**:2131–2139.

[12] Gibbs FA, Davis H, Lennox WG. The EEG in epilepsy and in conditions of impaired consciousness. *Arch Neurol Psychiat* 1935;**34**:1134–1148.

[13] Penry JK, Porter RJ, Dreifuss RE. Simultaneous recording of absence seizures with video tape and electroencephalography. A study of 374 seizures in 48 patients. *Brain* 1975;**98**:427–440.

[14] Engel J Jr. Report of the ILAE classification core group. *Epilepsia* 2006;**47**:1558–1568.

[15] Kurahashi H, Wang JW, Ishii A, *et al.* Deletions involving both KCNQ2 and CHRNA4 present with benign familial neonatal seizures. *Neurology* 2009;**73**:1214–1217.

[16] Coppola G. Malignant migrating partial seizures in infancy: an epilepsy syndrome of unknown etiology. *Epilepsia* 2009;**50**(Suppl. 5):49–51.

[17] Dravet C, Bureau M. Benign myoclonic epilepsy in infancy. In: Roger J, Bureau M, Dravet C, *et al.* (eds), *Epileptic Syndromes in Infancy, Childhood and Adolescence* 4th edition. London: John Libbey Eurotext, 2005; pp. 77–88.

[18] Dravet C, Bureau M, Oguni H, *et al.* Severe myoclonic epilepsy in infancy (Dravet syndrome). In: Roger J, Bureau M, Dravet C, *et al.* (eds), *Epileptic Syndromes in Infancy, Childhood and Adolescence* 4th edition. London: John Libbey Eurotext, 2005; pp. 89–114.

[19] Marini C, Mei D, Temudo T, *et al.* Idiopathic epilepsies with seizures precipitated by fever and SCN1A abnormalities. *Epilepsia* 2007;**48**:1678–1685.

[20] Narula S, Goraya JS. Febrile myoclonus. *Neurology* 2005;**64**:169–170.

[21] Covanis A, Ferrie CD, Koutroumandis M, *et al.* Panayiotopoulos syndrome and Gastaut type idiopathic childhood occipital epilepsy. In: Roger J, Bureau M, Dravet C, *et al.* (eds), *Epileptic Syndromes in Infancy, Childhood and Adolescence*. London: John Libbey Eurotext, 2005; pp. 227–254.

[22] Guerrini R, Parmeggiani L, Bonanni P, *et al.* (2005) Myoclonic astatic epilepsy. In: Roger J, Bureau M, Dravet C, *et al.* (eds), *Epileptic Syndromes in Infancy, Childhood and Adolescence*. London: John Libbey Eurotext, 2005; pp. 115–124.

[23] Loiseau P, Beaussart M. The seizures of benign childhood epilepsy with Rolandic paroxysmal discharges. *Epilepsia* 1973;**14**:381–389.

[24] Steinlein OK, Mulley JC, Propping P, *et al.* A missense mutation in the neuronal nicotinic acetylcholine receptor alpha 4 subunit is associated with autosomal dominant nocturnal frontal lobe epilepsy. *Nat Genet* 1995;**11**:201–203.

[25] Gastaut H. A new type of epilepsy: benign partial epilepsy of childhood with occipital spike-waves. *Clin Electroencephalogr* 1982;**13**:13–22.

[26] Bureau M, Tassinari CA. The syndrome of myoclonic absences. In: Roger J, Bureau M, Dravet C, *et al.* (eds), *Epileptic Syndromes in Infancy, Childhood and Adolescence*. London: John Libbey Eurotext, 2005; pp. 337–344.

[27] Hirsch E, Panayiotopoulos CP. Childhood absence epilepsy and related syndromes. In: Roger J, Bureau M, Dravet C, *et al.* (eds), *Epileptic Syndromes in Infancy, Childhood and Adolescence*. London: John Libbey Eurotext, 2005; pp. 315–335.

[28] Markand ON. Lennox–Gastaut syndrome (childhood epileptic encephalopathy). *J Clin Neurophysiol* 2003;**20**:426–441.
[29] Patry G, Lyagoubi S, Tassinari CA. Subclinical "electrical status epilepticus" induced by sleep in children. A clinical and electroencephalographic study of six cases. *Arch Neurol* 1971;**24**:242–252.
[30] Tassinari CA, Rubboli G, Volpi L, *et al*. Electrical status epilepticus during slow sleep (ESES or CSWS) including acquired epileptic aphasia (Landau–Kleffner syndrome). In: Roger J, Bureau M, Dravet C, *et al*. (eds), *Epileptic Syndromes in Infancy, Childhood and Adolescence*. London: John Libbey Eurotext, 2005; pp. 295–314.
[31] Wheless JW, Kim HL. Adolescent seizures and epilepsy syndromes. *Epilepsia* 2002;**43** (Suppl. 3):33–52.
[32] Pennacchio LA, Lehesjoki AE, Stone NE, *et al*. Mutations in the gene encoding cystatin B in progressive myoclonus epilepsy (EPM1). *Science* 1996;**271**:1731–1734.
[33] Minassian BA, Lee JR, Herbrick JA, *et al*. Mutations in a gene encoding a novel protein tyrosine phosphatase cause progressive myoclonus epilepsy. *Nat Genet* 1998;**20**:171–174.

3 Initiating and withdrawing medical management

David T. Hsieh[1] and Bhagwan Indur Moorjani[2]

[1]San Antonio Military Medical Center, Division of Child Neurology, Wilford Hall Medical Center, Lackland AFB, TX, USA
[2] Hope Neurologic Center, La Quinta, CA, JFK Memorial Hospital, Indio, CA , USA

The fundamental questions regarding the medical management of children and adolescents with epilepsy are when and in which patients to initiate treatment with antiepileptic drugs, and when and in which patients to discontinue treatment. The principles that shape these decisions are discussed, to include a thorough understanding of the risks and benefits of each option, providing a foundation upon which to have a partnering interchange with the patient and their family. The individualized decision to initiate or to discontinue antiepileptic drug therapy for a patient is usually focused upon preventing the occurrences of epileptic seizures, but is ultimately centered around minimizing morbidity and mortality, and maximizing quality of life for both the patient and their family.

3.1 Initiating medical management

Once a child or adolescent has been evaluated for and diagnosed with one or more epileptic seizures, the focus of care subsequently shifts toward treatment considerations. Although other treatment options are available, including different non-surgical (Box 3.1) and surgical options, in almost all patients the initial treatment to be considered is antiepileptic drug (AED) therapy.

Epilepsy in Children and Adolescents, First Edition. Edited by James W. Wheless.

Box 3.1 Available non-surgical treatment options for childhood epilepsy

Antiepileptic drug therapy

Behavioral changes

- Sleep hygiene
- Abstaining from alcohol
- Avoiding sensory triggers (e.g., flashing lights, heat)

Dietary modification therapy

- Ketogenic diet
- Atkins diet
- Modified Atkins diet
- Low glycemic index diet

Hormonal or immune-modulating therapy

- Adrenocorticotropin hormone (ACTH)
- Oral steroids
- Intravenous immunoglobulin (IVIG)
- Contraceptives

Vitamin deficiency supplementation

- Pyridoxine
- Folinic acid
- Pyridoxal phosphate
- Biotin

As a point of clarification, the term *antiepileptic drug* has become standard nomenclature to refer to those drugs that are used to decrease the risk of future occurrences of epileptic seizures, and will be used in this reference. It should not be misinterpreted that antiepileptic drugs possess the ability to prevent the development of epilepsy as an *antiepileptic*.

Whether or not to initiate antiepileptic drug therapy in a child or adolescent is a decision-making process that is led by the physician but should include active participation by the parents and other care-takers, and in older children and adolescents, by the patients themselves. This decision should be based upon an understanding of the treatment goals:

- Minimizing morbidity and mortality.
- Maximizing quality of life for both the patient and their family.

The decision of whether or not to initiate antiepileptic drug therapy should be individualized to each patient, based upon an understanding of several key questions (Box 3.2).

Box 3.2 Key questions to understand when considering initiation of antiepileptic drug therapy

What is the natural history of the disorder being treated (i.e., what are the chances of seizure recurrence if the patient is not initiated on antiepileptic drug therapy)?
What are the possible adverse effects of seizure recurrence on the individual patient and family?
What are the risks of initiating antiepileptic drug therapy?
What are the benefits of initiating antiepileptic drug therapy?

Thus, there is a need to understand the natural history of the disorder being treated, in particular, the chances of seizure recurrence, along with the possible adverse effects of seizure recurrence on the individual patient and family. This understanding is then balanced against the benefits and the risks of adverse effects associated with antiepileptic drugs to help each patient make an individualized decision for or against initiating antiepileptic drug therapy.

3.2 The chances of seizure recurrence after the first unprovoked seizure

The chances of seizure recurrence following a first unprovoked seizure have been reported in the literature to range from approximately 25% to 70% [1,2]. This wide range of recurrence rates can in part be attributed to differences in study methods. Specifically, the bias of studies including patients with a history of prior seizures at the time of study recruitment, as opposed to prospectively following patients from the time of their first seizure, tends to favor a higher rate of recurrence. In a prior meta-analysis pooling data from studies using first-seizure criteria [1], the following key points can be surmised:

- The overall estimated recurrence risk of a second seizure by 2 years is approximately 40%. Thus, the majority of children who have a first unprovoked seizure will not have a future seizure recurrence.
- This cumulative risk of seizure recurrence does continue to increase slightly with continued follow-up past 2 years; however, the large majority of recurrences will occur within the first 1–2 years.

When assessing the risk for seizure recurrence for an individual patient, however, there are certain factors to consider drawn from each patient's individual clinical presentation that can modulate this risk calculation (Box 3.3).

The most consistent factors

The two most consistent factors that can modulate an individual patient's seizure recurrence risk include seizure etiology and electroencephalogram (EEG) findings. Appropriately, the American Academy of Neurology guidelines are supportive of obtaining an EEG on all children after their first afebrile seizure, and obtaining other studies, to include neuroimaging, depending on the clinical circumstances [3].

Box 3.3 Factors that can modulate the recurrence risk after a first unprovoked seizure

Most consistent factors

- Seizure etiology
- EEG findings

Less consistent factors:

- Sleep state at the time of the first seizure
- Seizure type
- A family history of epilepsy

Inconsistent factors:

- Age
- Duration of the first seizure

Seizure etiology

In discussing seizure etiology, the most commonly used definitions [4] include remote symptomatic, idiopathic, and cryptogenic (Box 3.4).

- Children with a first seizure of remote symptomatic etiology tend to have higher rates of seizure recurrence, with an approximately 65% chance of recurrence [1,2]. Among those with a remote symptomatic etiology, patients with brain dysfunction since birth tend to have the highest rates of seizure recurrence.
- In contrast to patients with a remote symptomatic etiology, children with a first seizure of idiopathic or cryptogenic etiology tend to have lower rates of recurrence, with approximately a 35% chance of recurrence [1,2].

Box 3.4 Definitions of seizure etiology

A *remote symptomatic* etiology refers to those patients in whom seizures do not have an immediate provoking factor, but occur in patients with a prior static brain injury (i.e., cerebral dysgenesis, prior trauma, prior central nervous system infection, prior stroke), or known brain dysfunction (i.e., mental retardation).

An *idiopathic* etiology refers to normal patients whose seizure semiology, usually with supportive EEG findings, is suspected or confirmed to be of genetic origin.

A *cryptogenic* etiology refers to normal patients whose seizures are of uncertain cause.

EEG findings

Children with EEG abnormalities after a first seizure also tend to have higher rates of seizure recurrence [1,2]. When differentiating between types of EEG abnormalities, epileptiform abnormalities, such as spike waves and sharp waves, are more predictive of recurrence than non-epileptiform abnormalities, such as focal or generalized slowing [1,2]. However, the effect of EEG abnormalities on recurrence risk is partially dependent upon etiology, reflecting more of an increased risk of seizure recurrence in patients with either idiopathic or cryptogenic seizure etiologies, but not reflecting a significant change in recurrence risk in patients with remote symptomatic etiologies:

- The two-year seizure recurrence rate in children with idiopathic or cryptogenic etiologies with any EEG abnormality is approximately 50% [1,2]. On the other hand, a normal EEG can help identify patients who have lower risks of recurrence, as those children with a cryptogenic etiology and a normal EEG have a more favorable recurrence rate of approximately 25% [1,2].
- EEG abnormalities tend to have lesser or no significant effects on recurrence risk calculations in patients with a remote symptomatic etiology [1,2].

The less consistent factors

Sleep state

Two-year recurrence rates in children who have their first seizure while asleep have been reported to be approximately 50%, compared with approximately 30% for those who have their initial seizure while awake [2].

Seizure type

Some studies in children report a higher recurrence rate with a partial seizure semiology when compared with a generalized seizure semiology, while others do not. Once the effects of etiology and EEG abnormalities are controlled for, however, partial seizure semiology has less of an effect on recurrence risk [1,2].

Family history

For most children a positive family history of epilepsy is not predictive of recurrence [2]. In the subset of patients with a cryptogenic etiology and an abnormal EEG, however, a positive family history for epilepsy may be significant, exerting an increased risk of recurrence [2].

Unrelated factors

Age

Age at presentation of the first seizure does not appear to affect recurrent risk.

Seizure duration

A long duration of the initial seizure, to include a first seizure presentation in status epilepticus, does not significantly increase the risk for seizure recurrence in children [2].

3.3 Seizure recurrence

Although the majority of children do not have a recurrence after their first unprovoked seizure, those who do will incur an even higher risk of further recurrence:

- The cumulative risk of further seizure recurrence after having the second seizure is 71% after 5 years [5].
- However, the cumulative risk of further seizure recurrence does not increase significantly after the third seizure, with a cumulative risk for further recurrence of 81% at 5 years, lending support to the clinical definition of epilepsy after the second seizure [5].

As a note of clarification, although the occurrence of a second seizure predicts a higher rate of further seizure recurrence, when this second seizure occurs within 24 hours of the first seizure, it is generally accepted to be considered a single seizure event [4]. Most studies in children predefine multiple seizures within 24 hours as a single seizure event, but this definition is also supported by studies showing similar rates of seizure recurrence between those with a single seizure and those with multiple seizures in 1 day at initial presentation [2]. It should be noted, however, that one study in children supports the diagnosis of epilepsy even when the first two seizures occur within 24 hours of each other, based upon their results showing similar rates of seizure recurrence between those with two or more seizures on the same day, and those with two or more seizures separated by at least 24 hours [6].

For those patients who do have a seizure recurrence, the factors that can increase this risk of further recurrence include [5]:

- A remote symptomatic etiology.
- A time interval between the first and second seizure of less than 6 months.

An additional issue to consider is the fact that the initial presentation for neurological care may not actually be after the first seizure. Most studies [1,2] in children exclude patients with the seizure semiologies that tend to be recurrent before initial presentation (Box 3.5). However, even patients presenting for medical care after a first generalized tonic-clonic seizure can have prior unrecognized seizures, usually of complex partial semiology.

3.4 The possible adverse effects of seizure recurrence

Although the chance of seizure recurrence is usually the focus of whether or not to initiate treatment with antiepileptic drugs, an understanding, in the context of each individual

Box 3.5 Seizure types that tend to be recurrent before initial presentation

Absence
Myoclonic
Spasms
Atonic

Box 3.6 Possible adverse effects of seizures

Psychosocial reactions
Effects on learning and behavior
Effects on sleep
Risks of injury to the body
Risks of injury to the brain
Risks of death

patient, of the possible adverse effects of seizure recurrence (Box 3.6) is of comparable relevance. These adverse effects are not always substantiated in the literature in the pediatric population, thus furthering the need for open discussion with the patient and their family.

Psychosocial reactions

Witnessing a seizure in a family member can be a frightening event. However, there is a wide spectrum of seizure presentations, and in turn a wide range of tolerance among different families.

- On one end of the spectrum, an episode of convulsive status epilepticus can be an especially frightening event to witness as a parent.
- On the other end of the spectrum, brief, infrequent, partial, nocturnal seizures occurring in the safety of one's own bed in many patients with benign rolandic epilepsy may be better tolerated.

Although it is known that an initial seizure presentation in status epilepticus incurs no significant additional risk for recurrence, those that do recur have approximately a 20% chance of recurring in status epilepticus [2]. Despite the low morbidity of status epilepticus in children – if treated aggressively, and in the absence of acute or progressive neurological injury [7] – the fear of such a recurrence may weigh heavily on a family's decision regarding the initiation of antiepileptic drug therapy.

On the contrary, many patients with benign rolandic epilepsy choose not to initiate antiepileptic drug treatment. This is especially true when the seizures are brief and non-generalized, and occur only at night. Thus, the severity and setting of seizures, in the context of their psychosocial effects within the family, can be important considerations in the decision of whether or not to initiate antiepileptic drug therapy in a child.

Effects on learning, behavior, and sleep

Although less conspicuous than the immediate effects of a witnessed seizure, the insidious effects of uncontrolled epilepsy on a child's behavior and learning should also be factored into the decision-making process.

- On the one hand, evidence is supportive of the fact that risks for behavioral and learning difficulties may be an inherent part of the disease process of epilepsy [8].

- However, it is also evident that recurrent seizures are further predictive factors for behavioral and learning difficulties [9]. Furthermore, seizure occurrence is associated with abnormal sleep patterns, which can in turn promote behavioral difficulties during the day [10].

Risks of injury to the brain or body, and the risks of death

A point that often needs reassuring emphasis in discussion with families is that seizures in children are more frightening than they are physically harmful.

- Regarding bodily injury, this is rarely seen with seizures in children, especially injuries necessitating medical care [11]. Tonic-clonic and myoclonic seizures are more apt to cause injury than other types, due to sudden falls.

There is also a lack of evidence that non-prolonged seizures are injurious to the brain:

- Even when considering patients presenting with status epilepticus, the majority of children do not have a poor outcome. In one study of children aggressively treated for status epilepticus, mortality within 3 months was 3%, with new neurological deficits in 10% of the remaining survivors [7]. The prognosis in status epilepticus is related more to the provoking etiology than to the duration of the seizure.
- In addition, there is also no convincing evidence in humans that seizure recurrence itself harms the brain by altering the long-term prognosis of epilepsy [12]. Thus, the evidence does not support the initiation of antiepileptic drug therapy in order to prevent epileptogenesis. In studies involving first unprovoked seizure presentations, long-term prognosis is not significantly affected by whether a patient is initiated on antiepileptic drug therapy after the first seizure or after the first seizure recurrence [13].

Finally, although the risk of death in children with epilepsy is higher than in the general population, sudden unexplained death is rare in children with epilepsy, with a pooled estimate of one in 10 000 patient-years [14]. The risk of death is more closely related to a patient's underlying neurological deficits, as patients with idiopathic epilepsy have similar risks of death as the general population [14]. In addition, a higher frequency of seizures and a generalized convulsive semiology are reported to be risk factors for sudden death in patients with epilepsy [14].

3.5 The risks of initiating antiepileptic drug therapy

In addition to the risks of seizure recurrence and the possible adverse effects should seizures recur, the decision whether to initiate treatment is also dependent on the risks (Box 3.7) and the benefits of the antiepileptic drug therapy. The risks of idiosyncratic and allergic reactions are particular to the initiation of drug therapy. However, patients started on antiepileptic drugs are often maintained on treatment for years, and the risks of long-term adverse effects are also relevant concerns. Of particular concern with many antiepileptic drugs in children are their effects on behavior and learning. All of the antiepileptic drugs have their own side-effect profile, and the clinician should be familiar with the possible adverse effects associated with each of them, especially as newer drugs become available for use. Overall, the newer antiepileptic drugs may offer similar efficacy as the older generation antiepileptic drugs and appear to be better tolerated.

Box 3.7 Risks of antiepileptic drug therapy

Psychosocial stigma of taking a daily medication
Allergic reactions
Idiosyncratic reactions
Side effects and chronic toxicity:

- AED-specific side effects
- Adverse effects on behavior and learning
- Adverse effects on bone health

3.6 The benefits of initiating antiepileptic drug therapy

The primary benefit of initiating antiepileptic drug therapy is a reduction in the risk of seizure recurrence. Studies in which patients were randomized to either immediate treatment with antiepileptic drugs after the initial seizure or had treatment deferred report that treatment can reduce the risk of subsequent seizures by approximately 50% over the next 2 years [13]. However, it is important to note that early treatment with antiepileptic drugs does not affect long-term prognosis in terms of epilepsy remission rates [13]. Although there is proven benefit in reducing the rate of seizure recurrence, it is still uncertain whether initiating antiepileptic drug therapy will in turn result in additional benefits of improvements in behavior and learning, or in reducing the chances of sudden unexplained death.

3.7 How to initiate treatment with antiepileptic drugs

Choosing an appropriate antiepileptic drug is the key to successful medical management of epilepsy in children. Although the number of antiepileptic drugs available continues to increase on a near-yearly basis, not all AEDs are routinely used as initial therapy in the pediatric population. The antiepileptic drugs that are most commonly used in the initiation of treatment for children are listed in Table 3.1. The choice of antiepileptic drug depends on several factors, of which the most important is accurate seizure classification. Seizure classification ideally involves accurate epilepsy syndrome diagnosis; however, classification into a partial versus a generalized epilepsy may be sufficient to appropriately choose and initiate treatment:

- Patients with a partial, or localization-related, epilepsy can be treated with either a narrow-spectrum or broad-spectrum antiepileptic drug.
- Patients with either a generalized epilepsy or epilepsy with varying seizure types should be initiated on treatment with a broad-spectrum antiepileptic drug.

Once it is decided to use either a narrow-spectrum or a broad-spectrum antiepileptic drug, the other factors used to choose an appropriate antiepileptic drug include:

- The side-effect profile of the drug.
- The available age- and patient-appropriate preparations of the drug.
- Whether therapeutic levels are needed quickly or not (depending on the frequency and severity of the patient's seizures).
- Consideration of the patient's comorbidities.

Table 3.1 Antiepileptic drugs used commonly as initial therapy in children.

Anticonvulsant drug	Availability	Indications: seizure type and syndrome	Suggested initiating dosing for children*
Carbamazepine	Tabs: 100, 200 mg	Partial	Start: 5–10 mg/kg/day
(Tegretol)	XR tabs: 100, 200, 400 mg Liquid: 100 mg/5 mL	BRE	Increase: every 5–7 days, by 5 mg/kg/day
(Carbatrol)	ER caps: 100, 200, 300 mg		Initial goal: 15–20 mg/kg/day
Ethosuximide	Caps: 250 mg	Generalized	Start: 10 mg/kg/day
(Zarontin)	Liquid: 250 mg/5 mL	CAE without GTC	Increase: every 5 days, by 5 mg/kg/day Initial goal: 15–20 mg/kg/day
Lamotrigine†	Tabs: 25, 100, 150, 200 mg	Partial and generalized	Start: 0.5 mg/kg/day
(Lamictal)	Chewable tabs: 2, 5, 25 mg XR tabs: 25, 50, 100, 200 mg	CAE, JME	Increase: every 2 weeks, by 0.5–1 mg/kg/day Initial goal: 3–5 mg/kg/day
Levetiracetam	Tabs: 250, 500, 750, 1000 mg	Partial and generalized	Start: 5–10 mg/kg/day
(Keppra)	XR tabs: 500, 750 mg Liquid: 100 mg/mL	CAE, JME	Increase: every 5–7 days, by 5–10 mg/kg/day Initial goal: 20–30 mg/kg/day
Oxcarbazepine	Tabs: 150, 300, 600 mg	Partial	Start: 5–10 mg/kg/day
(Trileptal)	Liquid: 300 mg/5 mL	BRE	Increase: every 5–7 days, by 5 mg/kg/day Initial goal: 15–20 mg/kg/day

Phenobarbital (Phenobarbital)	Tabs: 15, 30, 60, 100 mg Liquid: 20 mg/5 mL	Partial and generalized	Start: oral load 4 mg/kg every 12 hours × 4 doses Initial goal: 4 mg/kg/day
Phenytoin (Dilantin)	Caps: 30, 100 mg Chewable tabs: 50 mg Liquid: 125 mg/5 mL	Partial	Start: oral load 6 mg/kg every 8 hours × 3 doses Initial goal: 5 mg/kg/day
Topiramate (Topamax)	Tabs: 25, 50, 100, 200 mg Sprinkles: 15, 25 mg	Partial and generalized	Start: 0.5–1 mg/kg/day Increase: every 1–2 weeks, by 1–2 mg/kg/day Initial goal: 5 mg/kg/day
Valproic acid (Depakote) (Depakene)	Tabs: 125, 250, 500 mg ER tabs: 250, 500 mg Sprinkles: 125 mg Liquid: 250 mg/5 mL	Partial and generalized CAE, JME	Start: 5–10 mg/kg/day Increase: every 5–7 days, by 5–10 mg/kg/day Initial goal: 15–25 mg/kg/day
Vigabatrin (Sabril)	Powder: 500 mg/packet mixed in 10 mL of water Tabs: 500 mg	Infantile spasms	Start: 50 mg/kg/day Increase: every 3 days by 25–50 mg/kg/day Goal: 100–150 mg/kg/day
Zonisamide (Zonegran)	Caps: 25, 50, 100 mg	Partial and generalized	Start: 2 mg/kg/day Increase: every 2 weeks, by 2 mg/kg/day Initial goal: 8–10 mg/kg/day

*Consider adult dosing in patients >50 kg.

†Dosing is for lamotrigine monotherapy (see Chapter 11 for exact dose instructions).

BRE, benign rolandic epilepsy; CAE, childhood absence epilepsy; Caps, capsules; GTC, generalized tonic-clonic seizures; JME, juvenile myoclonic epilepsy; SR, sustained release; Tabs, tablets; XR, extended release.

Once an antiepileptic drug is chosen with discussion and input from the patient and their family, the general principle in initiating treatment is to use the lowest possible dose and increasing the dose to therapeutic levels or until side effects that prevent increasing the dose further. Suggested initial dosing is also listed in Table 3.1; however, individual variations may be based upon physician experience and upon individual patient circumstances.

3.8 Special circumstances

Antiepileptic drug therapy is the initial treatment considered for almost all patients with epilepsy. Exceptions, however, can be made in special circumstances, including:

- Specific epilepsy syndrome diagnoses.
- Specific metabolic disorders.

An example of a specific epilepsy syndrome diagnosis with alternative initial treatment options is infantile spasms. Due to a paucity of prospective, randomized, masked, controlled studies, first-line treatment of infantile spasms can include either standard antiepileptic drugs or hormonal therapy:

- The American Academy of Neurology guidelines state that adrenocorticotropic hormone (ACTH) is "probably effective" for the treatment of infantile spasms [15]. However, recent caution has occurred in the use of ACTH due to the side-effect profile and cost, although ACTH remains a first-line therapy.
- Evidence is re-emerging that oral steroids, specifically high-dose oral prednisolone (40–60 mg/day), may have similar efficacy and fewer adverse effects than ACTH [16].
- In addition, some families may choose an initial trial of the ketogenic diet for infantile spasms, with a plan for conversion to a first-line antiepileptic drug or hormonal therapy if warranted by unsuccessful outcome within the first 2 weeks of treatment [17].

In addition, for some epilepsy syndromes, behavioral and environmental modifications are just as important as the antiepileptic drugs prescribed:

- For juvenile myoclonic epilepsy, consistent sleep hygiene and abstention from alcohol.
- For Dravet syndrome (severe myoclonic epilepsy of infancy), avoidance of high environmental temperatures and aggressive fever control.

Specific metabolic disorders are also recognized to have alternative first-line treatment options other than standard antiepileptic drugs:

- Specific vitamin supplementation is used to treat patients with deficiencies in pyridoxine, folinic acid, pyridoxal phosphate, or biotin.
- The ketogenic diet is the first-line treatment for patients with glucose transporter type 1 deficiency.

3.9 Summary: initiating medical management

In general practice, initiation of treatment with antiepileptic drugs in children is deferred after the first seizure and initiated after the first seizure recurrence. Exceptions can be made to treat after the first seizure in:

- Patients with a high risk of recurrence.
- Patients in whom the consequences of recurrence might be overwhelmingly distressing.

This necessitates having a good understanding of the preferences and expectations of the patient and family. The American Academy of Neurology (AAN) has published guidelines [18] on the treatment of the child with a first unprovoked seizure (Box 3.8).

Box 3.8 AAN guidelines on the treatment of the child with a first unprovoked seizure

After the first seizure in a child, treatment with antiepileptic drug therapy may be considered in circumstances where the benefits of reducing the risk of a second seizure outweigh the risks of pharmacological and psychosocial side effects.

If treatment with antiepileptic drug therapy is to be initiated, the indication should not be for the prevention of the development of epilepsy.

Conversely, exceptions to continue to defer treatment after the first seizure recurrence can be made when:

- The risks of recurrence are low.
- The consequences of recurrence are tolerable to the family.

Whether future seizures will continue to be tolerable may be difficult to predict in some situations; for some patients, identification of a specific seizure syndrome will help to guide treatment decisions. The decision to defer initiation of treatment should remain a fluid decision, readdressed as the clinical course shifts, being receptive to the fact that patient and family preferences and expectations may change over time.

In summary, the decision to initiate antiepileptic drug therapy should be a decision specific for each patient and their family, balancing the recurrence risk of future seizures against the risks and benefits realized by initiating antiepileptic drug therapy. This is a decision-making process that is led by the physician but should include active participation by the parents and other care-takers, and in older children and adolescents, by the patients themselves. Finally, this decision should be based upon an understanding of the treatment goals: minimizing morbidity and mortality, and maximizing quality of life for both the patient and their family.

3.10 Withdrawing medical management

Although the discussion of antiepileptic drug discontinuation is distinctly separate from that of treatment initiation, it is almost invariably inquired about by patients and families at the time of antiepileptic drug therapy initiation. Active participation should be promoted in the care of the patient by the family unit. Thus, discussion of the following should be integral to the ongoing education for patients with epilepsy and their families from the time of diagnosis, and should not be confined to the time period when treatment discontinuation is being considered:

- The long-term prognosis of childhood-onset epilepsy.
- When to consider discontinuing antiepileptic drug therapy.

Box 3.9 Scenarios to consider withdrawing antiepileptic medications

After a successful time period of being seizure-free on antiepileptic drug therapy.
After successful non-medication treatments:

- Epilepsy surgery
- Vagus nerve stimulator implantation
- Dietary therapy implementation

The long-term prognosis for remission in childhood-onset epilepsy is generally favorable for most patients. Thus, the most common scenario encountered (Box 3.9) is to determine what constitutes a sufficient length of time of seizure remission on antiepileptic drug therapy before treatment discontinuation is considered. Likewise, a working knowledge of additional risk factors for seizure recurrence will help the physician make an individualized decision for each patient.

3.11 The long-term prognosis of childhood-onset epilepsy

The majority of patients are able to achieve seizure freedom with antiepileptic drug therapy [19]:

- At the initiation of epilepsy treatment, approximately 50% of patients will become seizure-free with the first prescribed antiepileptic drug.
- Another 15% will achieve seizure freedom with treatment with a second or third drug.

It is also known that the majority of children do not need to take antiepileptic drugs for the remainder of their lifetime. In other words, childhood-onset epilepsy is, in most cases, not an enduring chronic disease. In fact, the overall long-term prognosis of childhood-onset epilepsy is favorable. Patients followed long term have rates of remission of approximately 65% [20].

In studies in which seizure freedom with antiepileptic drug treatment is achieved for at least one or two years, the chance of remaining seizure free after treatment discontinuation is approximately 70% [21–23]. Thus, there is a point at which the natural history of epilepsy, which is supportive of eventual remission, might allow discontinuation of antiepileptic drug therapy; deciding when and in which patients to consider discontinuing antiepileptic drug therapy then becomes the focus of the decision-making process. This decision is based upon an understanding of several key questions (Box 3.10). This physician-led decision-making process should encourage active participation and feedback from the patient and their family, as their perceptions about risk may be different from that of the physician [24]. This risk of seizure recurrence may be acceptable to some families seeking to discontinue possibly unnecessary antiepileptic drugs, while some families that are more risk averse might not be willing to discontinue therapy for a 25% risk of seizure recurrence [24].

Box 3.10 Key questions to understand when considering discontinuation of antiepileptic drug therapy

What is the natural history of the disorder being treated (i.e., what are the chances of seizure recurrence if antiepileptic drug therapy is discontinued?)?
What are the possible adverse effects of seizure recurrence on the individual patient and family?
What are the risks of discontinuing antiepileptic drug therapy?
What are the benefits of discontinuing antiepileptic drug therapy?

3.12 When to consider discontinuing antiepileptic drug therapy

The majority of studies are supportive of considering discontinuation of antiepileptic drug therapy after a seizure-free period of at least 2 years [21–23]. Children tend to have better seizure-free rates after antiepileptic drug discontinuation than adults [22]. Two years seizure-free seems to be a reasonable length of time because:

- Most studies do not statistically support prolonging antiepileptic drug therapy for durations of seizure-freedom longer than 2 years, as children in whom antiepileptic drugs are discontinued after 4 years without seizures have similar seizure-free rates [21].
- On the contrary, most studies in which treatment is discontinued after shorter seizure-free periods of 1 year or less tend to report lower rates of successful discontinuation [25].

3.13 Risk factors for seizure recurrence after discontinuation

Although the literature supports a discussion of antiepileptic drug discontinuation after achieving and maintaining seizure remission for 2 years, there are other risk factors involved that may alter the risk calculations in this decision-making process (Box 3.11). Etiology, the age of onset of seizures, and EEG findings are the most consistently reported of these factors. In addition, epilepsy syndrome classification can render a consistent prognosis and response to therapy.

The most consistent factors

Seizure etiology

In general the long-term prognosis for patients with a remote symptomatic etiology is relatively less favorable than idiopathic or cryptogenic etiologies [20]. Consistent with this less favorable long-term prognosis, there is a lower likelihood of remaining seizure-free after discontinuing treatment in children with a remote symptomatic etiology versus idiopathic and cryptogenic etiologies [21–23].

- Patients with a remote symptomatic etiology have seizure-free rates of approximately 50% after discontinuation of antiepileptic drug therapy [22,23].

Box 3.11 Factors that can modulate the recurrence risk after antiepileptic drug discontinuation

Most consistent factors

- Etiology
- Age at onset of seizures
- EEG findings
- Epilepsy syndrome classification

Less consistent factors

- Seizure type
- Number or duration of seizures prior to control
- Antiepileptic drug type

- Patients with idiopathic or cryptogenic etiologies have seizure-free rates of approximately 70% [22,23].

Although their outlook is relatively less favorable compared to other etiologies, patients with a remote symptomatic etiology still have a good chance of remaining seizure free after discontinuation of therapy, albeit some subgroups moreso than others. As an example, in children with cerebral palsy and epilepsy who discontinue antiepileptic drug therapy after two seizure-free years, those with spastic hemiplegic cerebral palsy have approximately a 40% chance of remaining seizure-free, compared to those with spastic diplegic cerebral palsy, who have an 85% chance of remaining seizure-free [26].

Age at onset of seizures

Patients whose onset of epilepsy is during adolescence, as opposed to onset during childhood, tend to have a less favorable chance of remaining seizure free after discontinuation of antiepileptic drug therapy [21–23]:

- Patients with epilepsy onset in adolescence have seizure-free rates of approximately 30% after discontinuation of antiepileptic drug therapy [23].

EEG findings

Most, but not all, studies report that EEG findings prior to antiepileptic drug discontinuation are helpful in predicting the risk of recurrence [21–23,25]. When differentiating between types of EEG abnormalities, most studies find that epileptiform findings are more predictive of recurrence [25], but it is also reported that slowing, whether generalized or focal, is more predictive than epileptiform abnormalities [23]. Patients with an abnormal EEG prior to AED discontinuation tend to have less favorable rates of maintaining seizure freedom. This is especially true for patients with idiopathic or cryptogenic etiologies, but there is less of an effect with patients with remote symptomatic etiologies [23].

- Overall, patients with an abnormal EEG have seizure-free rates of less than 60% [21–23].
- Patients with a normal EEG have slightly more favorable seizure-free rates of more than 70% [21–23].

Epilepsy syndrome

EEG findings can also be helpful in assessing recurrence risk after antiepileptic drug discontinuation by facilitating epilepsy syndrome diagnosis (Box 3.12):

- There are certain childhood epilepsy syndromes for which the natural history is remission by late childhood or during adolescence, thus predicting eventual success with antiepileptic drug discontinuation.
- In contrast, some epilepsy syndromes are classically known to have a low likelihood of remitting.

The recurrence risk after 1–3 years of seizure-freedom on antiepileptic drug therapy in patients with benign rolandic epilepsy is low, and it can almost be certain that repeated trials of AED discontinuation will result in eventual remission for all patients with classic benign rolandic epilepsy.

The majority of patients with juvenile myoclonic epilepsy (JME) are traditionally treated with antiepileptic drug therapy indefinitely. It should be noted, however, that more recent evidence has found that not all patients with JME will necessarily relapse with antiepileptic drug discontinuation, and for some patients only myoclonus persists [27]. Thus, even patients with epilepsy syndromes that are traditionally thought not to remit, like JME, can be given the opportunity to at least discuss the possibility of a trial of treatment discontinuation. However, this decision should be made with caution and based upon individualized circumstances and risk tolerance, as the chances for seizure freedom are

Box 3.12 Prognosis of selected epilepsy syndromes

Tend to remit by late childhood or adolescence

- Benign epilepsy of childhood with central-temporal spikes (benign rolandic epilepsy).
- Early-onset benign childhood seizures with occipital spikes (Panayiotopoulos syndrome).

Tend not to remit

- Early infantile epileptic encephalopathy with suppression bursts (Ohtahara syndrome).
- Early myoclonic epilepsy.
- Juvenile myoclonic epilepsy.
- Lennox–Gastaut syndrome.
- Severe myoclonic epilepsy of infancy (Dravet syndrome).

not favorably high, and it is unclear how long patients with JME should be treated before consideration of treatment discontinuation.

The less consistent factors

Seizure type

For patients with single seizure types, studies differ on whether a partial or generalized seizure semiology is more predictive of remaining seizure-free, but those with multiple seizure types tend to have less favorable chances.

The number or duration of seizures prior to control

A few studies report that the number of seizures a patient has before obtaining control with antiepileptic drug therapy, or the initial duration of having seizures prior to control with AED therapy, can be less favorable predictors.

Antiepileptic drug type

Finally, there are no consistent data to show that the antiepileptic drug type being discontinued is predictive of recurrence risk.

3.14 The risks of discontinuing antiepileptic drug therapy

The risks of discontinuing antiepileptic therapy are principally related to the risks associated with seizure recurrence (see Box 3.6). The possible adverse effects of seizure recurrence can include the psychosocial reactions to a seizure, effects on learning and behavior, effects on sleep, and the risks of injury to the brain or the body, including the possibility of sudden death. The psychosocial reaction to seizure recurrence is related to both the severity and setting of the previous seizures – which may have evolved from the patient's semiology at initial presentation. As previously discussed, the severity and setting of a patient's seizures, and the patient and family's psychosocial reactions are important considerations in the decision of whether or not to discontinue antiepileptic drug therapy in a child. The literature on the incidence of status epilepticus after discontinuation of antiepileptic drugs is scarce, but fortunately it appears to be a rare event. In addition, death due to seizure recurrence appears to be a rare event after discontinuation of antiepileptic drugs.

- If seizure recurrence does occur, it is most likely to occur early, with 60% occurring within the first 6 months and 90% of seizure recurrences occurring within the first 2 years after treatment discontinuation [23].
- Late recurrence, 3 years or more after treatment discontinuation, is rare.

If seizure recurrence does occur, reinitiation of antiepileptic drug therapy should be considered in most cases, once again balancing the risks and benefits, and in consideration of the individual patient's circumstances. If the decision is made to initiate therapy again, seizure control is re-established in the majority of patients, although this may not occur in all cases immediately [23,28]. The scenario in which reinitiation of antiepileptic drug therapy is unable to eventually resume seizure control is rare, seen in less than 5% of patients after discontinuation of antiepileptic drug therapy [28].

3.15 The benefits of discontinuing antiepileptic drug therapy

The benefits of discontinuing antiepileptic drug therapy are mostly related to the relief of possible side effects:

- The effects on behavior and cognition are especially important in children. Evidence suggests that cognitive function, especially speed of complex cognitive processing, can improve after withdrawal of antiepileptic drug therapy. But it should be noted, however, that cognitive function may be more closely related to the underlying etiology and the extent of seizure control [29] rather than the effects of antiepileptic drug therapy.
- For patients on long-term treatment, the chronic adverse effects of each individual antiepileptic drug are particularly pertinent. The issue of bone health is also of special importance in children and adolescents because this is the time that is most vital for skeletal mineralization. Antiepileptic drugs are thought to have adverse effects on bone health, although the long-term effects on bone mineralization of the newer generation antiepileptic drugs are not as well studied [30].
- For females, especially those approaching or having reached adolescence, the known teratogenicity of antiepileptic drugs and future pregnancy become issues of concern.
- Finally, the positive psychosocial impact of not having to take a daily medication for a chronic disorder that has remitted may be one of the most significant benefits of being able to discontinue antiepileptic drug therapy for many patients – and also for their families.

3.16 How to discontinue antiepileptic drugs

The ideal rate at which to taper antiepileptic drugs is uncertain. In antiepileptic drug discontinuation studies, reported rates of tapering range from 1 to 12 months, with the majority of studies tapering AEDs within 4–6 months. Studies comparing drug tapering over differing time periods found that tapering antiepileptic drugs over a period of less than 6 months versus longer periods results in an increased risk of seizure recurrence. However, in the only randomized study, children were randomized to either a 6-week taper versus a 9-month taper, and no difference in seizure recurrence rates was found [31]. In regards to medication type, although patients on benzodiazepine and barbiturate classes of antiepileptic drugs are generally tapered in a more conservative fashion, withdrawal seizures during their gradual tapers are rare [32].

3.17 Special circumstances

Other scenarios in which one can consider discontinuing antiepileptic drug therapy include after successful interventions with other non-medication treatments for epilepsy, such as epilepsy surgery or dietary therapy implementation. Whether and when to discontinue antiepileptic drugs after epilepsy surgery is often a decision made in conjunction with the neurosurgeon, along with the patient and family. These discussions are usually carried out before the surgery or dietary therapy implementation, as one of the goals of these other treatments is often to decrease or discontinue the need for antiepileptic drugs.

- The timing of when after successful epilepsy surgery to discontinue treatment is not clear. However, it appears that seizure freedom 6 months postoperatively is a good predictor of seizure-free outcome, and thus without continued antiepileptic drug therapy [33].

- An alternative surgical treatment for epilepsy for children is implantation of a vagus nerve stimulator. Due to a paucity of literature, especially in children, the timing and method of antiepileptic drug tapering is unclear, but patients with vagus nerve stimulators implanted appear to have the possibility of either antiepileptic drug discontinuation or, more likely, dose reduction.
- The optimal timing of when to consider tapering or discontinuing antiepileptic drugs after successful dietary therapy implementation with the ketogenic diet is unclear, but is traditionally considered after 6 months of successful diet implementation [34]. However, earlier tapering of antiepileptic drugs (during diet initiation or within the first month) may be considered in individual circumstances, specifically for patients for whom the adverse effects of their antiepileptic drugs are of major concern [34].

3.18 Summary: withdrawing medical management

In general practice, discontinuation of treatment with antiepileptic drugs in children is considered after 2 years of seizure freedom. Exceptions can be made to discontinue treatment sooner based upon individual patient circumstances. These circumstances can include:

- Patients with benign seizures.
- Patients with lower risks of recurrence.
- Patients with an epilepsy syndrome known to have eventual remittance.

This necessitates having a good understanding of the preferences and expectations of the patient and family. Conversely, there may be some patients and their families who are content to continue taking their medications, and this may be an acceptable choice for:

- Patients and families that prefer stability and are risk-averse.
- Adolescents who do not want to risk losing their driver's license.
- Patients who are well controlled at present, but have unfavorable risk factors for seizure recurrence.
- Patients for whom antiepileptic drug side effects are not a concern. It should be discussed, however, that even if current side effects are not a concern to the patient, antiepileptic drugs carry with them risks for long-term side effects (i.e., adverse effects on bone health) and, of special importance for females, the risks for teratogenicity.

For these patients, the decision to defer discontinuation of treatment should remain a fluid decision, keeping open the possibility of discontinuing antiepileptic drug treatment in the future.

The American Academy of Neurology (AAN) guidelines [35] state that drug withdrawal should be offered to patients who meet a specific profile (Box 3.13):

Box 3.13 AAN guidelines for patients considering antiepileptic drug withdrawal

Seizure-free for 2–5 years on antiepileptic drug therapy.
A single type of either partial or generalized seizures.
A normal neurological examination and a normal intelligence quotient.
An EEG that is normalized with treatment.

However, the American Academy of Neurology guidelines also state that treatment discontinuation may be appropriate for patients who do not meet this profile.

In summary, the decision to discontinue antiepileptic drug therapy should be a decision specific for each patient and their family, balancing the risks of future recurrences of seizures against the benefits realized by discontinuing antiepileptic drug therapy. This is a decision-making process that is led by the physician but should include active participation by the parents and other care-takers, and, in older children and adolescents, by the patients themselves, realizing that the perceptions of the patients and their families about risk may be different from that of the physician [24]. Finally, this decision should be based upon an understanding of the treatment goals: minimizing morbidity and mortality, and maximizing quality of life for both the patient and their family.

3.19 Disclaimer

The views expressed are those of the authors and do not reflect the official policy or position of the United States Air Force, Department of Defense, or the US Government.

References

[1] Berg AT, Shinnar S. The risk of seizure recurrence following a first unprovoked seizure: A quantitative review. *Neurology* 1991;**41**:965–972.

[2] Shinnar S, Berg AT, Moshe SL, *et al.* The risk of seizure recurrence after a first unprovoked afebrile seizure in childhood: An extended follow-up. *Pediatrics* 1996;**98**:216–225.

[3] Hirtz D, Ashwal S, Berg A, *et al.* Practice parameter: Evaluating a first nonfebrile seizure in children: Report of the Quality Standards Subcommittee of the American Academy of Neurology, the Child Neurology Society, and the American Epilepsy Society. *Neurology* 2000;**55**:616–623.

[4] Commission on Epidemiology and Prognosis, International League Against Epilepsy. Guidelines for epidemiologic studies on epilepsy. *Epilepsia* 1993;**34**:592–596.

[5] Shinnar S, Berg AT, O'Dell C, *et al.* Predictors of multiple seizures in a cohort of children prospectively followed from the time of their first unprovoked seizure. *Ann Neurol* 2000;**48**:140–147.

[6] Camfield P, Camfield C. Epilepsy can be diagnosed when the first two seizures occur on the same day. *Epilepsia* 2000;**41**:1230–1233.

[7] Maytal J, Shinnar S, Moshe SL, Alvarez LA. Low morbidity and mortality of status epilepticus in children. *Pediatrics* 1989;**83**:323–331.

[8] Austin JK, Harezlak J, Dunn DW, *et al.* Behavior problems in children before first recognized seizures. *Pediatrics* 2001;**107**:115–122.

[9] Austin JK, Dunn DW, Caffrey HM, *et al.* Recurrent seizures and behavior problems in children with first recognized seizures: A prospective study. *Epilepsia* 2002;**43**:1564–1573.

[10] Cortesi F, Giannotti F, Ottaviano S. Sleep problems and daytime behavior in childhood idiopathic epilepsy. *Epilepsia* 1999;**40**:1557–1565.

[11] Appleton RE, Mersey Region Paediatric Epilepsy Interest Group. Seizure-related injuries in children with newly diagnosed and untreated epilepsy. *Epilepsia* 2002;**43**:764–767.

[12] Berg AT, Shinnar S. Do seizures beget seizures? An assessment of the clinical evidence in humans. *J Clin Neurophysiol* 1997;**14**:102–110.

[13] First Seizure Trial Group. Randomized clinical trial on the efficacy of antiepileptic drugs in reducing the risk of relapse after a first unprovoked tonic-clonic seizure. *Neurology* 1993;**43**:478–483.

[14] Camfield P, Camfield C. Sudden unexpected death in people with epilepsy: A pediatric perspective. *Semin Pediatr Neurol* 2005;**12**:10–14.
[15] Mackay MT, Weiss SK, Adams-Webber T, *et al.* Practice parameter: medical treatment of infantile spasms: Report of the American Academy of Neurology and the Child Neurology Society. *Neurology* 2004;**62**:1668–1681.
[16] Kossoff EH, Hartman AL, Rubenstein JE, Vining EP. High-dose oral prednisolone for infantile spasms: An effective and less expensive alternative to ACTH. *Epilepsy Behav* 2009;**14**:674–676.
[17] Kossoff EH, Hedderick EF, Turner Z, Freeman JM. A case-controlled evaluation of the ketogenic diet versus ACTH for new-onset infantile spasms. *Epilepsia* 2008;**49**:1504–1509.
[18] Hirtz D, Berg A, Bettis D, *et al.* Practice parameter: treatment of the child with a first unprovoked seizure: Report of the Quality Standards Subcommittee of the American Academy of Neurology and the Practice Committee of the Child Neurology Society. *Neurology* 2003;**60**:166–175.
[19] Kwan P, Brodie MJ. Early identification of refractory epilepsy. *N Engl J Med* 2000;**342**:314–319.
[20] Sillanpaa M, Jalava M, Kaleva O, Shinnar S. Long-term prognosis of seizures with onset in childhood. *N Engl J Med* 1998;**338**:1715–1722.
[21] Shinnar S, Vining EPG, Mellits ED, *et al.* Discontinuing antiepileptic medications in children with epilepsy after two years without seizures. *N Engl J Med* 1985;**313**:976–980.
[22] Berg AT, Shinnar S. Relapse following discontinuation of antiepileptic drugs: A meta-analysis. *Neurology* 1994;**44**:601–608.
[23] Shinnar S, Berg AT, Moshe SL, *et al.* Discontinuing antiepileptic drugs in children with epilepsy: A prospective study. *Ann Neurol* 1994;**35**:534–545.
[24] Gordon K, MacSween J, Dooley J, *et al.* Families are content to discontinue antiepileptic drugs at different risks than their physicians. *Epilepsia* 1996;**37**:557–562.
[25] Peters ACB, Brouwer OF, Geerts AT, *et al.* Randomized prospective study of early discontinuation of antiepileptic drugs in children with epilepsy. *Neurology* 1998;**50**:724–730.
[26] Delgado MR, Riela AR, Mills J, *et al.* Discontinuation of antiepileptic drug treatment after two seizure-free years in children with cerebral palsy. *Pediatrics* 1996;**97**:192–197.
[27] Camfield CS, Camfield PR. Juvenile myoclonic epilepsy 25 years after seizure onset: A population-based study. *Neurology* 2009;**73**:1041–1045.
[28] Camfield P, Camfield C. The frequency of intractable seizures after stopping AEDs in seizure free children with epilepsy. *Neurology* 2005;**64**:973–975.
[29] Aldenkamp AP, Alpherts WC, Sandstedt P, *et al.* Antiepileptic drug-related cognitive complaints in seizure-free children with epilepsy before and after drug discontinuation. *Epilepsia* 1998;**39**:1070–1074.
[30] Sheth RD. Bone health in pediatric epilepsy. *Epilepsy Behav* 2004;**5**(Suppl. 2):S30–S35.
[31] Tennison M, Greenwood R, Lewis D, Thorn M. Discontinuing antiepileptic drugs in children with epilepsy. A comparison of a six-week and a nine-month taper period. *N Engl J Med* 1994;**330**:1407–1410.
[32] Chadwick D. Does withdrawal of different antiepileptic drugs have different effects on seizure recurrence? Further results from the MRC Antiepileptic Drug Withdrawal Study. *Brain* 1999;**122**:441–448.
[33] Lachwani DK, Loddenkemper T, Holland KD, *et al.* Discontinuation of medications after successful epilepsy surgery in children. *Pediatr Neurol* 2008;**38**:340–344.
[34] Kossoff EH, Pyzik PL, McGrogan JR, Rubenstein JE. The impact of early versus late anticonvulsant reduction after ketogenic diet initiation. *Epilepsy Behav* 2004;**5**:499–502.
[35] Practice parameter: A guideline for discontinuing antiepileptic drugs in seizure-free patients – Summary Statement. *Neurology* 1996;**47**:600–602.

4 Common genetic and neurocutaneous disorders in childhood epilepsy

Dewi Frances T. Depositario-Cabacar[1], William McClintock[1], and Tom Reehal[2]

[1]*Neurology and Pediatrics, George Washington University Medical Center, Children's National Medical Center, Washington, DC, USA*
[2]*University of Sheffield School of Medicine, Dentistry, and Health, Sheffield, UK*

Genetic studies of epilepsy play a significant role in improving early diagnosis, avoiding ordering of unnecessary tests, selecting the appropriate antiepileptic medication, and providing information on prognosis and recurrence risk.

The International Classification of Epileptic Syndromes has divided epilepsies based upon their underlying cause as either idiopathic or symptomatic [1].

- *Symptomatic* is used when there is an acquired cause of epilepsy (e.g., stroke, tumors) and/or when there are associated neurological deficits, such as cognitive delay and motor weakness.
- *Idiopathic* epilepsies are often referred for syndromes with a genetic cause, where there are no other neurological and neuroimaging findings.
- The term *cryptogenic* has been used for epilepsies for which an etiology cannot be identified.

Idiopathic epilepsies are assumed to be mainly genetic and comprise about 30% of cases [2]. Genetic studies have identified more than 20 genes with a major association to the

Epilepsy in Children and Adolescents, First Edition. Edited by James W. Wheless.

Box 4.1 Importance of genetic studies in epilepsy

- Provide for early diagnosis.
- Avoid ordering unnecessary expensive or invasive tests once the diagnosis is made.
- Help select the appropriate antiepileptic medications.
- Provide information on prognosis and recurrence risk for seizures.
- Facilitate genetic counseling.
- Enable monitoring of other organ involvement associated with the genetic syndrome.

idiopathic epilepsies [3]. Although not as common, some of the symptomatic epilepsies also have a genetic basis.

Genetic studies of epilepsy play a significant role in facilitating earlier diagnosis and avoiding unnecessary laboratory work-up once the diagnosis is made. Genetic testing can also provide information regarding prognosis and the need for genetic counseling (Box 4.1). Clues to a genetic etiology would include dysmorphic features, multiple congenital anomalies, history of consanguinity, and multiple miscarriages [4]. It is therefore crucial in a routine epilepsy evaluation to obtain a detailed family history that also includes a pedigree analysis.

A guide to the appropriate genetic testing associated with epilepsy can be obtained at the GeneTests website (http://www.ncbi.nlm.nih.gov/sites/GeneTests). This resource provides a list of both clinical and research laboratories that offer specific genetic tests. The website also contains educational materials and reviews on specific disorders [3]. Despite these advances in knowledge, genetic testing is mostly available for monogenetic epilepsies and is limited in the diagnosis of epilepsy syndromes that have a complex inheritance pattern [5].

This chapter will discuss some of the more common genetic causes of idiopathic epilepsies. A few of the symptomatic epilepsies with a genetic basis, which include the neurocutaneous disorders, chromosomal anomalies, metabolic and mitochondrial disorders, and disorders of malformations of cortical development, will also be reviewed.

4.1 Idiopathic epilepsies

With the breakthroughs in the field of genetics over the past two decades, genetic studies have identified more than 20 genes with a major association with idiopathic epilepsies [3]. Some of the common idiopathic epilepsies are summarized in Table 4.1. Note that most of the genetic mutations involve an ion channel (sodium or potassium) or a neurotransmitter receptor (acetylcholine, or gamma-aminobutyric acid). Commonly seen idiopathic epilepsies are discussed in detail in this chapter.

In infancy, the three common familial focal epilepsies occurring are benign familial neonatal seizures (BFNS), benign familial neonatal-infantile seizures (BFNIS), and benign familial infantile seizures (BFIS) (Table 4.2). All of these focal epilepsies have an autosomal dominant inheritance pattern and are known to occur in previously normal infants. These epilepsies tend to have similar clinical characteristics but differ in age of onset and gene

Table 4.1 Genes identified in some common idiopathic epilepsy syndromes

Syndrome	Chromosome	Gene	Defect
Benign familial neonatal seizures	20q13.3 8q24	*KCNQ2* *KCNQ3*	Potassium channel Potassium channel
Benign familial neonatal-infantile seizures	2q23-q24.3	*SCN2A*	Sodium channel
Benign familial infantile seizures	19q12-q13.11		
Dravet syndrome (severe myoclonic epilepsy of infancy)	2q24	*SCN1A*	Sodium channel
Generalized epilepsy with febrile seizure plus (GEFS+)	2q24 19q13.1 5q34	*SCN1A* *SCN1B* *GABRG2*	Sodium channel Sodium channel $GABA_A$ receptor
Childhood absence epilepsy	5q31-33 3q26 5q34-35	*GABRG2* *CLCN2* *GABRA1*	GABA receptor Chloride channel GABA receptor
Juvenile myoclonic epilepsy	5q34-q35 6p12-p11	*GABRA1* *EFHC1*	$GABA_A$ receptor EH-hand motif protein
Rolandic epilepsy	15q23		
Autosomal dominant nocturnal frontal lobe epilepsy	20q13.2-q13.3 1q21 8p21	*CHRNA4* *CHRNB2* *CHRNA2*	Acetylcholine receptor Acetylcholine receptor Acetylcholine receptor
Autosomal dominant lateral temporal lobe epilepsy (also called autosomal dominant partial epilepsy with auditory features)	10q24	*LGI1*	Leucine-rich repeat epilepsy protein

Adapted from Ottman *et al.* (2010).

defect [5]. Mostly the seizures resolve without treatment and developmental outcome is usually normal.

Generalized epilepsy with febrile seizure plus (GEFS+)

Generalized epilepsy with febrile seizure plus (GEFS+) is a genetic epilepsy syndrome characterized by a large phenotypic heterogeneity, which includes typical febrile seizures

Table 4.2 Neonatal seizures

Seizure type	Seizure onset	Seizures	Gene	Defect
BFNS	2 to 3 days of life	Tonic, focal, clonic apnea, autonomic features	*KCNQ2* *KCNQ3*	Potassium channel
BFNIS	2 days to 7 months	Occur in cluster	*SCN2A*	Sodium channel
BFIS	4 to 8 months	Focal seizures, occur in cluster	Unknown	Unknown

BFNS, benign familial neonatal seizures; BFNIS, benign familial neonatal-infantile seizures; BFIS, benign familial infantile seizures.

(FS) and a variety of childhood-onset generalized epilepsy phenotypes [6]. GEFS+ occurring in families may have a variable phenotype even with the same genetic mutation [4].

- Patients typically present with febrile seizures that extend beyond 6 years of age, or have accompanying afebrile seizures that are mainly generalized but in some cases are focal.
- The seizures are of multiple types and include absence, myoclonic, atonic, or the more generalized epilepsy syndrome of myoclonic-astatic epilepsy (MAE) [6]. The most severe end of the spectrum is Dravet syndrome, which will also be discussed.
- GEFS+ has been caused by mutations in three genes, namely *SCN1B* [7], *SCN1A* [8], and *GABRG2* [9].

Dravet syndrome

Dravet syndrome, or severe myoclonic epilepsy in infancy (SMEI), represents the most severe form of the GEFS+ spectrum and is a rare epileptic syndrome affecting approximately 1 in 40 000 [5].

- It usually starts in the first year of life (peak age 5 months).
- Seizures consist of early infantile clonic febrile convulsions (seen initially in the mild period), followed by refractory myoclonic jerks, atypical absences, and complex focal seizures (seen in the aggressive period). These are followed by residual mental and neurological abnormalities (the static period), such as psychomotor delay and ataxia [10].
- Around 70% individuals have a mutation of *SCN1A* [11].
- The interictal EEG may show generalized spike and waves, polyspike and waves, and focal abnormalities [5].
- Elevated body temperature due to fever, hot baths, or a warm environment may precipitate more seizures. Photic stimulation, gazing at visual patterns, and eye closure precipitate generalized discharges, myoclonias, and absences [10].
- Seizures are refractory. Valproate, topiramate, and stiripentol may be therapeutic. Lamotrigine and carbamazepine may exacerbate seizures.

Autosomal dominant nocturnal frontal lobe epilepsy

Autosomal dominant nocturnal frontal lobe epilepsy (ADNFLE) is the first syndrome of idiopathic focal epilepsy with a single gene inheritance [12].

- Seizures consist of clusters of brief motor seizures that occur in sleep. The seizures have hyperkinetic or tonic manifestations that arise from the frontal lobes [12].
- It is an autosomal dominant epilepsy linked to chromosome 20q and 15q. Mutations have been identified in the *CHRNA4* gene, which encodes the $\alpha4$ subunit of the neuronal nicotinic acetylcholine receptor (nAChR) [13], and in *CHRNB2*, also an acetylcholine receptor gene [14].
- Treatment of choice is either carbamazepine or oxcarbazepine.

Autosomal dominant lateral temporal lobe epilepsy

Autosomal dominant lateral temporal lobe epilepsy (ADLTE) is also called autosomal partial epilepsy with auditory features. It is characterized by auditory hallucinations or auras.

- Onset is usually during adolescence or early adulthood.
- Mutations of leucine-rich, glioma-inactivated 1 gene (*LGI1*) on chromosome 10q22-24 have been reported [15]. The leucine-rich protein is responsible for neuronal migration and adhesion.
- This syndrome is generally responsive to antiepileptic medications and has a good prognosis.

Juvenile myoclonic epilepsy

Juvenile myoclonic epilepsy (JME), also called Janz syndrome, accounts for 5–10% of all epilepsies.

- The age of onset is from 8 to 26 years and it typically presents with early morning myoclonus. The vast majority have generalized tonic-clonic seizures, and one-third have absence [16].
- The interictal EEG consists of bilateral, symmetrical 3.5–6 Hz spike or polyspike and wave, with bifrontal predominance and photosensitivity.
- Valproic acid, lamotrigine and topiramate have been used for therapy.

4.2 Symptomatic epilepsies

Symptomatic epilepsies are generally secondary to an acquired central nervous system injury. The patients usually have neurological deficit, cognitive delay, developmental delay, and abnormal neuroimaging findings.

Focal and symptomatic generalized epilepsies are thought less likely to have a genetic basis compared to the idiopathic epilepsies, However, there are also some epilepsies thought of as acquired that have a genetic etiology. These include the neurocutaneous disorders, neuronal migration disorders, chromosomal abnormalities, inborn errors of metabolism, and mitochondrial disorders. A few examples of these symptomatic epilepsies with prominent seizures are also reviewed in this chapter.

4.3 Epilepsy in common chromosomal abnormalities

Chromosomal anomalies are known to carry an increased risk of seizures compared to the general population. The loss or abnormal function of the genetic loci on the chromosome may lead to increased seizure susceptibility, cortical irritability, or changes in neurotransmitters [17]. A few of these chromosomal anomalies that are associated with epilepsy are discussed (Table 4.3).

Wolf–Hirschhorn syndrome

Wolf–Hirshhorn syndrome is a contiguous gene syndrome caused by a deletion in the terminal band of the short arm of chromosome 4.

- Typical features include distinct facial features, severe growth retardation with delayed bone age, mental retardation, and microcephaly. Typically patients have the “Greek warrior helmet” profile (broad, beaked nose, prominent glabella, and frontal bossing).

Table 4.3 Common epilepsies associated with chromosomal abnormalities

Epilepsy syndrome	Chromosome involved
Wolf–Hirschhorn syndrome	Deletion in short arm of chromosome 4p
Angelman syndrome	Chromosome 15q11-q13
Miller–Dieker syndrome	Deletion in chromosome 17p13.3
Trisomy 21	Chromosome 21
Ring 20 syndrome	Chromosome 20
Rett syndrome	Mutation in *MECP2* gene in chromosome Xq28

- Seizures occur in about 70–100%, with most cases occurring in the first year of life. They may be partial motor or unilateral seizures, generalized tonic-clonic seizures, or myoclonic seizures. Interictal EEG consists of high-voltage slow waves, occasionally appearing paroxysmally, as irregular 3–4 Hz high voltage slow waves [18].

Angelman syndrome

This is a classic disorder of genetic imprinting that is caused by the deletion or inactivation of genes on the maternally inherited chromosome 15q11-q13 (causing defective *UBE3A* gene expression).

- Patients present with moderate to severe mental retardation, ataxia, tremulousness, and a characteristic behavior that is described as a "happy puppet."
- Onset of seizures occurs from age 18 to 24 months [19].
- Seizures are described as being either tonic-clonic, complex partial, atypical absence, myoclonic, or atonic.
- Interictal EEG patterns are characteristic and consist of high-amplitude bilateral spike and wave activity at ∼2 Hz [20].
- Initially the seizures are refractory but they improve in later childhood [19].

Rett syndrome

Rett syndrome is caused by a mutation in the gene encoding methyl-CpG-binding protein-2 (MeCP2) located in chromosome Xq28. MECP2 is a transcription factor that binds to methylated CpG and silences transcription.

- Clinical features include developmental regression and deceleration of brain growth leading to microcephaly during the first year of life. Ataxia, hypotonia, seizures, and autistic behavior are also seen.
- The hallmark is repetitive hand-wringing movements and the loss of purposeful hand use.
- Typical seizures are generalized tonic-clonic seizures (66% of patients). Video electroencephalography is recommended in differentiating non-epileptic events from true seizures [20].
- Interictal EEG may show multifocal centrotemporal discharges with a slow background for age [20].
- Seizures respond to most antiepileptic medications.

Ring chromosome 20

Ring chromosome 20 is a rare condition associated with refractory epilepsy.

- Patients typically have mild to moderate learning difficulties, behavioral disorders, and epilepsy, often without significant dysmorphism [21]. The lack of dysmorphism suggests that the condition may be underdiagnosed.
- Patients may have frequent episodes of atypical absence or non-convulsive status, associated with diffuse slow rhythmic EEG changes [21]. Perioral and eyelid myoclonias may also be present.
- During non-convulsive status the EEG shows high-amplitude rhythmic slow activity at 2–3 Hz, with spike or spike waves predominant in the frontal areas [21].
- Seizures are often refractory.

Miller–Dieker syndrome (MDS)

Miller–Dieker syndrome is caused by defective neuronal migration resulting in lissencephaly. It is an autosomal disorder that is caused by a deletion of chromosome 17p involving multiple genes, including neuronal migration genes *LIS1* and *YWHAE* (14-3-3 epsilon protein) [22]. Because of the associated lissencephaly, the syndrome can also be categorized as symptomatic epilepsy.

- Patients typically have characteristic facial dysmorphism, which includes a high forehead with furrows and vertical ridges, indentation of the temples, a small upturned nose, upslanting eyes, a small mouth, a thick, broad upper lip with a thin border, and low-set ears.
- Epileptic seizures in MDS are refractory to treatment. Some improvement may be achieved with ACTH or benzodiazepines [18].

4.4 Epilepsy in metabolic and mitochondrial disorders

Inborn errors of metabolism are congenital disorders associated with an abnormality or disruption of a metabolic pathway. These would include disorders of carbohydrate, amino acid, or organic acid metabolism as well as lysosomal storage and peroxisomal disorders. Metabolic and mitochondrial disorders should always be considered in a child with seizures with no known etiology, especially if there are other symptoms present, such as developmental delay or regression, and other organ involvement. In a few of these disorders, seizures are a prominent symptom, especially myoclonic seizures (Table 4.4).

The metabolic disorders tend to present in the neonate or infant. Pyridoxine dependency presents with severe refractory seizures in the first few days of life, which may have been noted *in utero*. The genetic defect has been mapped to chromosome 5q31 [23]. Recent research has disclosed deficiency of antiquitin in the lysine degradation pathway as the primary metabolic defect in at least some patients. Administration of pyridoxine, typically 100 mg intravenously, with concomitant EEG, is of both diagnostic and therapeutic value.

Biotinidase deficiency is an autosomal recessive inherited metabolic disorder that leads to multiple carboxylase deficiency. It presents with refractory seizures of multiple seizure types and is treated with high doses of biotin. The gene locus has been mapped to chromosome 3p25.

Table 4.4 Genetically defined epileptic syndromes – metabolic and mitochondrial disorders

Disorder	Chromosome/gene	Defect
Metabolic disorders		
Pyridoxine dependency	5q31.2-q31.3	Lysine degradation (antiquitin deficiency)
Glycine encephalopathy	9p22	Glycine cleavage
Glut-1 deficiency	*GLUT1* gene chromosome 1	Glucose transport
Biotinidase deficiency	3p25	Deficient biotinidase
Progressive myoclonic epilepsies		
Unverricht–Lundborg	21q22.2	Cystatin B
Lafora disease	6q24	Protein phosphatase
MERRF syndrome	tRNA-lysine mutation	

Glycine encephalopathy (non-ketotic hyperglycinemia), a defect in the glycine cleavage system at gene locus 9p22, also presents with neonatal and sometimes *in utero* seizures.

Glucose transporter-1 deficiency results from a defect in glucose transport into the brain and has been mapped to chromosome 1p [24]. Seizures usually respond to the ketogenic diet, which provides an alternative fuel to glucose for cerebral metabolism.

Progressive myoclonus epilepsies are a group of disorders that are characterized by myoclonus, mental deterioration, and ataxia. These disorders can be due to lysosomal disorders or mitochondrial disorders. Lafora disease is an autosomal recessive disorder with a mutation in the protein tyrosine phosphatase gene on chromosome 6q24 [25]. Unverricht–Lundborg disease is an autosomal recessive disorder that is secondary to mutations in the cystatin B gene causing abnormal function of the cysteine protein inhibitor. Myoclonic epilepsy with ragged red fibers (MERRF syndrome) is a rare mitochondrial disease that presents with progressive myoclonic epilepsy, lactic acidosis, hearing problems, and short stature.

4.5 Epilepsy in malformations of cortical development

Central nervous system malformations account for a significant cause of symptomatic epilepsies. A causative gene has been identified in some of these cortical malformations. As shown in Table 4.5, these conditions range from neuronal migration disorders, such

Table 4.5 Epilepsy associated with malformations of cortical development

Malformation	Locus	Gene
Periventricular nodular heterotopia	Xq28	Filamin A
Isolated lissencephaly	17p13.3	*LIS1*
Subcortical band/double cortex	X21-24	*XLIS* or *DCX*; doublecortin gene
Autosomal recessive lissencephaly with cerebellar hypoplasia	7q22	*RELN*
Lissencephaly with abnormal genitalia		*ARX*
Schizencephaly	10q26.1	*EMX2*
Tuberous sclerosis	9q34	Hamartin
	16p13.3	Tuberin

as lissencephaly and schizencephaly, to heterotopias to tuberous sclerosis, a multi-organ neurocutaneous disorder in which epilepsy is often the major morbidity.

4.6 Neurocutaneous disorders

Neurocutaneous disorders, or the phakomatoses, are a special category of epilepsy-associated genetic disorders that all share the following characteristics:

- Cerebral involvement (with or without seizures).
- Dermatological or ocular involvement.
- Typically a genetic etiology.

The genetics are variable and include autosomal dominant, autosomal recessive, X-linked, and sporadic inheritance (Table 4.6).

A diagnosis can often be made with simple examination of the skin or eyes, or by characteristic findings on neuroimaging studies. Although each of these disorders is rare; as a group they are common. Early recognition and diagnosis of this group reduces the need for further diagnostic work-up and allows prompt genetic counseling to be given. Another important factor is that these disorders often have multi-organ involvement, which requires monitoring protocols to prevent complications (see Table 4.1). Many of these disorders have variable expressivity and prognosis, even within families.

Tuberous sclerosis complex (TSC) has well-documented clinical and imaging manifestations (Table 4.7). It is associated with various seizure types in the majority of patients. Multi-organ monitoring is required (Table 4.8). While it is listed as having autosomal dominant inheritance, many cases are sporadic new mutations, and germline mosaicism may occur where siblings are affected but parents are not. There is also considerable phenotypic heterogeneity within the same families.

Epilepsy associated with TSC is often very disabling and difficult to control. There is a close association of TSC and infantile spasms (IS), with 10% of children presenting with IS having TSC, and 25% of children with the diagnosis of TSC experiencing IS [26].

Table 4.6 Inheritance pattern of common neurocutaneous syndromes

Inheritance	Disorder
Autosomal dominant	Neurofibromatosis 1 Neurofibromatosis 2 Tuberous sclerosis complex Basal cell nevus syndrome Epidermal nevus syndrome (linear sebaceous nevus syndrome)
Autosomal recessive	Ataxia telangiectasia Xeroderma pigmentosum
X-linked	Incontentia pigmenti Menkes disease
Sporadic	Sturge–Weber syndrome POEMS* syndrome

*Polyneuropathy, organomegaly, endocrinopathy, M-protein, skin abnormalities.

Table 4.7 Clinical manifestations of tuberous sclerosis complex

Category	Features
Skin manifestations	Hypomelanotic macules Facial angiofibromas Shagreen patch Periungual and ungual fibroma Gum fibroma and dental pits Forehead plaque Skin tags
Eye manifestations	Achromic macule Retinal hamartoma
Neuroimaging manifestations	Subependymal nodule Subcortical tubers Subependymal giant cell astrocytoma (SEGA) Radial glia lines Focal cortical dysplasia

A comprehensive skin exam is important with any infant presenting with IS. There is a more guarded prognosis for infants with TSC presenting with IS. Also children with these two conditions seem to be much more responsive to treatment with vigabatrin than other children with IS [27]. Multiple other seizure types are seen with TSC, and the treatment is similar to treating epilepsy in general. Choice of antiepileptic medication depends on seizure type. Other treatment options include the ketogenic diet, vagus nerve stimulation, and epilepsy surgery.

Renal involvement is the leading cause of morbidity in adults with TSC. Regular monitoring is needed for renal angioleiomyomas and rare renal cell cancer [28]. This can often be accomplished with regular renal magnetic resonance imaging (MRI) examinations. Younger children should also be monitored for a subependymal giant cell astrocytoma (SEGA) [29], a tumor that can cause obstructive hydrocephalus and occurs in about 10% of patients.

Table 4.8 Monitoring in tuberous sclerosis complex

Organ	Lesion	Monitoring required
Kidney	Angiomyolipomas renal cysts, renal cell cancer	Renal ultrasound or MRI
Heart	Rhabdomyomas Arrhythmias	Cardiac echocardiogram EKG
Lungs	Lymphangiomyolioma	Chest imaging (adolescents/ adult women)
Brain	SEGA Cognitive deficits	Brain MRI or CT Neuropsychological studies

CT, computed tomography; EKG, electrocardiogram; MRI, magnetic resonance imaging; SEGA, subependymal giant cell astrocytoma.

SEGAs tend to grow during childhood and especially during puberty. Many patients with TSC have learning difficulties, even if they do not have autism or cognitive deficiency.

There are multiple neurocutaneous conditions associated with an increased incidence of epilepsy [30]. Some of these conditions are more common but are associated with just a small incidence of epilepsy, for example, neurofibromatosis 1. Other conditions are rare, but have a high incidence of epilepsy. Besides TSC, other neurocutaneous conditions that are strongly associated with epilepsy are described below.

Sturge–Weber syndrome

The main features are:

- Hemangioma (port-ine stain) involving V1 distribution on the face, and may also involve V2 and V3. May be unilateral or bilateral, or have no facial hemangioma (5%) [31].
- Ipsilateral leptomeningeal angioma.
- Partal seizures emanating from the side of the angioma.
- Progressive atrophy and hemiparesis.
- Some mental deficiency is common.
- Often presents at birth with the port-wine stain.
- An angioma of the choroid of the eye leads to glaucoma and vision loss and must be monitored [32].

An MRI during infancy can often demonstrate the leptomeningeal angioma [33]. The facial hemangioma can be isolated.

Incontinentia pigmenti

The main features can be summarized thus:

- X-linked dominant seen primarily in females. NEMO gene encoding NFκB [34].
- Manifest as a rash with four stages: starting with a bullous eruption, followed by crusting over, then hyperpigmentation in a swirling pattern, and finally resolving in adulthood.
- Epilepsy is frequently seen.
- Mental retardation is common.
- Eye involvement is very frequent and includes optic atrophy, retinal artery occlusion and other retinal vasculopathy, strabismus, cataracts, coloboma, and blindness.
- Vasculopathy with perivascular infiltration and strokes.
- CNS manifestations include MR, hydrocephalus, seizures, spasticity, ataxia, and cerebral edema.
- Dental abnormalities.
- Malignancies including leukemia, kidney tumors, retinoblastoma, and rhabdomyosarcoma.

Linear sebaceous nevus syndrome

This is included with the autosomal dominant disorder of "epidermal nevus syndrome," but is more restricted to patients with typical midline nevus.

- May affect every organ system.
- CNS is most often affected with mental retardation (MR) and epilepsy.

- Relatively high frequency of 1 in 1000 live births [35].
- The nevus usually appears on the face or scalp and is present at birth or in early childhood. The course consists of three stages. Initially the nevus is small and hairless. At puberty there is enlargement and it becomes verrucose. In stage three possible malignant transformation may occur.
- Skeletal abnormalities including skull defects and scoliosis.
- Ocular abnormalities in ~70% with strabismus most often seen [36].
- Neurological findings include brain dysgenesis, cortical dysplasia, glial hamartomas, and low-grade gliomas. Strong correlation with hemimegalencephaly [37].
- Epilepsy in 75% of patients. Early-onset syndromes such as infantile spasms seen [38].

4.7 Summary

Genetic studies in epilepsy play a significant role in improving early diagnosis, avoiding ordering of unnecessary tests, selecting the appropriate antiepileptic medication, and providing information on prognosis and recurrence risk. Specifically, the genes identified in some of the more common idiopathic epilepsy syndromes have been discussed. Some of the more common epilepsy syndromes associated with neurocutaneous disorders, neuronal migration disorders, chromosomal abnormalities, inborn errors of metabolism, and mitochondrial disorders have also been considered in this chapter.

References

[1] Commission on Classification and Terminology of the International League against Epilepsy. Proposal for revised classification of epilepsies and epileptic syndrome. *Epilepsia* 1989;**30**:389–399.

[2] Hauser WA, Kurland LT. Incidence of epilepsy and unprovoked seizures in Rochester, Minnesota: 1935–1984. *Epilepsia* 1993;**34**:453–468.

[3] Ottman R, Hirose S, Jain Lerche H, *et al.* Genetic testing in the epilepsies – Report of the ILAE Genetics Commission. *Epilepsia* 2010;**51**:655–670.

[4] Gupta A, Scheffer IE. Genetics aspects of epilepsy and genetics of idiopathic epilepsy. In: Wylie E, Gupta A, Lachhwani DK (eds), *The Treatment of Epilepsy: Principles and Practice*, 4th edn. Lippincott Williams & Wilkins, Philadelphia, 2006.

[5] Deprez L, Jansen A, De Jonghe P. Genetics of epilepsy syndromes starting in the first year of life. *Neurology* 2009;**72**:273–281.

[6] Picard F, Scheffer IE. Recently defined genetic epilepsy syndrome. In: Roger J, Bereau M, Dravet C, Genton P, Tassinari CA, Wolf P (eds), *Epileptic Syndromes in Infancy, Childhood and Adolescence*. London: John Libbey & Co., 2005; pp. 519–535.

[7] Wallace R, Scheffer IE, Parasivam G, *et al.* Generalised epilepsy with febrile seizures plus: mutation of the sodium channel subunit SCN1B. *Neurology* 2002;**58**:1426–1429.

[8] Escayg A, MacDonald BT, Meisler MH, *et al.* Mutations of SCN1A, encoding a neuronal sodium channel, in two families with GEFS+. *Nat Genet* 2000;**24**:343–345.

[9] Baulac S, Huberfeld G, Gourfinkel-An I, *et al.* First genetic evidence of GABA(A) receptor dysfunction in epilepsy: a mutation in the gamma1-subunit gene. *Nat Genet* 2001;**28**:46–48.

[10] Panayiotopoulos CP. A Clinical Guide to Epileptic Syndromes and their Treatment. Oxford: Bladon Medical Publishing, 2002; p. 63.

[11] Mulley JC, Scheffer IE, Petrou S, *et al.* SCN1A mutations and epilepsy. *Hum Mutat* 2005;**25**:535–542.

[12] Derry CP, Davey M, Johns M, *et al.* Distinguishing sleep disorders from seizures: diagnosing bumps in the night. *Arch Neurol* 2006;**63**:705–709.
[13] Combi R, Dalprà L, Tenchini ML, Ferini-Strambi L. Autosomal dominant nocturnal frontal lobe epilepsy; a critical overview. *J Neurol* 2004;**251**:923–924.
[14] Phillips HA, Favre I, Kirkpatrick M, *et al.* CHRNB2 is the second acetylcholine receptor subunit associated with autosomal dominant nocturnal frontal lobe epilepsy. *Am J Hum Genet* 2001;**68**:225–231.
[15] Ottman R, Rosenberger L, Bagic A, *et al.* Altered language processing in autosomal dominant partial epilepsy with auditory features. *Neurology* 2008;**71**:1973–1980.
[16] Gardiner, M. Genetics of idiopathic generalized epilepsies. *Epilepsia* 2005;**46**:15–20.
[17] Varadkar S, Cross JH. Less common epilepsy syndromes and epilepsy associated with chromosomal abnormalities. In: Wylie E, Gupta A, Lachhwani DK (eds), *The Treatment of Epilepsy: Principles and Practice*, 4th edn. Philadelphia: Lippincott Williams & Wilkins, 2006; pp. 478–486.
[18] Gobbi, G, Genton P, Pini A, Gurrieri F, Livet MO. Epilepsies and chromosomal disorders. In: Roger J, Bereau M, Dravet C, Genton P, Tassinari CA, Wolf P (eds), *Epileptic Syndromes in Infancy, Childhood and Adolescence*. London: John Libbey & Co, 2005; pp. 467–492.
[19] Pelc K, Boyd SG, Cheron G, Dan B. Epilepsy in Angelmann Syndrome. *Seizure* 2008;**17**:211–217.
[20] Moser S, Weber P, Lütschg J. Rett syndrome: clinical and electrophysiologic aspects. *Pediatr Neurol* 2007;**36**:95–100.
[21] Ville D, Kaminska A, Bahi-Buisson N, *et al.* Early pattern of epilepsy in the ring chromosome 20 syndrome. *Epilepsia* 2006;**47**:543–549.
[22] Toyo-Oka K, Shionoya A, Gambello MJ, *et al.* 14-3-3epsilon is important for neuronal migration by binding to NUDEL: a molecular explanation for Miller–Dieker syndrome. *Nat Genet* 2003;**34**:274–285.
[23] Cormier-Daire V, Dagoneau N, Nabbout R, *et al.* A gene for pyridoxine-dependent epilepsy maps to chromosome 5q31. *Am J Hum Genet* 2000;**67**:991–993.
[24] Leen WG, Klepper J, Verbeek MM, *et al.* Glucose transporter-1 deficiency syndrome: the expanding clinical and genetic spectrum of a treatable disorder. *Brain* 2010;**133**:655–670.
[25] Lohi H, Turnbull J, Zhao XC, *et al.* Genetic diagnosis in Lafora disease: Genotype-phenotype correlations and diagnostic pitfalls. *Neurology* 2007;**68**:996–1001.
[26] Holmes GL, Stafstrom CE, the Tuberous Sclerosis Study Group. Tuberous sclerosis complex and epilepsy: recent developments and future challenges. *Epilepsia* 2007;**48**:617–630.
[27] Osborne JP, Merrifield J, O'Callaghan FJK. Tuberous sclerosia; what's new? *Arch Dis Child* 2008;**93**:728–731.
[28] Rosser T, Panigrahy A, McClintock W. The diverse clinical manifestations of tuberous sclerosis complex: a review. *Semin Pediatr Neurol* 2006;**13**:27–36.
[29] Franz DN, Leonard J, Tudor C, *et al.* Rapamycin causes regression of astrocytomas. *Ann Neurol* 2006;**59**:490–498.
[30] Barbagallo JS, Kolodzieh MS, Silverberg NB, Weinberg JM. Neurocutaneous disorders. *Dermatol Clin* 2002;**20**:547–560.
[31] Thomas-Sohl K, Vaslow D, Maria B. Sturge–Weber syndrome: A review. *Pediatr Neurol* 2004;**30**:303–310.
[32] Abdulaziz H. Awad MD, Mullaney PB, *et al.* Glaucoma in Sturge–Weber syndrome. *J Am Assoc Pediatr Ophthalmol Strabismus* 1999;**3**:40–45.
[33] Hu J, Yu Y, Juhasz C. MR susceptibility weighted imaging (SWI) complements conventional contrast enhanced T1 weighted MRI in characterizing brain abnormalities of Sturge–Weber syndrome. *J Magn Reson Imaging* 2008;**28**:300–307.
[34] Smahi A, Courtois G, Vabres P, *et al.* Genomic rearrangement in NEMO impairs NF-B activation and is a cause of incontinentia pigmenti. *Nature* 2000;**405**:466–472.

[35] Menascu S, Donner EJ. Linear nevus sebaceous syndrome: Case reports and review of the literature. *Pediatr Neurol* 2008;**38**:207–210.

[36] Katz B, Wiley CA, Lee VW. Optic nerve hypoplasia and the syndrome of nevus sebaceous of Jadassohn. *Ophthalmology* 1987;**94**:1570–1576.

[37] Domingo J, Helwig EB. Malignant neoplasms associated with nevus sebaceous of Jadassohn. *J Am Academic Dermatol* 1979;**1**:545–56.

[38] Holden KR, Dekaban AS. Neurological involvement in nevus unis lateralis and nevus linearis sebaceus. *Neurology* 1972;**22**:879–87.

Section 2

Diagnostic evaluation of childhood epilepsies

David F. Clarke

5 Evaluating the child with seizures

Kristen Park and Susan Koh

Children's Hospital Colorado, Aurora, CO, USA

Seizures are paroxysmal alterations in neurological function caused by abnormal, rhythmic, neuronal discharges within the brain. Clinical manifestations of this dysfunction usually coincide with the anatomical substrate of the area affected by the discharge. Symptoms can range from posturing of the limbs, visual phenomena, sudden loss of muscle tone, jerking or twitching, to loss of consciousness and generalized convulsions. The annual incidence of seizures for children in the United States is 25 000 to 40 000 per year [1], resulting in significant healthcare utilization in a variety of settings. Seizures can be further divided by etiology to include provoked and unprovoked events. Provoked seizures are considered to be temporally related to a known cause, which can include minor head trauma, central nervous system infections, metabolic derangements, or toxic insults. Unprovoked seizures, on the other hand, do not have an apparent provocative cause. Epilepsy is defined as the occurrence of more than two unprovoked seizures and has an estimated incidence of 35–124 per 100 000, depending on the population cited and the ages included [2]. In children, many other conditions can mimic the appearance of seizures and require careful consideration to avoid inappropriate treatment (see Chapter 8). It is therefore important to outline a strategy for evaluation of seizures that includes a discussion of accurate diagnosis,

Epilepsy in Children and Adolescents, First Edition. Edited by James W. Wheless.

etiology, and assessment of recurrence risk in order to determine appropriate management and counseling.

Evaluating the child with seizures is a complex process that often involves a variety of different care providers in several settings, including pediatricians, emergency room personnel, teachers, and parents along with the neurologist who may be ultimately responsible for the diagnosis and management of the patient. This chapter will attempt to discuss the tools and diagnostic tests involved in this process, and current practice parameters regarding emergent evaluation and initial assessment. Many of these issues will also be discussed in more detail in subsequent chapters.

5.1 Emergent diagnosis and management

Initial presentation is most often determined by the type of seizure. Convulsive or complex partial seizures usually result in the family or child receiving emergency room care. Smaller or repetitive events such as myoclonic seizures, infantile spasms, or absence seizures, which can appear less like seizures to the family or caregiver, may result in visits to the pediatrician or neurological consultation as an outpatient. They may also often be misdiagnosed and lead to a delay in treatment. Next, we will address the unique consideration of an initial seizure presenting to the emergency department, as significant research has been devoted to the appropriate management of this clinical scenario.

Practice parameters published by the American Academy of Neurology (AAN) exist regarding the emergency management of the first seizure in children; these address both diagnostic testing and treatment (Box 5.1). These recommendations are based on a review of available literature in addition to committee review and will form the evidence base for the following section. Although some recommendations still create a considerable amount of debate, they represent a thorough compilation and distillation of the current evidence. With regards to diagnostic evaluation, it should be stated that the practice parameter excludes neonatal seizures, status epilepticus, and febrile seizures. A separate practice parameter through the American Academy of Pediatrics addresses the unique situation of febrile seizures in children [3].

Recommendations are made regarding first-time seizures (complex partial, secondarily generalized, or convulsive seizures) in children ages 1 month to 21 years of age, excluding myoclonic and atonic seizures, which often do not present in an emergent fashion.

Routine blood work is often obtained in the setting of an unprovoked seizure to assess for electrolyte imbalances or infection. Several studies suggest limited utility for these measurements in children, with positive results usually expected on a clinical basis – history of lethargy or diarrhea, multiple seizures, or failure to return to baseline status. In children under 6 months of age, a Class II study did find a higher incidence of hyponatremia (33/47 = 70%); however, the data was collected in a manner retrospective [4]. In three studies involving a total of 400 adults, only 27 (<7%) had abnormal laboratory findings, and of these only three were unsuspected on a clinical basis. In a subset of adolescents from another study, no clinically significant laboratory abnormalities were found; however, it was limited by its sample size of 16 [5]. With a limited number of class I studies, 166 total subjects, limited conclusions can be shown the available data. Recommendations suggest that such testing be ordered on an individual basis based on clinical history. While routine chemistry and hematology studies may not disclose an etiology (unless clinically suspected), they serve as a baseline prior to starting antiepileptic drug therapy. No studies

Box 5.1 Evaluation of the first unprovoked seizure in childhood: summary of the American Academy of Neurology (AAN) practice parameter [1]

Laboratory studies

Laboratory tests should be ordered based on individual clinical circumstances that include suggestive historic or clinical findings such as vomiting, dehydration, or failure to return to baseline alertness.
Toxicology screening should be considered across the entire pediatric age range if there is any question of drug exposure or substance abuse.

Lumbar puncture (LP)

In the child with a first non-febrile seizure, LP is of limited value and should be used primarily when there is concern about possible meningitis or encephalitis.

Electroencephalogram (EEG)

The EEG is recommended as part of the neurodiagnostic evaluation of the child with an apparent first unprovoked seizure.

Neuroimaging

If a neuroimaging study is obtained, MRI is the preferred modality.
Emergent neuroimaging should be performed in a child of any age who exhibits a postictal focal deficit (Todd's paresis) not quickly resolving, or who has not returned to baseline within several hours after the seizure.
Non-urgent imaging studies with MRI should be seriously considered in any child with a significant cognitive or motor impairment of unknown etiology, unexplained abnormalities on neurological examination, a seizure of partial (focal) onset with or without secondary generalization, an EEG that does not represent a benign partial epilepsy of childhood or primary generalized epilepsy, or in children under 1 year of age.

systematically evaluated the utility of toxicology screening in the pediatric age group; however, positive results were found in two patients in this pooled data set. Given that this is an important diagnostic consideration, the recommendation was made to obtain clinical history regarding exposures and to consider screening if no alternative etiology is available. This may be especially true if medications are present in the home or if the child is a teenager.

While evidence exists regarding the use of lumbar puncture in the evaluation of febrile seizures, there are limited data regarding its diagnostic utility for unprovoked seizures. A single report in the emergency medicine literature was not supportive of this test with no children having central nervous system infection, but abnormalities were present in many of the samples obtained after seizures. Special consideration should be given to the child under 6 months who often falls into a "gray zone" with respect to the recommendations as signs and symptoms of infection in this age group can be limited. In addition, lumbar puncture should be considered in any child showing persistent encephalopathy or meningeal signs.

Considerably more literature exists regarding the utility of the electroencephalogram (EEG) after a single unprovoked seizure. Class I evidence exists to suggest that epileptiform abnormalities on EEG can be predictive of recurrence risk or may show evidence of an epileptic syndrome such as benign rolandic epilepsy with centrotemporal spikes (BRECTS) or juvenile myoclonic epilepsy (JME), which may influence treatment decisions [1]. A review of the literature by Gilbert and Buncher suggests that the predictive utility of this test is, in their opinion, more limited than expected. Citing low sensitivity and specificity in addition to factoring in pretest and post-test probability of recurrence, they found that the EEG does not have sufficient power to alter treatment decisions above a set threshold of 80%. This threshold was set based on the probability of recurrence after a second seizure when treatment is usually initiated [6]. Given that a number of epidemiological studies have suggested a pooled recurrence risk in children of 50% for recurrence after a single seizure [7], and that treatment after the first seizure has limited to no effect on eventual outcome, this appears to be an appropriate criterion. Others argue that EEG can be used to differentiate seizures from other events; however, this should be done largely by history, and the absence of EEG abnormalities cannot accurately exclude an epilepsy diagnosis. In addition, the EEG is only one of several predictive factors, others being the neurological examination and presumed etiology. Even when these other factors are considered, no algorithm has been able to accurately predict recurrence risk for an individual child to the degree that the risks of treatment can be comfortably pursued after a single seizure. With regards to the diagnosis of an epilepsy syndrome, this seems to be presumptuous after a single event. A study of 300 children and adults presenting after a single seizure allowed accurate syndrome diagnosis in only 14%, with more common findings being a description of possible generalized or partial seizure classifications [8]. Nonetheless, this is a controversial opinion and the EEG is the mainstay to assist in the diagnosis of seizures. Its role is less contested in the diagnosis, management, and classification of the epilepsies and this will be discussed further in Chapter 6.

Finally, the issue of neuroimaging should be addressed. Several Class I studies exist regarding the routine use of head computed tomography (CT) after a first seizure. In the study of new-onset seizures exclusively in children, there were abnormalities in 12/112 ($n = 156$) patients, none of whom had therapeutic consequences [9]. Class I and II studies for magnetic resonance imaging (MRI)/CT when combined showed a rate of 1.9% for lesions that altered or influenced management ($n = 2423$ with 1290 imaged). Neuroimaging studies were likely to be normal unless there was a known neurological diagnosis, a focal deficit, or the child was under 5 months of age. Emergent neuroimaging was suggested in children who had a persistent focal deficit or encephalopathy. In these cases, imaging would be used to detect cerebral edema, structural lesions, or hemorrhage, and CT was adequate. Once the diagnosis of epilepsy was established most clinicians would obtain a MRI with a specific epilepsy protocol (see Chapter 7).

Treatment in the emergency department should initially address medical stabilization of the actively seizing child by managing airway, breathing, and circulation needs. Most seizures last, on average, 1–2 minutes [10]; however, approximately 20% of children will present in status epilepticus and this is more common in children under 5 years of age [11]. In cases of convulsive status epilepticus, subtle seizures may be preceded by intermittent convulsions that become shorter and less prominent over time. In these children, and in children who present in complex partial or absence status, manifestations of seizure activity can be subtle and include disturbances of consciousness, increased oral secretions, eye deviation, or subtle clonic activity [12]. Therefore, the child who presents after seizures at home or en route should be assessed for the possibility of ongoing seizure activity. If there is concern over incomplete return to the child's baseline mental status or unresponsiveness to stimuli that exceeds the expected postictal lethargy, further assessment (e.g., EEG) and treatment are warranted.

5.2 Subsequent evaluation

History

Although an accurate assessment of the clinical history is no doubt important in the emergency room assessment of the child with seizures, a thorough history and examination should be undertaken at the time of neurological assessment. Clues to the etiology of seizures, risk factors for epilepsy, and syndrome classification, discovered during this process, will become the foundation for ongoing evaluation and management of the child with epilepsy. Historic details should be obtained about the child, the family, and the event/s.

The child's history should begin with the pregnancy and include questions regarding prior miscarriages or fetal losses, *in utero* drug exposure, prenatal care, prenatal laboratory results, growth of the baby, and fetal movements *in utero*. Perinatal risk factors for cerebral injury should also be discussed with questions regarding precipitous or emergent delivery, signs of fetal distress, abruption, or significant maternal blood loss. Postnatal factors to consider include resuscitation, prolonged hospitalization, or neonatal seizures. Hypoxic ischemic injury has been found to be a frequent cause of neonatal seizures, especially of those with onset during the first 24 hours of life. However, variability in the definition of this term should prompt further questions regarding the infant's Apgar scores, neurological examination, and any evidence of multi-organ system dysfunction. Literature regarding the risk of epilepsy and neurological sequelae after neonatal seizures is variable and cites an incidence anywhere between 9% and 50%, with a mortality of 15–30% [13].

Developmental history should also be addressed in the initial consultation and can provide valuable information regarding etiology, lateralization, and prognosis. Given that early developmental milestones have a narrow window of normalcy they can be easily assessed with verbal recall or the use of rapid screening tools. Handedness can also be an important diagnostic tool. Early handedness or significant hand preference prior to the age of 1 year can be an indicator of underlying cortical malfunction [14]. Although population data are limited, there is some evidence that people with epilepsy have a higher incidence of pathologic left-handedness or atypical handedness [15,16]. When questions of more subtle cognitive problems arise, additional testing and careful history from multiple sources, including those at school, may be necessary. The prevalence of epilepsy in children with intellectual disabilities, cerebral palsy, and autism spectrum disorders is much higher than in the general population and indicates that the symptoms of motor impairment, cognitive impairment, and seizures are intertwined [17]. Comorbidities such as intellectual disability and cerebral palsy have been shown to have a significant impact on treatment response and prognosis for remission. In addition, they are a large part of the psychosocial morbidity of this disease. This connection is discussed further in Chapter 1, which addresses the epidemiology and comorbidities of epilepsy.

In addition to perinatal and developmental risk factors for epilepsy, there are other intrinsic risks that should be assessed as part of the child's history. Febrile seizures have been shown to carry a slight increase in risk for the development of subsequent epilepsy; this is minimal in the case of simple febrile convulsions (2–10%) but can be substantial in some reports of long-term follow-up in complex febrile seizures. Several large cohort studies have examined this association and found a 6–50% risk for later epilepsy after complex febrile seizures, with variability being determined by the number and type of complex features [18]. Prior meningitis and encephalitis also have epilepsy as a frequent sequela. Population-based studies of children cite the development of post-infectious epilepsy with a range of 3–13%, and one study reporting late unprovoked seizures in 40–65% of patients with herpes simplex virus. Most studies are limited by methodological constraints but multiple risk factors have consistently been cited as modifiers of this risk (age, type of infection, acute symptomatic seizures, and persistent neurological deficits) [19–21]. Traumatic brain injury is also associated with pediatric epilepsy, with trauma cited as the cause for approximately 14% of epilepsies in children under 14 years of age [22]. All families will question whether their child's fall down the stairs or off a changing table resulted in seizures. However, these types of minor head traumas can usually be ignored as causes of significant post-traumatic epilepsy unless there was intracranial injury or significant loss of consciousness. Lastly, comorbid medical conditions should also be assessed as they may carry an increased risk for seizures related to involvement of or injury to the CNS (congenital heart disease, lupus, HIV, celiac, etc.) or due to medications that lower the seizure threshold.

Family history should also be obtained at initial consultation. Due to the historic stigma of epilepsy, some family history may be hidden and only apparent at subsequent visits after families have discussed the diagnosis. Thus, this question should be revisited during at least 1–2 subsequent visits. While there are some documented autosomally inherited epilepsy syndromes that have been extensively researched in multiply affected families, these are not felt to be responsible for the majority of sporadic epilepsies. However, population-based studies do document an increased risk of epilepsy among first-degree relatives of individuals with epilepsy [23]. Family history should include not only epilepsy but also febrile seizures and other neurological disorders as some phenotypes have variable presentations, and ongoing research in genetics is discovering connections between epilepsy and other paroxysmal disorders such as migraine, ataxia, and dystonia [24,25].

After patient-related contextual information has been obtained, attention can be turned to the event itself as this history can determine whether the spell truly represented a seizure and, if so, how it should be further categorized. Some weight should be given to the context in which the event occurred. Both seizures and non-epileptic events can have a characterized relationship to the sleep–wake cycle. Benign sleep myoclonus often occurs during light stages of sleep, whereas the myoclonus of JME is more often present after awakening in the morning hours. Sleep stage may also provide a clue to etiology, with seizures more often associated with stage 1–2 sleep and parasomnias with slow-wave or rapid eye movement sleep. Preceding events or provoking factors may also provide clues as to etiology. The first convulsion of JME often presents after sleep deprivation [26]. The sight of blood, injury, or prior dehydration and exertion may be suggestive of convulsive syncope. Stressful social situations or psychological trauma may indicate concern for pseudoseizures.

Specific provoking factors have been linked to particular epilepsy syndromes and linked to particular epilepsy syndromes and some maybe explored as a seizure trigger. If absence is expected hyperventilation may be performed during a clinic visit with the child taking slow, deep, regular breaths for approximately 3 minutes. In one review of children with idiopathic generalized epilepsies that included absence seizures, this maneuver occurred in up to 87% of children, depending on the syndrome [27]. Many idiopathic generalized epilepsies can have a photoconvulsive component, which can be triggered both by natural stimuli (light being filtered through the trees) and artificial flashes (such as video games or strobe lights). There also exists a rare category of seizures that are reflex mediated, being triggered by specific stimuli such as reading, a specific sound or piece of music, or hot water. While these considerations may not have high sensitivity or specificity for determining whether an event was epileptic or not, when combined with other elements of the history or diagnostic tools, they can be helpful in suggesting an alternative diagnosis. These considerations will be further discussed in Chapter 8, which addresses the diagnosis of non-epileptic paroxysmal events.

In addition to the context, events immediately preceding the seizure may provide useful information. Many parents report, often in retrospect, the presence of prodromal symptoms anywhere from hours to several days preceding a seizure. These can include irritability, fatigue, pallor, moodiness, or other non-specific signs and symptoms. There is little objective evidence to support this type of intuition and it has received limited attention by epilepsy researchers. Certain prodromal symptoms may also suggest an alternative etiology such as migraine. Currently, however, prolonged prodromal symptoms are of limited diagnostic and therapeutic utility except in the monitoring of children by parents or caregivers [28,29].

Initial symptoms preceding a convulsion or complex partial seizure may provide information regarding the ictal onset zone. A thorough discussion of seizure semiology and the tools used to distinguish between different regions of the brain, with specificities and sensitivities cited from the literature, is beyond the scope of this chapter. Suffice to say that this topic should be explored with the child and family in an attempt to localize the area of ictal onset. In many situations, this may be difficult to determine as parents report that non-verbal children will sometimes come to them with a fearful look or grab on to them as if they are aware that a seizure is about to occur. Even if children are able to provide a description of the aura, it is often non-specific such as a "strange feeling in my head." Though vague, if consistent, this can lend credence to the conclusion that a convulsion has partial onset with secondary generalization. In general, questions should be asked about abnormal sensations, visual symptoms (possibly suggestive of occipital onset), unusual smells, or an epigastric rising sensation (common in temporal lobe seizures), psychiatric symptoms (fear, *déjà vu*, *jamais vu*), uncontrolled movements (such as myoclonus, jacksonian march, or other focal clonic activity), or autonomic symptoms (tachycardia, flushing).

A description of the semiology of the event is also important for characterization of the seizure type and localization, if partial in onset. The most useful information is usually contained within the initial evolution of the seizure. This information is usually provided by witnesses as the patient is often amnesic for the event or unable to give an accurate description. It is often helpful to have the historian mimic the movements. Often in the clinic, parents can be reticent to perform this type of role play, and acting out various types of ictal symptoms may facilitate parents' willingness to perform this type of gesture. This may allow recognition of details not thought to be significant by the witness or enable the examiner to distinguish between clonic movements and the vibratory tremor associated with tonic posturing. If doubt remains regarding the diagnosis of seizures, families can be asked to videotape frequent events. The duration of the seizure should also be assessed with the understanding that parents may exaggerate this time frame due to the fear and panic that often accompanies the first seizure in a child. This information is important for future management as children who present with status epilepticus have a higher incidence of repeated prolonged seizures in the future [30,31]. Therefore, appropriate anticipatory guidance should be provided and emergency medication prescribed, if appropriate.

In evaluating the child with epilepsy, information should be obtained for potentially different seizure types specifically in order to understand the totality of the child's presentation. History should be obtained regarding the child's most recent seizure as this is likely to be vivid in the mind of the historian. In addition, recollection of the first seizure is also likely to contain important details. It may also provide clues to localization as it occurred prior to initiation of any treatment. A description of all seizure types witnessed by the family or school should also be obtained. Many epilepsy syndromes are characterized by more than one seizure type. Lay persons may also not recognize events as seizures unless direct inquiry is pursued – absence seizures, myoclonus, head drops. In many instances, the descriptions provided may not represent distinct seizure types but categorizations used by the family ("big ones," "staring," "jerking," etc.). Nonetheless, this provides an opportunity for education and can aid the physician in monitoring for treatment efficacy in language understood by the patient and family. Finally, a good seizure history should contain information about the most severe seizure. Again, this may allow for guidance regarding the risk of status epilepticus; however, it may also provide clues to localization as prolonged seizures can be associated with postictal symptoms not apparent with briefer events (Todd's paralysis, aphasia) [29]. A summary of these historical elements can be found in Box 5.2.

Assessment of comorbidities

Additional attention is now being paid to the so-called interictal dysfunction of epilepsy with a growing realization that the comorbidities associated with epilepsy can often be equally, if

Box 5.2 Epilepsy/seizure history

Epilepsy history

- Most recent seizure
- First seizure
- All seizure types witnessed by family
- Most severe seizure

Seizure history

- Provoking factors
- Context
- Prodromal symptoms
- Aura
- Initial symptoms and evolution

not more, debilitating than the seizures that have traditionally defined this condition. Recent literature has cited what is being termed the "epilepsy spectrum" to define this entity, which has support from both clinical and basic science research [32]. It is suspected that there are shared underpinnings between neuropsychiatric issues and epilepsy that are responsible for this co-occurrence. In this context, an assessment of comorbidities can be considered the "review of systems" for epilepsy. Significant literature exists regarding the incidence of several common comorbidities in children with epilepsy. This research cites a higher rate of attention-deficit/hyperactivity disorder (ADHD), learning disorders, mood disorders, and migraine [33]. These comorbidities may impact school functioning, medication choices, and coping mechanisms. They may also determine the degree to which epilepsy impacts the life of the child and family. Take the example of childhood absence epilepsy to illustrate this point. It was traditionally considered a benign epilepsy of childhood with high rates of remission and minimal effects on cognition and behavior; however, recent research has documented that this disorder is associated with a high incidence of attentional difficulties, as measured by a continuous performance task, that predate treatment [34]. In addition, these comorbidities are often underdiagnosed in children with epilepsy and may persist despite seizure control leading to poorer long-term vocational, educational, and social outcomes [35]. The assessment of a child with any epilepsy, even those without obvious problems, should therefore include at least some screening questions regarding these disorders. Parents should be questioned about their child's behavior at home and school, interactions with siblings and other children, attention or learning difficulties, general mood, and sleep habits [36]. Screening tools may also be valuable in this situation and can include such measures as the Child Depression Inventory [37], and Conners Parent Rating Scale for ADHD [38]. If significant concern develops in areas of school or behavior, additional assistance from neuropsychologists and/or psychiatrists may be needed. This can help to further outline areas to target for intervention in school and allow for appropriate strategies to be implemented. In addition, medical management and psychotherapy may be of benefit in some children. The epidemiology of common comorbidities in childhood epilepsies is further addressed in Chapter 1.

Physical examination

A comprehensive evaluation of the child with seizures should also include a thorough general medical and neurological examination. Many neurological syndromes can be associated with seizures, which represent a final common pathway in CNS dysfunction. The general medical examination should include an assessment of any dysmorphic facial features or other congenital anomalies as seizures can be associated with multiple congenital anomaly syndromes and particular genetic disorders with characteristic phenotypes [39,40]. Head circumference should also be measured as the presence of microcephaly may suggest a prior neurological insult or malformation of cortical development, while macrocephaly is associated with storage disorders and hydrocephalus, among other diagnostic considerations. Embryologically, the nervous system develops from the ectodermal layer, which is also responsible for the formation of skin, hair, and nails. For this reason, there is a close connection between cutaneous findings and neurological disorders. A thorough examination of the skin should be conducted with careful attention to areas of increased or decreased pigmentation, birthmarks, and abnormal hair whorls. This topic is discussed further in Chapter 4. The general medical examination should also assess for signs of systemic disease as these disorders can involve the CNS resulting in seizures. Examples include hepatomegaly or splenomegaly in storage disorders, and the malar rash of lupus, which can be associated with CNS vasculitis and seizures.

Neurological examination should include a careful assessment of all divisions of the nervous system. Careful examination of the visual fields may identify deficits associated with brain lesions and these are of localizing value. Special attention should be paid to assessment of the motor system. Asymmetries in size or bulk, reflexes, or tone can be clues to laterality of seizure onset. Subtle differences may require measurement of extremity girth, balancing on each leg, stressed gait, fine finger movements, or pronator drift testing.

5.3 Additional neurodiagnostic evaluation

Once all of these elements of history and physical evaluation have been obtained, attention can be turned to prognosis, treatment, and additional diagnostic testing. These divisions are somewhat arbitrary, however, as an understanding of the first contributes to decisions regarding the latter. The epidemiology and classification of childhood epilepsies is discussed more thoroughly in Section 1 of this book; however, discussions of additional evaluations to be considered are incomplete without a thorough understanding of the prognosis after a single seizure and for childhood epilepsy in general. As reviewed earlier, prognosis after a single seizure is not always relevant by the time the child arrives in the neurology clinic but will be reviewed nonetheless. Estimates of recurrence risk vary significantly across published studies. This is likely related to methodology, population selection, and the variables assessed. A systematic analysis by Berg and Shinnar addressed some of these issues by examining studies containing prospectively followed patients who presented with a first seizure for recurrence risk. Using these "first-seizure" methods, pooled recurrence risks for children were approximately 43%, with follow-up ranging from 1 to 4 years. Modifiers of this risk included an epileptiform EEG (especially when combined with etiology), partial seizures, and prior provoked seizures [7]. Treatment after the first seizure may decrease the risk of recurrent seizures in the short term but does not alter the long-term prognosis, and is not currently indicated in practice guidelines [41].

Once a child is diagnosed with epilepsy, there are a number of additional factors that determine prognosis and guide management. Epidemiological studies and other available evidence suggests that 70% of children with epilepsy enter remission. The most consistent modifiers of this risk are etiology, epilepsy syndrome, age of onset, seizure frequency, and early response to treatment. Children with idiopathic epilepsies or benign syndromes are repeatedly found to have the best prognosis for remission.

EEG

As discussed earlier, while recommended in the AAN practice parameter, the utility of the EEG after a single seizure remains a topic of some debate. However, for the classification and management of epilepsy it remains a valuable tool. Its main utility is in classification of the child's epilepsy syndrome, which can then be used to guide appropriate medication selection, management, and additional evaluation. Although not strictly "population-based," a study by Berg and Shinnar that was able to ascertain most of the cases of childhood epilepsy diagnosed in Connecticut between 1993 and 1997 was able to use medical records, a structured interview, and EEG to classify 609/613 children into an ILAE epilepsy syndrome.

They cited the EEG as clearly contributory to the diagnosis in 36% of patients. Factors cited for incomplete or non-specific categorization were largely related to lack of EEG data, highlighting the importance of conducting an EEG in combination with the elements of history and physical examination already discussed [42]. The sensitivity of the EEG varies by diagnostic syndrome, and repeat studies may increase the yield of this test. In addition, the EEG is a more powerful tool for classification when it is performed with provocative maneuvers such as hyperventilation, photic stimulation, and sleep deprivation [43]. A further discussion of the EEG in the diagnosis of childhood epilepsies is undertaken in Chapter 6.

Neuroimaging

As discussed earlier, few children who present with an initial unprovoked seizure have unsuspected neuroimaging abnormalities that require acute intervention. Therefore, the current AAN practice parameter recommends non-urgent imaging for several clinical situations: suspected symptomatic etiology, focal onset seizures, seizures or EEG not consistent with a benign epilepsy of childhood, and children less than 1 year of age. Consistent literature is available regarding the sensitivity of various neuroimaging tools, with MRI being more sensitive than CT for detecting abnormalities relevant to the treatment of the child with seizures (cortical dysplasia, hippocampal sclerosis, heterotopias, etc.). Therefore, MRI is recommended as the preferred modality for the non-urgent evaluation of children presenting with a first seizure [1]. The use of MRI for the evaluation and management of the child with epilepsy and findings on neuroimaging associated with seizure disorders will be further addressed in Chapter 7.

Laboratory testing

As discussed in the section on emergency management, seizures provoked by metabolic abnormalities in otherwise normal children are rare, therefore basic tests for electrolyte imbalances should be performed only when suspected by clinical history, as outlined in the AAN Practice Parameter [1]. More specialized testing related to potential underlying etiologies is usually pursued later in the diagnostic course and when indicated by suggestive features of the child's epilepsy. More than 200 inherited and metabolic disorders have been associated with seizures. Suspicion for one of these disorders is heightened when epilepsy is associated with developmental delays, microcephaly, or failure to thrive. In addition, certain types of seizures or epilepsy merit consideration of these disorders, including myoclonic seizures, infantile spasms, and early-onset tonic seizures (as can be seen in Ohtahara or Lennox–Gastaut syndromes). Finally, onset of seizures in the first month of life is suspicious for a metabolic or inherited disorder [44]. An exhaustive evaluation should also be undertaken when the course of epilepsy is felt to be progressive, as can be seen in the myoclonic epilepsies. Selected evaluations may also be indicated for intractable seizures in young children or if there is concern for developing intellectual disability or atrophy on MRI. Given the range of disorders associated with these scenarios, a full review of this type of evaluation is beyond the scope of this chapter. Box 5.3 outlines some of the metabolic and genetic disorders associated with severe epilepsies of childhood based on syndrome and age of onset. Most reviews recommend a tiered approach, with initial

Box 5.3 Genetic and metabolic etiologies of epilepsy in children

Neonatal seizures

Urea cycle defects
Organic acidurias
Disorders of biotin metabolism
Peroxisomal disorders
Other: molybdenum cofactor deficiency/sulfite oxidase deficiency, disorders of fructose metabolism, pyridoxine dependency

Early infantile epileptic encephalopathy (Ohtahara)

Non-ketotic hyperglycinemia
Propionic aciduria
D-glyceric acidemia
Leigh disease
Known Gene mutation: STXBP1, ARX

West syndrome/infantile spasms

Phenylketonuria/hyperphenylalaninemia
Pyruvate dehydrogenase deficiency
Pyruvate carboxylase deficiency
Carbohydrate-deficient glycoprotein syndrome (type III)
Organic acidurias
Amino acidurias
Known Gene mutation: ARX, CDKL5, TSC1 and 2

Other epileptic encephalopathies of infancy and childhood

GM1 and GM2 gangliosidoses
Infantile neuroaxonal dystrophy
GLUT1 deficiency
Late-onset multiple carboxylase deficiency
Disorders of folate metabolism
Arginase deficiency
Tetrahydrobioptrin deficiency
Tyrosinemia type 1
Genetic causes: SCN1A, PCDH19, chromosomal microdeletions

Progressive myoclonic epilepsies

Lafora disease
Unverricht–Lundborg disease

Myoclonic epilepsy with ragged red fibers (MERRF)/Mitochondrial encephalopathy, lactic acidosis and stroke like episodes (MELAS)
Dentatorubral-pallidoluysian atrophy
Neuronal ceroid lipofuscinosis
Sialidoses
Gaucher disease

Adapted from Nordli and DeVivo [45] and Deprez *et al.* [46].

screening metabolic labs to include serum amino acids, urine organic acids, and lactate. Additional evaluations can include a metabolic spinal tap and mitochondrial testing. For children with severe developmental abnormalities or epileptic encephalopathies, a referral to a metabolic or genetic specialist may be indicated.

References

[1] Hirtz D, Ashwal S, Berg A, *et al.* Practice parameter: evaluating a first nonfebrile seizure in children: report of the Quality Standards Subcommittee of the American Academy of Neurology, The Child Neurology Society, and The American Epilepsy Society. *Neurology* 2000;**55**:616–6-23.

[2] Hauser WA, Banerjee PN. Epidemiology of epilepsy in children. In: Pellock JM, Bourgeois BFD, Dodson WE (eds), *Pediatric Epilepsy: Diagnosis and Therapy*, 3rd edn. New York: Demos Medical Publishing, 2008; pp. 147–164.

[3] American Academy of Pediatrics. Provisional Committee on Quality Improvement, Subcommittee on Febrile Seizures. Practice parameter: the neurodiagnostic evaluation of the child with a first simple febrile seizure. *Pediatrics* 1996;**97**:769–72; discussion 73–75.

[4] Farrar HC, Chande VT, Fitzpatrick DF, Shema SJ. Hyponatremia as the cause of seizures in infants: a retrospective analysis of incidence, severity, and clinical predictors. *Ann Emerg Med* 1995;**26**:42–48.

[5] Turnbull TL, Vanden Hoek TL, Howes DS, Eisner RF. Utility of laboratory studies in the emergency department patient with a new-onset seizure. *Ann Emerg Med* 1990;**19**:373–377.

[6] Gilbert DL, Buncher CR. An EEG should not be obtained routinely after first unprovoked seizure in childhood. *Neurology* 2000;**54**:635–641.

[7] Berg AT, Shinnar S. The risk of seizure recurrence following a first unprovoked seizure: a quantitative review. *Neurology* 1991;**41**:965–972.

[8] King MA, Newton MR, Jackson GD, *et al.* Epileptology of the first-seizure presentation: a clinical, electroencephalographic, and magnetic resonance imaging study of 300 consecutive patients. *Lancet* 1998;**352**:1007–1011.

[9] Stroink H, Brouwer OF, Arts WF, Geerts AT, Peters AC, van Donselaar CA. The first unprovoked, untreated seizure in childhood: a hospital based study of the accuracy of the diagnosis, rate of recurrence, and long term outcome after recurrence. Dutch study of epilepsy in childhood. *J Neurol Neurosurg Psychiatry* 1998;**64**:595–600.

[10] Theodore WH, Porter RJ, Albert P, *et al.* The secondarily generalized tonic-clonic seizure: a videotape analysis. *Neurology* 1994;**44**:1403–1407.

[11] Hauser WA. Status epilepticus: frequency, etiology, and neurological sequelae. *Adv Neurol* 1983;**34**:3–14.

[12] Arzimanoglou A, Guerrini R, Aicardi J. Status epilepticus. In: Aicardi J (ed), *Aicardi's Epilepsy*, 3rd edn. Philadelphia: Lippincott Williams & Wilkins, 2004; pp. 241–261.

[13] Arzimanoglou A, Guerrini R, Aicardi J. Neonatal seizures. In: Aidari J (ed), *Aicardi's Epilepsy in Children*, 3rd edn. Philadelphia: Lippincott Williams & Wilkins, 2004; pp. 188–209.

[14] Fenichel GM. Hemiplegia. In: Fenichel GM (ed), *Clinical Pediatric Neurology: A Signs and Symptoms Approach*, 5th edn. Philadelphia: Elsevier Saunders; 2005; pp. 239–253.

[15] Slezicki KI, Cho YW, Yi SD, *et al.* Incidence of atypical handedness in epilepsy and its association with clinical factors. *Epilepsy Behav* 2009;**16**:330–334.

[16] Rasmussen T, Milner B. The role of early left-brain injury in determining lateralization of cerebral speech functions. *Ann N Y Acad Sci* 1977;**299**:355–369.

[17] Dodson WE. Epilepsy, cerebral palsy, and IQ. In: Pellock JM, Bourgeois BFD, Dodson WE (eds), *Pediatric Epilepsy: Diagnosis and Therapy*, 3rd edn. New York: Demos Medical Publishing, 2008; pp. 847–863.

[18] Knudsen FU. Febrile seizures: treatment and prognosis. *Epilepsia* 2000;**41**:2–9.

[19] Murthy JM, Prabhakar S. Bacterial meningitis and epilepsy. *Epilepsia* 2008;**49**(Suppl. 6):8–12.

[20] Misra UK, Tan CT, Kalita J. Viral encephalitis and epilepsy. *Epilepsia* 2008;**49**(Suppl. 6):13–18.

[21] Fowler A, Stodberg T, Eriksson M, Wickstrom R. Long-term outcomes of acute encephalitis in childhood. *Pediatrics* 2010;**126**:e828–835.

[22] Lowenstein DH. Epilepsy after head injury: an overview. *Epilepsia* 2009;**50**(Suppl. 2):4–9.

[23] Winawer MR, Shinnar S. Genetic epidemiology of epilepsy or what do we tell families? *Epilepsia* 2005;**46**(Suppl. 10):24–30.

[24] Dichgans M, Freilinger T, Eckstein G, *et al.* Mutation in the neuronal voltage-gated sodium channel SCN1A in familial hemiplegic migraine. *Lancet* 2005;**366**:371–377.

[25] Kullmann DM. Neurological channelopathies. *Annu Rev Neurosci* 2010;**33**:151–172.

[26] Vendrame M, Kothare SV. Epileptic and nonepileptic paroxysmal events out of sleep in children. *J Clin Neurophysiol* 2011;**28**:111–119.

[27] Sadleir LG, Scheffer IE, Smith S, Carstensen B, Farrell K, Connolly MB. EEG features of absence seizures in idiopathic generalized epilepsy: impact of syndrome, age, and state. *Epilepsia* 2009;**50**:1572–1578.

[28] Taylor DC. Whatever happened to the "epileptic prodrome"? *Epilepsy Behav* 2007;**11**:251–252.

[29] Moshe SL, Pedley TA. Overview: diagnostic evaluation. In: Engel J, Pedley TA (eds), *Epilepsy: A Comprehensive Textbook*. Philadelphia: Lippincott-Raven, 1997; pp. 801–811.

[30] Shinnar S, Berg AT, Moshe SL, Shinnar R. How long do new-onset seizures in children last? *Ann Neurol* 2001;**49**:659–664.

[31] Raspall-Chaure M, Chin RF, Neville BG, Bedford H, Scott RC. The epidemiology of convulsive status epilepticus in children: a critical review. *Epilepsia* 2007;**48**:1652–1663.

[32] Jensen FE. Epilepsy as a spectrum disorder: Implications from novel clinical and basic neuroscience. *Epilepsia* 2011; **52**(Suppl. 1):1–6.

[33] Pellock JM. Understanding co-morbidities affecting children with epilepsy. *Neurology* 2004;**62**(5 Suppl. 2):S17–23.

[34] Masur D, Shinnar S, Cnaan A, *et al.* Abstracts from the 2006 Annual Meeting of the American Epilepsy Society and the Canadian League against Epilepsy (1st North American Regional Epilepsy Congress). *Epilepsia* 2006;**47**(Suppl. 4):1–377.

[35] Caplan R, Siddarth P, Stahl L, *et al.* Childhood absence epilepsy: behavioral, cognitive, and linguistic comorbidities. *Epilepsia* 2008;**49**:1838–1846.

[36] Pellock JM. The challenge of neuropsychiatric issues in pediatric epilepsy. *J Child Neurol* 2004;**19**(Suppl. 1):S1–5.

[37] Kovacs M. The Children's Depression Inventory (CDI). *Psychopharmacol Bull* 1985;**21**:995–998.

[38] Conners CK, Sitarenios G, Parker JD, Epstein JN. The revised Conners' Parent Rating Scale (CPRS-R): factor structure, reliability, and criterion validity. *J Abnorm Child Psychol* 1998;**26**:257–268.

[39] Singh R, Gardner RJ, Crossland KM, Scheffer IE, Berkovic SF. Chromosomal abnormalities and epilepsy: a review for clinicians and gene hunters. *Epilepsia* 2002;**43**:127–140.

[40] Schinzel A, Niedrist D. Chromosome imbalances associated with epilepsy. *Am J Med Genet* 2001;**106**:119–124.

[41] Hirtz D, Berg A, Bettis D, *et al*. Practice parameter: treatment of the child with a first unprovoked seizure: Report of the Quality Standards Subcommittee of the American Academy of Neurology and the Practice Committee of the Child Neurology Society. *Neurology* 2003;**60**:166–175.

[42] Berg AT, Shinnar S, Levy SR, Testa FM. Newly diagnosed epilepsy in children: presentation at diagnosis. *Epilepsia* 1999;**40**:445–452.

[43] Pillai J, Sperling MR. Interictal EEG and the diagnosis of epilepsy. *Epilepsia* 2006;**47**(Suppl. 1):14–22.

[44] Jain SV, Morton LD. Evaluating the child with seizure. In: Pellock JM, Bourgeois BFD, Dodson WE (eds), *Pediatric Epilepsy: Diagnosis and Therapy*, 3rd edn. New York: Demos Medical Publishing, 2008; pp. 185–194.

[45] Nordli DR Jr, De Vivo DC. Classification of infantile seizures: implications for identification and treatment of inborn errors of metabolism. *J Child Neurol* 2002;**17**(Suppl. 3):3S1–7; discussion 3S8.

[46] Deprez L, Jansen A, De Jonghe P. Genetics of epilepsy syndromes starting in the first year of life. *Neurology* 2009;**72**:273–281.

6 The use of EEG in the diagnosis of childhood epilepsy

David F. Clarke

Dell Children's Comprehensive Epilepsy Program, Dell Children's Medical Center of Central Texas, Austin, TX, USA

Richard Caton, in his studies on rabbits and monkeys, was the first to identify electrical activity of the brain utilizing scalp electrodes. Hans Burger is credited with identifying similar electrical activity utilizing scalp electrodes in humans. In 1929 describing Caton's work he stated, "There were found distinct variations in currents which increased during sleep with the onset of death strengthened and after death became weaker and completely disappeared" [1]. This suggests that he saw the high-amplitude delta activity of slow-wave sleep, with the "onset of death" an encephalopathic state and "after death became weaker," electrocerebral silence. As the electroencephalogram (EEG) evolved it was not only able to identify abnormal electrical activity of the brain including seizures, but also offered great diagnostic and prognostic utility. With neuroimaging and genetic advances, the diagnostics utility outside of the field of epilepsy has become somewhat limited. It is still an inexpensive, widely available, and benign procedure, which in many instances may drive diagnostic decision-making. It still has great utility in defining encephalopathic states and prognosticating recovery. In this chapter, an evidence-based approach for the necessity of its use or the lack thereof will be discussed. The use of the electroencephalogram in identifying a seizure, risk of epilepsy, and identifying epilepsy syndromes will be outlined.

Epilepsy in Children and Adolescents, First Edition. Edited by James W. Wheless.

As Dr Ernst Neidermeyer clearly stated, one must always remember, EEG reading in epilepsy is more than simply "hunting spikes" [2]. Incorrect interpretation of the EEG may have negative psychosocial and management ramifications. EEG patterns and waveforms should be interpreted by professionals trained in the field, who are aware of benign and pathological variations but also aware of the ramifications of false interpretation.

6.1 Technical aspects of the EEG

Neuronal, transmembrane, ionic flow generates currents along the cell membranes inside the cell and in the extracellular space. The extracellular current is responsible for generating electrical field potentials. Thousands of these potential differences between neurons are amplified and correspond with waveforms depicted on the EEG. The time constant, number of electrodes, electrode placement, and filter parameters place limitations on the waveforms visualized by the interpreter. Gold and silver disk electrodes are often used due to their conducting ability. Electrodes from different neuroanatomical regions are grouped in arrangements called montages. Internationally recognized letter and number labels have been designated for electrodes placed over specific neuroanatomical regions. Fp, F, C, P, O, and T symbolize fronto-polar, frontal, central, parietal, occipital, and temporal placement, respectively. Electrodes placed over the left side of the scalp are labeled with odd numbers and those over the right side of the scalp with even numbers. F3, therefore, suggests that the electrode is placed over the left frontal region, and C4 over the right central area. A minimum number of electrodes should be placed according to the American EEG Society guidelines [3]. Potential difference between adjacent electrodes (bipolar) or all electrodes referred to a common electrode source (referential) are the montage types used during interpretation. An internationally standardized 10–20 electrode placement system is used to determine exact and consistent placement.

6.2 Methods used to increase EEG yield

Of patients with epilepsy, 29–55% have interictal epileptiform discharges with their first EEG [4]. Observing sleep when possible and carrying out the activating procedures of hyperventilation and photic stimulation are recommended and increase yield.

Seizures and interictal epileptiform discharges are more apt to be activated during non-rapid eye movement (NREM) sleep. There is a negative correlation between the degree of desynchronization of the EEG and interictal epileptiform discharges. Epileptiform activity is less frequent while the subject is fully awake, and suppressed during rapid eye movement (REM) sleep [5]. It is for this reason that sleep deprivation is requested prior to the EEG in capable individuals.

Hyperventilation is a recommended procedure except when it has the potential for exacerbating an underlying disease process such as asthma, cardiovascular diseases, or vaso-occlusion as seen in sickle-cell disease. It is standard to continue the process for approximately 3 minutes but it may be prolonged under special circumstances. A skilled technician has many strategies to produce this effect, with the blowing of a pin wheel being a favorite in many labs. It is most effective in exacerbating seizures or interictal epileptiform discharges in absence epilepsy and other generalized seizure types. Its true yield in focal epilepsies is controversial. Holmes *et al.* suggested a rare association, whereas Guaranher *et al.* found it to be both safe and effective [6,7]. Both authors found its use to be particularly effective during long-term studies in activating temporal lobe seizures. Hyperventilation may exacerbate pathological focal slowing. This slowing has to be interpreted with caution, especially in children, because of the normal age-related phenomenon of generalized, high-voltage, frequently rhythmic slowing seen during this procedure. This normal phenomenon has been theorized to be caused by metabolic or blood flow changes.

In 1934, Adrian and Matthews [8] were the first to describe the effect of intermittent photic stimulation on the human EEG. Four types of photoparoxysmal discharges during the procedure are described by Walter and colleagues (rhythmic occipital spikes, more anterior involvement of the parietal region with a biphasic slow wave, spread to the frontal region, or a more generalized response) [9]. During the procedure a strobe lamp applies flashes of high-intensity white light at frequencies ranging from 1 to 30 flashes per second. The lamp is placed 20–30 cm in front of the patient's eyes, often with the eyes closed (but it can be done with the eyes open). EEG labs follow different protocols with odd, even, or mixed numbers of flash frequencies used. Failure to respond is not abnormal. The typical physiological response consists of rhythmic activity time-locked to the light stimulator (photic driving). Variations of this response include simultaneous high-amplitude activity over the frontal area or more diffuse involvement. In a small percentage of individuals a photo-myoclonic response may be seen. This consists of repetitive muscle activity over the anterior head region. This finding is not predictive of seizure risk. The clinical significance of the variations described is unknown. Asymmetrical driving may indicate an underlying lesion/dysfunction from the unresponsive posterior quadrant.

The photoparoxysmal response, characterized by synchronized symmetrical spike and polyspike and slow-wave activity with or without associated myoclonus, may be seen in primary generalized epilepsies. It is particularly observed in individuals with juvenile myoclonic epilepsy (JME), absence and eyelid myoclonia with or without absence. It rarely occurs in individuals with focus seizures but may be sometimes seen in individuals with a posterior epileptogenic focus. A low-frequency, high-amplitude response is characteristic of neuronal ceroid lipofuscinosis, but may be seen in other epilepsy syndromes such as Dravet syndrome and other progressive myoclonic epilepsies at varying frequencies.

6.3 When should an EEG be ordered?

EEGs are requested appropriately for many clinical scenarios, but unfortunately in some cases it may be unjustified or cause unnecessary antiepileptic drug usage. The yield of the EEG in several common clinical scenarios will be discussed below.

Febrile seizures

An EEG is frequently requested for febrile seizures, yet many physicians have not explored if it is helpful or necessary. The classifications of abnormalities, case selection, and time from convulsion to carrying out the EEG are inconsistent between studies. One of the most rigorous studies was carried out by Frantzen *et al.* [10]. They followed 218 children with febrile seizures who were hospitalized for 2 weeks, a scenario unlikely to be justified or accomplished in present-day practice. EEGs were done at <1 week, week 2 prior to discharge, and at intervals of 3 months, 6 months, and then yearly. One-third of acute EEGs had focal or occipital slowing. Positive predictors were seizures lasting longer than 30 minutes, and higher temperatures, or if EEGs were done less than 36 hours after the seizure. Only 1.4% of acute EEGs had epileptiform activity, and neither slowing nor epileptiform activity predicted seizure recurrence. Shinnar and Glauser found that older children with complex febrile seizures and neurodevelopmental abnormalities were more likely to have EEG abnormalities [11]. However, they suggested that there was no evidence that abnormalities predicted recurrence or development of subsequent epilepsy. The American Academy of Pediatrics and its Provisional Committee on Quality Improvement, after reviewing over 200 journals, suggested that EEGs are not required in simple febrile seizures [12]. The yield of performing EEGs after complex febrile seizures is still unclear and likely dependent on the clinical scenario.

Non-febrile seizures

The International League Against Epilepsy suggests that an EEG be done after all initial unprovoked seizures. Practice parameters by the American Academy of Neurology (AAN), Child Neurology Society (CNS), and American Epilepsy Society (AES) concur with this recommendation [13]. Their practice parameter guidelines reviewed five studies and found epileptiform activity and focal slowing to be predictive of recurrence. Fifty-four percent of individuals with an abnormal EEG had seizure recurrence versus 25% with normal EEGs. Recurrence was highest if the EEG finding was consistent with an idiopathic (genetic) generalized epilepsy predisposition. There is an increased yield if the EEG is completed within the first 24 hours of the seizure; however, the practice parameter guidelines warned of transient abnormalities and cautioned about over-interpretation of acute EEGs. It is suggested that if the individual returns to baseline in a timely manner post-seizure, an acute EEG is not required and need not be done acutely prior to hospital discharge. An EEG after the first non-febrile seizure is helpful in defining seizure type, syndrome, and recurrence risk.

Emergent EEGs in the hospital setting have been found to have low diagnostic yield in the adult population, with a diagnosis of subclinical seizures in only 10.7% [14]. EEG yield is higher when done in unresponsive children. Hosain *et al.* found non-convulsive status epilepticus in 33% of children studied [15]. The CNS and AAN (endorsed by American College of Emergency Physicians (ACEP), American Academy of Pediatrics (AAP), and AES) reviewed diagnostic assessment in children with status epilepticus. Six Class 3 studies with EEGs done hours to days after status epilepticus, found abnormalities in 66% to 100% of patients. Practice parameters for the diagnostic assessments of child with status epilepticus suggests considering an EEG in status epilepticus to determine focal versus generalized abnormalities, influence diagnosis and treatment, and to exclude pseudo-status epilepticus [16].

6.4 EEG findings in epilepsy and epilepsy syndromes

There are many EEG waveform variations that the electroencephalographer has to be aware of when attempting to predict epileptogenicity and seizure risk. Normal patterns such as the slow alpha variant, posterior slow waves of youth, and hypersynchronous states seen during drowsiness in children (such as hypnogogic hypersynchrony) must be differentiated from pathological slowing. The sharply contoured activity of small sharp spikes, 14 and 16 hertz positive bursts, and 6 Hz phantom spike and wave must be differentiated from focal and generalized interictal discharges. More prolonged rhythmic bursts of activity such as rhythmic temporal theta burst of drowsiness, (psychomotor variant pattern) (Figure 6.1), midline theta rhythm, and the frontal arousal rhythm should not be mistaken for clinical or subclinical seizures.

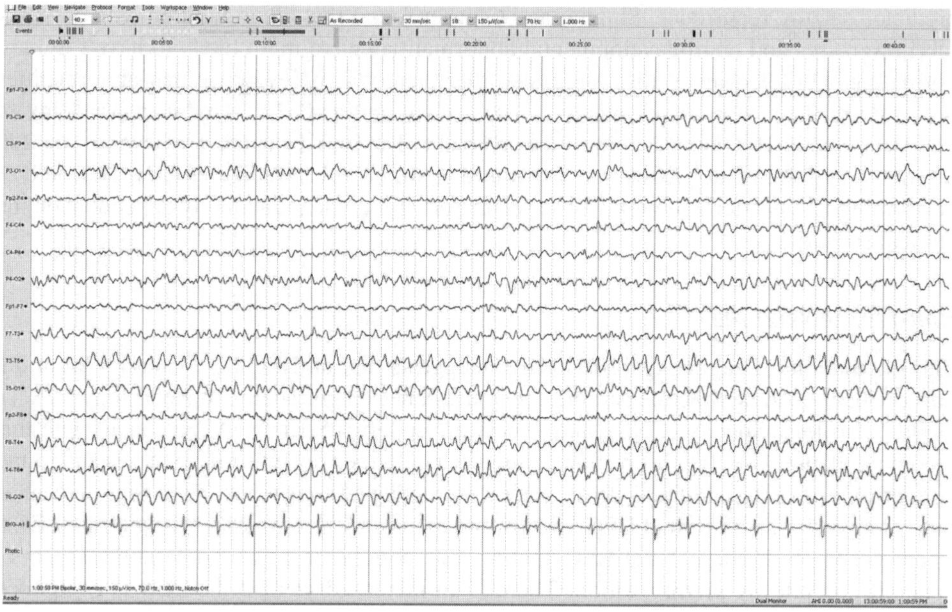

Figure 6.1 Electroencephalogram depicting bilateral rhythmic mid-temporal theta bursts of drowsiness (psychomotor variant or mid-temporal discharges) in a teenager with no prior definitive history of seizures.

There are also physiological and non-physiological artifacts that require differentiation from cortical activity. Some of these such as eye movements and electrocardiographic artifacts require specific electrode placement and additional monitoring devices for better differentiation. Others such as glossokinetic artifacts and galvanic skin responses require a keen eye and knowledge of the EEG. All instrument artifacts and electrode artifacts should be clearly documented by the EEG technologist.

Spikes and sharp waves are the only definitive interictal epileptiform discharges. The spike or sharp wave, with durations of 20–70 ms or 70–200 ms respectively, represent a hyperexcitable state of a synchronized group of neurons, the depolarization shift. The following hyperpolarization is represented by a slow wave. They are infrequently seen in the normal patient population, and hence their presence may not always translate to a seizure diagnosis. They are, however, highly predictive of seizures and epilepsy risk, and their morphology, distribution, and mode of activation (such as 3 Hz spike and wave activation with hyperventilation) may help to define specific seizure types or epilepsy syndromes. Multifocal, temporal, and vertex waves while awake are the most indicative of future epilepsy risk, whereas central and occipital spikes carry significant but lower risk of future epilepsy.

6.5 Neonatal EEGs

Of all EEG interpretations, that of the neonate may be the most critical yet most difficult. If interpreted correctly, however, it is one of the few functional methods of evaluating the evolving maturation in the first weeks of life. The preconceived notion of normal and abnormal EEG findings in children and adults could lead to misdiagnosis and incorrect prognosis and management in neonates. What is perceived to be burst suppression may be a normal finding at 28 weeks gestational age. Sharp waves (positive and negative) do not necessarily predict seizure risk, but may be more suggestive of underlying neuronal dysfunction.

The EEG technologist should be experienced in neonatal studies, noting every situation – rocking, feeding, and movements such as chewing, eye rolling, hiccups, etc. The activity of concern should be documented, and auditory and somatosensory stimuli applied to show EEG reactivity. It is ideal to capture sleep states during the EEG recording. Secondary to immature myelination and maturation of pathways, truly generalized seizures are rare in neonates and infants. Independent focal seizures evolving from both hemispheres (Figure 6.2) are not unheard of in neonates with diffuse neuronal insult. It has been shown clinically that focal motor activity (tonic, clonic, or myoclonic) is more indicative of neonatal cortical seizure than more subtle movements such as chewing and eye movements or generalized stiffening. The ictal EEG reveals variations in frequency and amplitude but activity does not always spread to contiguous electrodes or follow the pathways and distribution of seizures in older children and adults. A seizure may be isolated to one region and often there may be ongoing independent seizures evolving from different regions of the same hemisphere or from both hemispheres. Persistent electroencephalographic seizures are frequent after

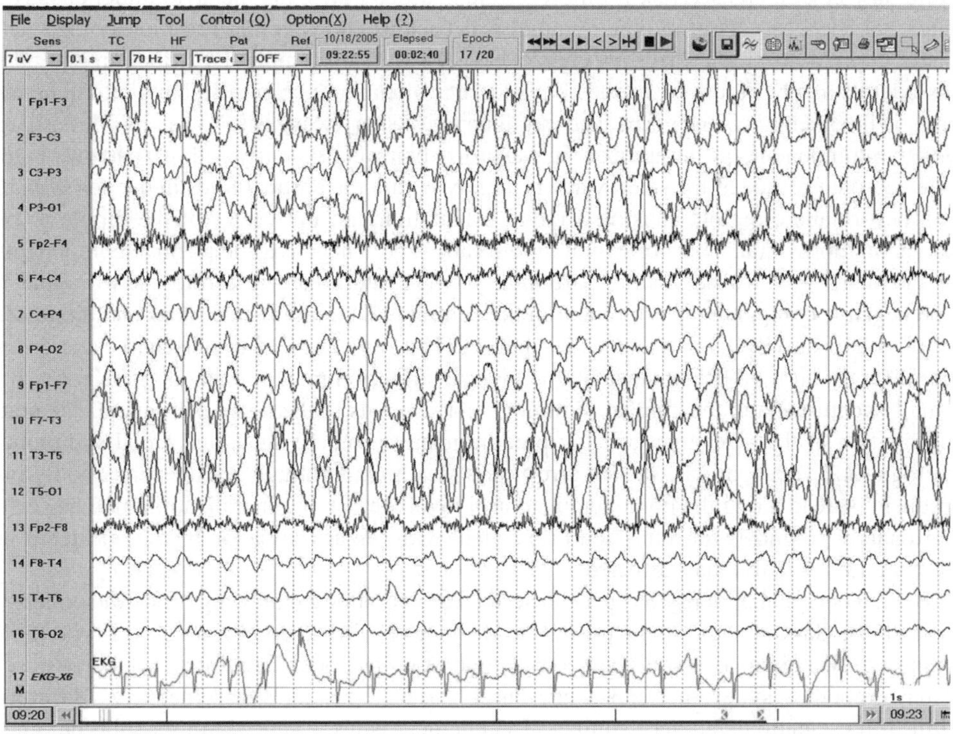

Figure 6.2 Electroencephalographic depiction of seizures involving both hemispheres in a neonate diagnosed with hypoxic ischemic encephalopathy. The waveforms are of different amplitude, frequency, and rhythmicity.

cessation of clinical seizures, mandating continuation of the EEG after control of clinical seizures or a repeat EEG study.

6.6 The EEG in focal epilepsy

The specificity of the ictal scalp EEG in identifying a seizure focus is limited by multiple variables including, but not limited to, the depth of the discharge from the scalp, cortical volume involved, underlying pathology, age, and lobe involved. Optimal localization and laterality are both noted in less than 66% of individuals [17]. Seizure onset may seem to involve one section, lobe, region, or hemisphere, or may appear bilateral or generalized. Frequency at onset also ranges from a slow delta to faster beta or gamma, spike and wave activity, or abrupt attenuation of the EEG, Although the interictal EEG has similar limitations it is often more specific to the site of seizure origin.

Idiopathic (genetic) focal epilepsy

Benign childhood epilepsy with centrotemporal spikes (BECTS) is an age-related genetic focal epilepsy whose seizure course is often benign. The age of onset of BECTS ranges from approximately 3 to 13 years. Although the neurological exam is often normal, the affected child may be at increased risk for more subtle neurocognitive and behavioral deficits. The interictal EEG reveals a normal, symmetrical background rhythm. The morphology and distribution of the sharp waves are characteristic. The centrotemporal distribution gives the disorder its name (Figure 6.3). One hemisphere is often more prominent but bilateral hemispheric involvement is the norm. The initial negative sharp wave is followed by a less sharp positive component, the duration of the waveform being consistently within a narrow range. The neuronal source of the sharp wave is largely within the cortical folds in the perisylvian and peri-rolandic region, causing a radial orientation and the vector of the dipole to be tangential/horizontal. This horizontal dipole causes both negative and positive components of the sharp wave to be visible, particularly when interpreted in a referential montage. The negative component is prominent in the central and temporal electrodes and the lower amplitude positivity has a frontal distribution. The frequency of the discharge increases significantly during NREM sleep and a wider distribution may be seen [18]. Seizures are usually nocturnal and the clinical semiology corresponds to the neuroanatomical, rolandic distribution of the discharge, causing predominantly oropharyngeal and facial symptoms with guttural vocalizations, speech arrest, and drooling. Although seizures are usually infrequent, spread along the homunculus to arm involvement or generalization may be seen. Fortunately prognosis for remission is excellent with seizure cessation by the mid-teens in the majority of individuals affected.

Benign occipital epilepsy has been described as everything that benign rolandic epilepsy is not [19]. Gastaut suggests that it has no distinctive clinical course or seizure type [20]. This said, two distinctive subtypes of this condition have been identified. The early-onset Panayiotopoulos syndrome, and a late-onset variant (Gastaut syndrome) have different clinical presentations but very similar EEG characteristics. The early-onset subtype often begins between ages 3 and 5 years but as old as 8 years of age, and presents clinically as eye deviation and ictal emesis with or without alteration of consciousness. The late subtype starts a few years later, 7–9 years, with visual phenomena lasting a few seconds, without

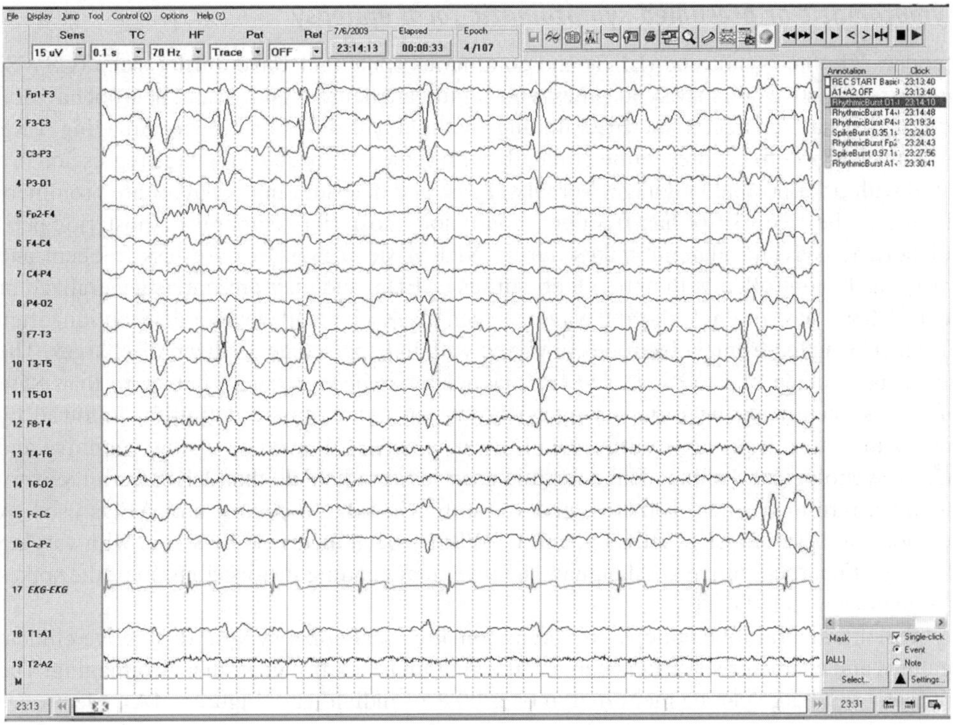

Figure 6.3 Left centrotemporal sharp waves during NREM sleep, in a 7-year-old child diagnosed with benign epilepsy with centrotemporal spikes.

alteration of consciousness, often with a postictal headache, nausea, and vomiting. The classic EEG signature is that of runs of occipital spikes, which are reduced or disappear with eye opening. Distribution of the discharge may encompass a wider field or may be generalized, especially in Panayiotopoulos syndrome. The latter often follows a benign course that is outgrown, but Gastaut syndrome is less predictable.

Autosomal dominant nocturnal frontal lobe epilepsy is a relatively rare familial condition with variable penetrance and expressivity. The interictal EEG reveals rare to no discharges and the ictal EEG may be even less helpful. It has no distinctive associated seizure pattern at onset, and may be normal or riddled with movement or myogenic artifact during the event. A prolonged Video EEG (VEEG) may, however, be helpful in identifying the stereotypic movements seen during the seizure. As in most frontal lobe seizures, the frequency is increased at night, making a prolonged overnight study optimal.

Autosomal dominant partial epilepsy with auditory features often presents during adolescence with the individual experiencing simple or complex auditory phenomena (buzzing, ringing, or hearing a specific song or voice) or receptive aphasia (an abrupt onset and end of inability to understand requests or commands). Consciousness is often retained. Mid to posterior temporal epileptiform discharges have only been described in one-third of individuals affected, and the ictal EEG may be negative. Seizure and family history is often the driving force for genetic testing and identification.

Symptomatic or presumed symptomatic focal epilepsy

Landau–Kleffner syndrome (LKS) and continuous spike and wave during sleep (CSWS) are two distinctive epilepsy syndromes with significant neurocognitive and neurobehavioral effects that have characteristic EEG findings without a clear lesion on neuroimaging. LKS is more clearly defined, presenting clinically with acute or subacute language regression in a child with prior normal language. Verbal agnosia and deteriorating behavior are prominent findings. The sleep EEG has frequent, continuous posterior temporal or posterior peri-rolandic/perisylvian bilateral spikes during NREM sleep. Seizures are less frequent and fairly easily controlled with antiepileptic drugs (AEDs) and may present as generalized or focal. CSWS has similar spike and waves as seen in LKS but with a wider distribution, often also involving the frontal electrodes or mixed with indispersed generalized discharges. The actual percentage of EEG involved for diagnosis has been debated, but more than 85% of spikes occupying the EEG during NREM sleep is the classic definition followed by most authorities. It presents initially with focal seizures followed by a slow cognitive and neuropsychological decline. The course is even less predictable than LKS, with recovery in some, rare to frequent seizures, and variability in seizure control and AEDs used. A relationship between LKS, BECTS, and CSWS has been theorized by some, with varying degrees of neurocognitive and language involvement pending the distribution of the spikes and regions affected [21].

Medial temporal lobe epilepsy is a symptomatic focal epilepsy with distinctive clinical features and characteristic EEG changes. It can often be confirmed with neuroimaging. The interictal discharge can be identified in over 90% of individuals (Figure 6.4A). Electrodes placed close to the anterior and basal temporal region are most active and sensitivity may be

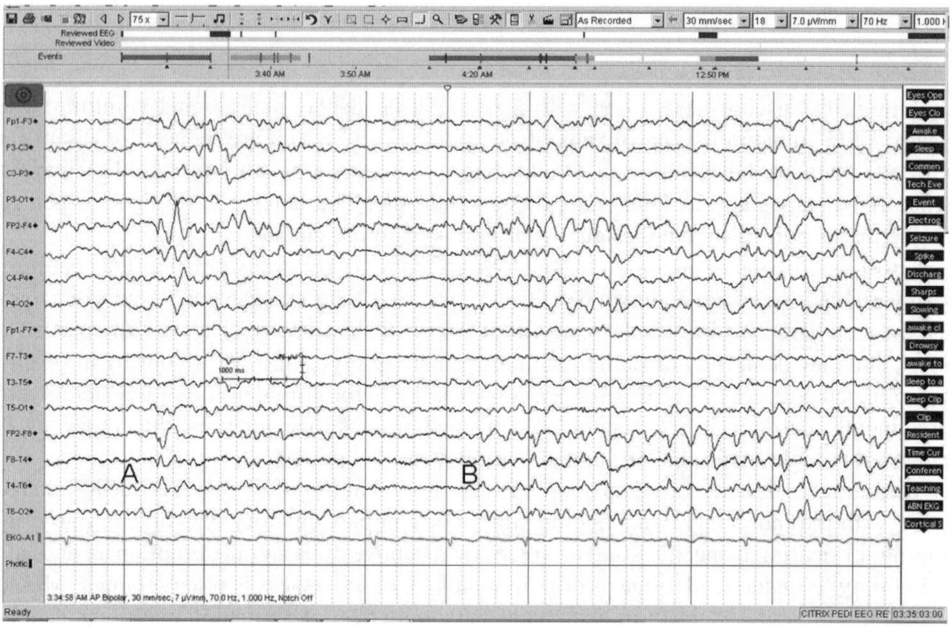

Figure 6.4 A right temporal epileptiform discharge (A) followed several seconds later by right temporal seizure onset (B) in a 16-year-old female with magnetic resonance imaging (MRI)-confirmed mesial temporal sclerosis.

increased by placing T1, T2 electrodes or sphenoidal electrodes [22]. Intermittent rhythmic delta is often seen over the affected temporal lobe, and some patients may have less frequent sharp waves over the unaffected side. The ictal pattern often involves primarily the temporal region at onset (Figure 6.4B). The patient frequently describes a preceding aura (usually a gastric rising sensation or discomfort) prior to alteration of consciousness followed by staring and oral and/or appendicular automatisms.

Lateral temporal and neocortical ictal and interictal activity, interpreted in isolation, are not predictive of the underlying pathology. Lateral temporal seizures often have more posterior displaced epileptiform discharges than mesial temporal seizures, and the seizures usually spread more quickly to the frontal lobe or become secondarily generalized. Frontal lobe seizures are often frequent and nocturnal, and those originating from the orbitofrontal or mesial frontal regions are seldom seen until spread or may be missed on scalp EEG. Parietal seizures are easily missed because symptoms and ictal and interictal EEGs may be particularly elusive and may represent the area of spread (to the temporal or frontal lobes) and not the region of origin. Occipital spikes are often prominent but if close to the midline, as in all midline structures affected, may appear to have a contralateral origin, because of volume conduction, rapid spread, and the vector of the discharge. True hemispheric or multilobar involvement may be seen in situations where the entire hemisphere is involved such as hemimegaloencephaly, or syndromes affecting multiple lobes such as tuberous sclerosis.

6.7 The EEG of generalized epilepsy

Idiopathic (genetic) generalized epilepsy

Benign myoclonic epilepsy in infants and early childhood (BME), childhood absence epilepsy (CAE), juvenile absence epilepsy (JAE), juvenile myoclonic epilepsy (JME), and epilepsy with grand mal on awakening (EGMA) are a spectrum of disorders that share some overlap in their phenotype and genotype and for the most part have a favorable outcome. Affected individuals are usually neurocognitively normal. Juvenile myoclonic epilepsy, childhood absence epilepsy, and juvenile absence epilepsy are the most prevalent. Absence, myoclonic, and generalized tonic-clonic are the three seizure types associated with these conditions. Although there is significant overlap, their nomenclature describes both the relative age of onset and the predominant seizure type.

Typical absence epilepsy is characterized by an abrupt onset of impairment of consciousness without a prior aura with resumption of baseline activity immediately after. Tone is often preserved and a duration of 5 to 15 seconds is the norm, rarely longer than 20 seconds. It may be missed if the child is not closely observed. Accompanying features may include subtle clonic activity, especially of the upper limbs, head, or neck area, eye blinking or rolling, automatisms, eyelid myoclonia, or subtle loss in tone without falls. The frequency is greatest in CAE, with seizures occurring multiple times per day; they are prominent but less frequent in JAE, being experienced in less than one-third of children with JME; they are rarely if ever seen in BME or EGMA. The classic interictal EEG described (found in most patients with CAE) comprises bilateral, synchronous, often frontally dominant 3 Hz spike and slow-wave runs of similar amplitude and morphology (Figure 6.5). The ictal discharge is similar to the inter-ictal bursts, often ranging in frequency from 2.5 to 4 Hz, and is of longer duration than the interictal bursts. In the absence seizures of JME, unlike those of CAE, disorganized, slightly higher frequency generalized polyspikes

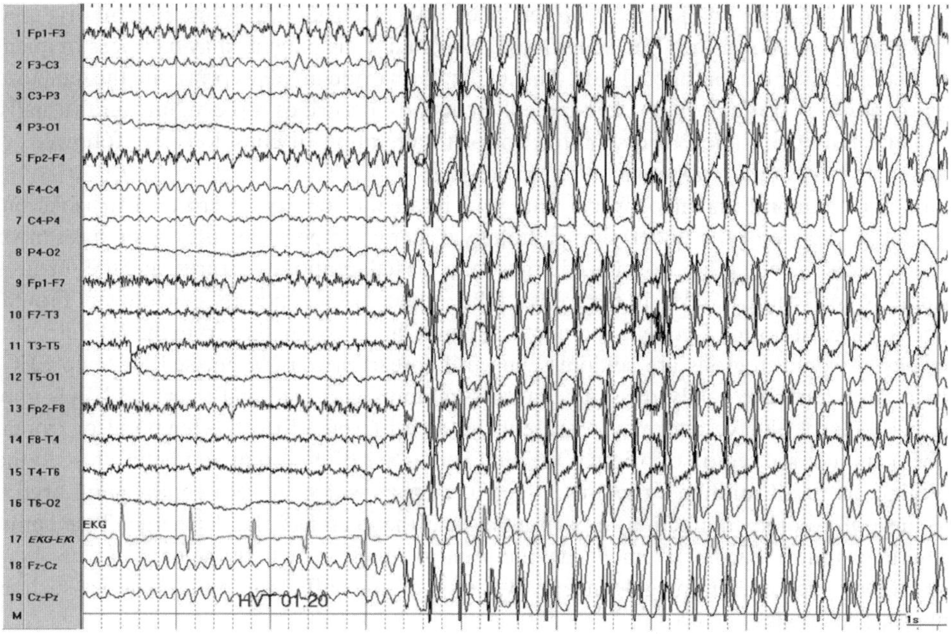

Figure 6.5 An absence seizure induced after 1.2 minutes of hyperventilation in an 8-year-old child.

may be more prominent, but features of both JME and CAE may be seen in the absence seizures of JAE [23]. Hyperventilation frequently induces both ictal and interictal responses (CAE > JAE > JME), and a similar response is less frequently seen when photic stimulation is applied (JME > JAE > CAE).

Two other often self-limiting epilepsy syndromes with prominent absence features are worth mentioning. Eyelid myoclonia with or without absence is characterized by eye rolling and rapid eyelid myoclonia with or without alteration in consciousness, often induced by flashing light precipitated by the child's actions (waving of open fingers in front of the face or opening and closing blinds). Facial twitching or jerking also may be seen with this seizure type. The EEG maybe identical to that seen in CAE [24]. Even after the EEG pattern clears, the obsessive-type seizure-inducing behaviors and tic-like blinking may persist. Micturition absence is similar clinically and electroencephalographically to childhood absence with the unfortunate addition of detrusor muscle contraction and urination during attacks. It is also a social problem because with frequent seizures the child is constantly wet. This absence variant is pharmacoresistant to the typical absence medications, but like CAE, is often outgrown [18].

Myoclonic seizures are the hallmark of JME but may also be seen in isolation in JAE. Clinically it is characterized by lightning like contractions of a muscle or group of muscles. Myoclonus varies in severity of amplitude of the movement and parts of the body involved. The classic EEG pattern is generalized 4–6 Hz polyspike and slow-wave activity, and it is activated by photic stimulation (Figure 6.6). In JME the myoclonic seizures are more prominent in the morning, and both the seizures and electroencephalographic abnormalities are exacerbated by lack of sleep and by alcohol. As in individuals with most seizure types, interictal activity is activated by NREM sleep. The ictal activity of the less frequently

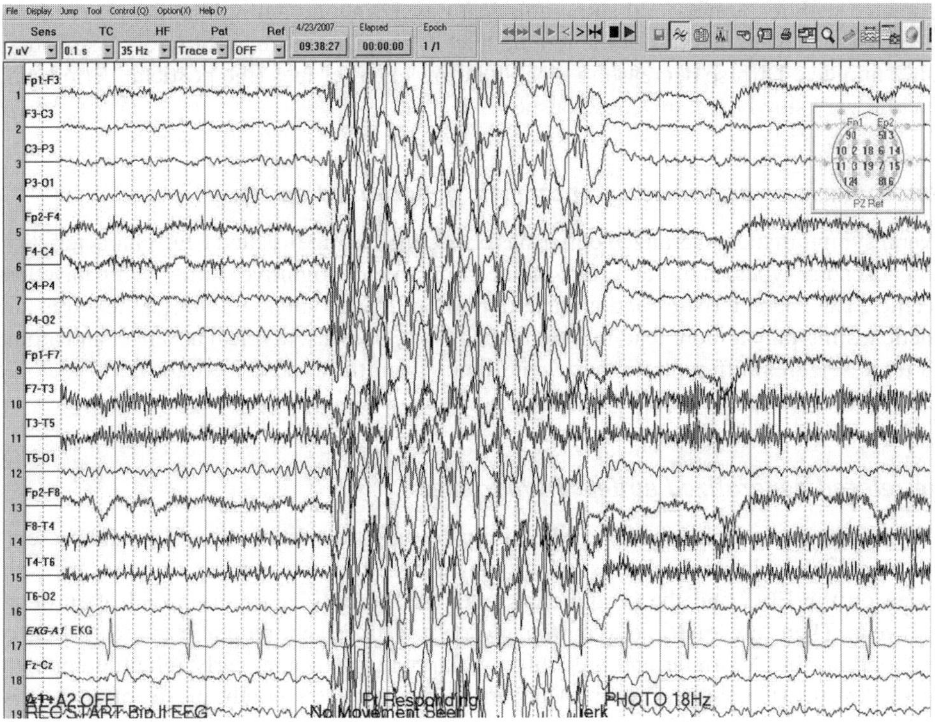

Figure 6.6 A photoparoxysmal response (at 18 Hz photic stimulation) in a 16-year-old male with a clinical picture suggestive of juvenile myoclonic epilepsy (JME).

encountered BME may have a slower spike and wave frequency with the moclonic jerks time-locked to the discharge. The myoclonus seen in JME often affects the distal extremities, with prominent extension movements occurring in succession, whereas those in BME have prominent proximal flexion of the limbs or upper trunk [25]. Myoclonic seizures sometimes crescendo to generalized tonic-clonic activity.

Generalized tonic-clonic seizures (GTC; grand mal seizures) are experienced in EGMA, may be seen in JME and JAE, but have a reduced incidence in CAE. There are no known classic characteristics of the GTC seen in various epilepsy syndromes. EEG onset is heralded by abrupt attenuation or rhythmic generalized spike/polyspike and slow-wave activity. Alpha frequency spike and slow-wave activity during the tonic phase follows, which is frequently obscured by myogenic artifact. As the clonic phase ensues, the spike and slow-wave activity slows, with concurrent time-locked slowing of the clonic jerks. Finally spikes or sharps of 1 Hz or less succeed to often prolonged postictal slowing or diffuse attenuation before gradual resumption of baseline activity. Clinically there is an acute loss of consciousness with or without an accompanying guttural sound (forced expiration). The following tonic stiffening is often symmetric with flexion or extension of the limbs and clenching of the fist. The jaw is also clenched shut with eyes rolling upwards (this phase often last less than 30 seconds). The clonic phase follows with rhythmic jerking or convulsions of the limbs, initially starting out fast and low in amplitude but gradually decreasing in frequency and increasing in amplitude of the movements prior to the end of the seizure. It is often associated with respiratory and autonomic features. Urination during the event is common and biting the cheek or sides of the tongue may occur. The entire event rarely lasts longer than 2 minutes. Diffuse decrease in tone and drowsiness ensues (the postictal period) and the child very slowly regains consciousness.

Symptomatic or presumed symptomatic generalized epilepsy

Several symptomatic generalized epilepsies are defined by age-related EEG characteristics, clinical seizure types, and their effect on the child's neurocognitive status. Many have less specific EEG characteristics and clinical definition. Underlying pathological features and genetic testing play a more leading role in diagnosis. Spasms, atypical absence, and atonic and tonic seizures differentiate these syndromes from those described above. Myoclonic and GTC seizures are seen in both. Clonic seizures in isolation are rare.

Age-related generalized epilepsy syndromes

Early myoclonic encephalopathy (EME) occurs during the first month of life and presents with myoclonic or partial seizures, which may evolve to tonic spasms. Burst suppression is seen on the EEG and the prognosis is poor with rapid deterioration and often death by 1 year. There are multiple symptomatic or presumed symptomatic causes, often of metabolic origin. A similar and arguably overlapping syndrome, early infantile epileptic encephalopathy (Ohtahara syndrome), occurs within the first 3 months of life, often the first 2 weeks. It is also characterized by a burst suppression pattern on EEG. The seizures are primarily tonic or tonic spasms, but focal and myoclonic seizures may be seen. Prognosis is poor with neurocognitive regression and mental retardation in most children. The underlying cause varies greatly and is often accompanied by structural dysgenesis. Both conditions, especially Ohtahara syndrome, may progress to West syndrome.

West syndrome consists of a triad of a hypsarrhythmic EEG, infantile spasms, and neurocognitive delay/regression. Two of three are necessary to make the diagnosis. The seizures may be very subtle at onset, most beginning between 3 months and 1 year. Hypsarrhythmia has a distinctive disorganized pattern with high-voltage, asynchronous waveforms and mutifocal independent spike foci (Figure 6.7). During NREM sleep a burst suppression pattern may be the first to appear and the last to disappear. Well-formed background rhythm and sleep features are seldom seen. Modification of this pattern, with focal epileptiform discharges, sleep features, or a less disorganized background, does not negate the diagnosis, but may alter management. Kallaway *et al.* found 11 different types of ictal EEG patterns, but most consist of generalized attenuation, generalized bursts of spike/polyspike or slow wave followed by attenuation, or low-amplitude faster frequency activity, or variations of the three themes. Immediate treatment may alter the clinical course, with adrenocorticotropic hormone (ACTH) and vigabatrin being the medications most often used. In children with focal hypsarrhythmia or an identifiable focal structural or functional (PET, SPECT) lesion, surgery may be an option. Epilepsy surgery is also an option for those children in whom functional studies such as Positron Emission tomography (PET) and Single-photon emission computed tomography (SPECT) define a focal region responsible for seizure onset. There are multiple structural, infectious, inflammatory, metabolic, and mitochondrial causes. West syndrome often evolves to other seizure types or Lennox–Gastaut syndrome.

The EEG hallmark of Lennox–Gastaut syndrome (LGS) is generalized slow-spike and slow-wave activity at a frequency of 1.5–2.5 Hz (Figure 6.8). The epileptiform discharge

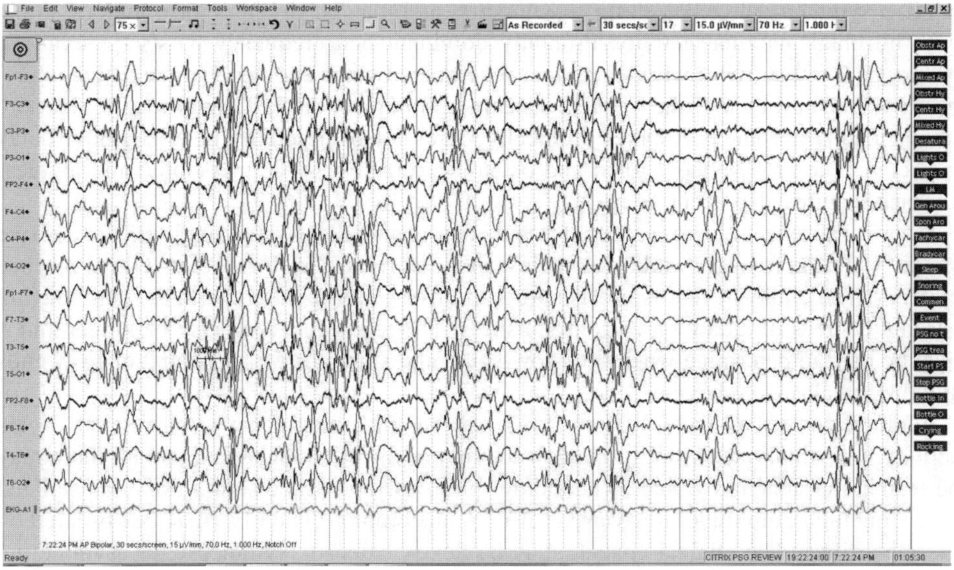

Figure 6.7 Hypsarrythmia in a 10-month-old child presenting with flexor spasms. The EEG reveals independent multifocal and generalized spikes/polyspikes as well as generalized discharges followed by relative attenuation.

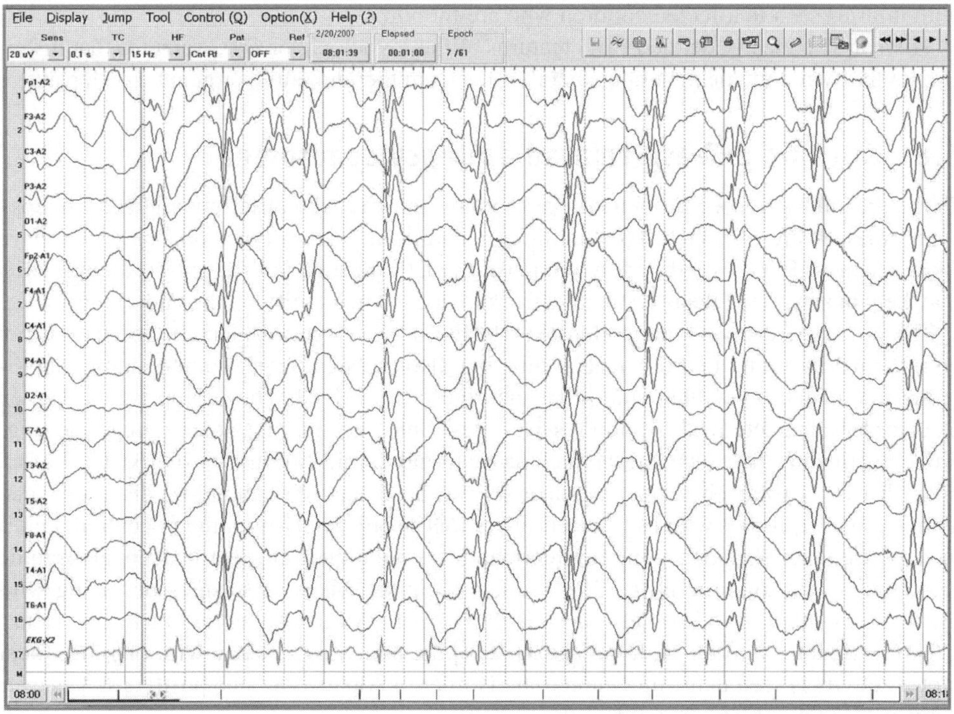

Figure 6.8 The electroencephalographic slow-spike and slow-wave pattern of Lennox–Gastaut syndrome seen in a 9-year-old child.

is often symmetrical or has shifting symmetry, and may be rhythmic or pseudorhythmic with bifrontal maximal activity. Frontally dominant beta-frequency bursts (generalized paroxysmal fast activity) without clinical accompaniment is another characteristic feature. NREM sleep may change the frequency and morphology of the EEG abnormalities to more frequent, polymorphic polyspikes. Clinically regression or significant neurocognitive delay is accompanied by frequent tonic and or atonic seizures. GTC, myoclonic and atypical absence seizures also occur often.

Atypical absence seizures seen in this and other generalized symptomatic epilepsies have slower 1–2.5 Hz frequency bilateral but less monomorphic waveforms than typical absence epilepsy. The clinical event is not as abrupt in onset or termination, with the child having varying degrees of alteration of consciousness. The ictal event may also be longer and it may be hard to determine where the slow-spike and slow-wave background of LGS ends and the actual seizure begins.

Tonic seizures may have different EEG patterns including paroxysmal fast 10–25 Hz activity, low-amplitude faster frequency activity, or diffuse attenuation, and all three may be seen in the same individual. A heralding spike, polyspike, and slow wave or an isolated preceding high-amplitude slow wave is also not uncommon. The EEG may be obscured by muscle artifact. The clinical episode may be flexor, extensor, symmetric, or asymmetric. There is usually rapid resumption to baseline activity after the seizure.

In atonic seizures an initial generalized polyspike is followed by a large-amplitude slow wave with the atonic component of the seizure occurring during the slow wave. It may be preceded by a myoclonic jerk or brief tonic stiffening. These seizures are often frequent, with injuries seen in affected children who are mobile.

There are no clearly defined EEG features of the myoclonic or GTC seizures that differentiate the symptomatic generalized epilepsies from the idiopathic or genetic epilepsies.

6.8 Specific disease-related epilepsy syndromes

There are multiple specific genetic, metabolic, and mitochondrial generalized epilepsy syndromes, many of which have multiple generalized seizure types and may also have focal seizures. Rarely do they rely on a specific EEG feature for diagnosis, though EEG may help in narrowing the investigative workup needed in identifying the underlying cause.

The progressive myoclonic epilepsies (PMEs) deserve special mention because of not only their devastating neurological decline but also the significant, compounding, debilitating role of the myoclonic and other seizure types involved. They comprise a complex of disorders characterized by progressive myoclonus, ataxia, and neurological and cognitive decline. Well-known causes include neuronal ceroid lipofuscinosis (NCL), Lafora body disease, Unverricht–Lundborg disease, sialidosis, and mitochondrial disorders such as myoclonic epilepsy with ragged-red fibers (MERRF). High-amplitude occipital spikes in response to low-frequency intermittent photic stimulation is an electroencephalographic signature of late infantile NCL [26]. Similar occipital spikes or seizures occurring with photic stimulation have been also described in other PMEs such as Lafora Body disease [27]. Continuous anterior high-voltage 1–3/s spike and wave activity with ongoing focal motor activity is seen in the mitochondrial disorder of Alpers [28], and positive spikes over the vertex are described in sialidosis type 1 [29].

Myoclonic seizures play a prominent role during the evolution of other conditions such as severe myoclonic epilepsy of infancy (Dravet syndrome). This condition, first described in

France in 1978, is characterized by focal or generalized febrile seizures (often prolonged) in the first year of life, evolving to generalized seizure types including frequent GTCs, myoclonic seizures, and atypical absence. It is often caused by a cortical sodium channel mutation, and a small percentage of females have a mutation in protocadherin 19 gene (*PCDH19*) on the X-chromosome. The EEG starts out normal but evolves to generalized and multifocal spike and slow-wave activity with a positive response to intermittent photic stimuli often observed. This must be differentiated from idiopathic myoclonic epilepsy of infancy with GTCs, described by Doose, which often carries a better prognosis, although there is likely some overlap. Generalized epilepsy with febrile seizure plus (GEFS+) is another compilation of disorders caused by a defect in a neuronal gated sodium channel. It is an autosomal dominant condition, and clinical symptoms range from simple and complex febrile seizures to different types of generalized and sometimes focal non-febrile seizures with varying degrees of pharmacoresistance. It has been theorized that Dravet syndrome is a severe form of GEFS+, although some regard them as separate. GEFS+ does not have a clearly defined EEG signature.

6.9 Conclusion

The EEG has many limitations, but remains the gold standard for determining seizure risk and seizure type and for identifying epilepsy syndromes. It may prognosticate and determine the urgency and type of seizure management required. History and exam should determine when it is necessary and should assist in its interpretation, which should be undertaken by an expert in the field. EEG still also has utility in directing investigative flow as to when newer genetic and neuroimaging studies are warranted for diagnostic confirmation. The EEG also has uses outside of diagnosing seizures and epilepsy syndromes, such as quantifying cerebral dysfunction and defining prognosis.

References

[1] Berger H. Über das Elektroenkephalogramm des Menschen. *Arch Psychiatr* 1929;**87**:527–570.
[2] Niedermeyer E. The clinical relevance of EEG interpretation. *Clin Electroencephalogr* 2003;**34**:93–98.
[3] American Electroencephalographic Society. Guidelines in EEG and evoked potentials. *J Clin Neurophysiol* 1986;**3**(Suppl. 1):1–152.
[4] Salinsky M, Kanter R, Dasheiff RM. Effectiveness of multiple EEGs in supporting the diagnosis of epilepsy: an operational curve. *Epilepsia* 1987;**28**:331–334.
[5] Foldvary-Schaefer N, Grigg-Damberger M. Sleep and epilepsy: what we know, don't know, and need to know. *J Clin Neurophysiol* 2006;**23**:4–20.
[6] Holmes MD, Dewaraja AS, Vanhatalo S. Does hyperventilation elicit epileptic seizures? *Epilepsia* 2004;**45**:618–620.
[7] Guaranha MS, Garzon E, Buchpiguel CA, *et al.* Hyperventilation revisited: physiological effects and efficacy on focal seizure activation in the era of video-EEG monitoring. *Epilepsia* 2005;**46**:69–75.
[8] Adrian E, Matthews B. The Berger rhythm: potential changes from the occipital lobes in man. *Brain* 1934;**57**:355–384.
[9] Waltz S, Christen H-J, Doose H. The different patterns of the photoparoxysmal response – a genetic study. *Electroencephalogr Clin Neurophysiol* 1992;**83**:138–145.

[10] Frantzen E, Lennox-Buchthal M, Nygaard A. Longitudinal EEG and clinical Study of children with febrile convulsions. *Electroenceph Clin Neurophsiol* 1968;**24**:197–212.

[11] Shinnar S, Glauser T. Febrile seizures. *J Child Neurol* 2002;**17**;S44.

[12] Steering Committee on Quality Improvement and Management, Subcommittee on Febrile Seizures of the American Academy of Pediatrics. Febrile seizures: clinical practice guideline for the long-term management of the child with simple febrile seizures. *Pediatrics* 2008;**121**:1281–1286.

[13] Hirtz D, Berg A, Bettis D, *et al*. Practice parameter: treatment of the child with a first unprovoked seizure: Report of the Quality Standards Subcommittee of the American Academy of Neurology and the Practice Committee of the Child Neurology Society. *Neurology* 2003;**60**:166–175.

[14] Varelas PN, Spanaki MV, Hacein-Bey L. Emergent EEG: indications and diagnostic yield. *Neurology* 2003;**61**:702–704.

[15] Hosain SA, Solomon GE, Kobylarz EJ. Electroencephalographic patterns in unresponsive pediatric patients. *Pediatr Neurol* 2005;**32**:162–165.

[16] Riviello JJ, Aswal S, Hirtz D, *et al*. Practice Parameter: Diagnostic assessment of the child with status epilepticus (an evidence-based review) *Neurology* 2006;**67**:1542–1550.

[17] Foldvary N, Klem G, Hammel J, *et al.* The localizing value of itcal EEG in focal epilepsy. *Neurology* 2001;**57**:2022–2028.

[18] Graf M, Lischka A. Topographical EEG analysis of rolandic spikes. *Clin Electroencephalogr* 1988;**29**:132–137.

[19] Camfield P, Camfield C. Epileptic syndromes in childhood: Clinical features, outcomes and treatment. *Epilepsia* 2002;**43**(Suppl. 3):27–32.

[20] Gastaut H. Benign partial epilepsy with occipital paroxysms. In: Roger J, Dravet C, Bureau M, *et al.* (eds). *Epileptic Syndromes in Infancy, Childhood and Adolescence*. London: John Libbey, 1992; pp. 201–208.

[21] Deonna T, Roulet-Perez E. Early-onset acquired epileptic aphasia (Landau–Kleffner syndrome, LKS) and regressive autistic disorders with epileptic EEG abnormalities: the continuing debate. *Brain Dev* 2010;**32**:746–752.

[22] Mintzer S, Nicholl JS, Stern JM, Engel J. Relative utility of sphenoidal and temporal surface electodes for localization of ictal onset in temporal lobe epilepsy. *Clin Neurophysiol* 2002;**113**:911–916.

[23] Sadleir LG, Scheffer IE, Smith S, *et al*. Factors influencing clinical features of absence seizures. *Epilepsia* 2008;**49**:2100–2107.

[24] Ducan JS, Panayiotopoulos CP. *Eyelid Myoclonia with Absences*. London: John Libbey & Co. Ltd, 1966.

[25] Hirano Y, Oguni H, Funatsuka KI, Osawa M. Differentiation of myoclonic seizures in epileptic syndromes: A video-polygraphic study of 26 patients. *Epilepsia* 2009;**50**:1525–1535.

[26] Green JB. Neurophysiological Studies in Batten's Disease. *Dev Med Child Neurlo* 1971;**13**:477–498.

[27] Satishchandra P, Sinha S. Progressive myoclonic epilepsy. *Neurol India* 2010;**58**:514–522.

[28] Brick JF, Westmoreland BF, Gomex MR. The electroencephalogram in Alper's disease. *Electroencepahlor Clin Neurophysiol* 1984;**58**:3 P (abst).

[29] Engel J Jr, Rapin I, Giblin DR. Electrophysiological studies in two patients with cherry red spot myoclonus syndromes. *Epilepsia* 1977;**18**:73–87.

7 Imaging of pediatric epilepsy

Asim F. Choudhri

Departments of Radiology and Neurosurgery, University of Tennessee Health Science Center, Memphis, TN, USA; Le Bonheur Neuroscience Institute, Le Bonheur Children's Hospital, Memphis, TN, USA

7.1 Introduction

Modern neuroimaging techniques have improved the ability to detect underlying structural abnormalities in children with epilepsy. Using imaging to aid in the diagnosis and treatment of epilepsy requires an understanding of congenital, neoplastic, acquired, and idiopathic brain abnormalities that may be encountered, as well as an appreciation for the imaging techniques themselves to help understand the strengths, weaknesses, and risks of each modality.

Multidisciplinary expert panels have come up with guidelines to help determine the possible role of different imaging modalities in children with seizures [1,2] (Box 7.1).

7.2 Imaging considerations

Computed tomography

Computed tomography (CT) is a rapid and widely available way to image the brain, with few contraindications. As it can be performed rapidly, it typically does not require sedation.

Epilepsy in Children and Adolescents, First Edition. Edited by James W. Wheless.

Box 7.1 Summary of imaging modalities

- *CT without contrast:* Emergent evaluation (particularly in cases of suspected acute hemorrhage and/or trauma).
- *MRI without contrast:* Gold standard for non-invasive structural evaluation of the brain.
- *MRI without and with contrast:* When there is a concern for infection or inflammation, or to characterize a known structural lesion.
- *SPECT perfusion:* To evaluate the perfusion pattern profile of a known structural lesion, or an area with suspicious EEG findings (anticipating hyperemia of epileptogenic areas on ictal imaging and hypoperfusion of epileptogenic areas on interictal imaging).
- *FDG-PET:* For spatial localization of epileptogenic foci (anticipating hypometabolic activity of epileptogenic areas on interictal imaging and hypermetabolic activity of epileptogenic areas on less common ictal imaging).
- *Magnetoencephalography (MEG):* For spatial localization of epileptogenic foci as well as localization of cortex activated by sensory stimuli.
- *Functional MRI (fMRI):* Surgical planning to define lesion location relative to eloquent cortex (speech, motor cortices).
- *Head ultrasound:* Neonatal seizure evaluation.
- *Cerebral angiography:* To define suspected complex vascular anomalies as well as to confirm the lateralization of language and memory (Wada testing).

CT is excellent at detecting acute abnormalities such as hemorrhage, hydrocephalus, and herniation, and is the gold standard for assessing osseous structures and for parenchymal mineralization. The soft tissue detail of CT does not match that of magnetic resonance imaging (MRI); however, CT remains an important tool for evaluation of acute emergencies in children with seizures. CT is performed using ionizing radiation, approximately 100 times that from a chest radiograph, so caution is warranted prior to initiating this technique [3].

Children with chronic seizures or hydrocephalus may have frequent emergency department visits. At each visit the child must be carefully evaluated and a determination made whether a CT scan is warranted, keeping in mind the patient's cumulative radiation exposure. CT may not be appropriate after each seizure in a child with a known seizure disorder if there are no new or concerning symptoms. Given that CT is typically used for rapid emergent evaluation, scans performed without intravenous contrast ("unenhanced" scans) are the most common. Performing additional scans after the administration of intravenous contrast typically has little role unless patients have a contraindication to a subsequent MRI.

Magnetic resonance imaging

Magnetic resonance imaging (MRI) is the gold standard for structural evaluation of the brain in children with seizures (Box 7.2). MRI makes use of a magnetic field, and the image quality improves with a higher field strength. Most modern clinical MRI is performed on 1.5 T (1.5 tesla) or 3.0 T scanners.

Box 7.2 Sample magnetic resonance imaging (MRI) seizure protocol

Sagittal T1 weighted.
Axial T2 weighted.
Axial T2-FLAIR.
Axial DWI with apparent diffusion coefficient (ADC).
Coronal thin-section T2-FLAIR of temporal lobes.
Coronal thin-section inversion recovery of temporal lobes.
Axial T1 weighted (optional, however helpful if patient is not completely myelinated or if post-contrast imaging will be performed).
Axial and coronal T1 weighted images post-gadolinium administration (optional).

While MRI provides excellent structural detail, it presents several challenges. Individual imaging sequences typically take 2 to 8 minutes, and are sensitive to motion. Depending upon the sequences selected, and whether intravenous contrast is administered, imaging can take 30–50 minutes for an entire brain. Many children, in particular those under 8 years of age, will require some degree of sedation for the procedure. Patients with implanted medical devices will often have relative and/or absolute contraindications to MRI scanning, and careful patient screening prior to performing a study is imperative. Just as anaphylactic reactions cannot be predicted in patients with drug allergies, the successful completion of a scan without complications does not mean that a patient (or device) can be safely scanned.

The basic MRI sequences are T1 and T2 weighted sequences. T1 weighted sequences (Figure 7.1A) have excellent anatomical detail, including depiction of gray-white differentiation. Substances such as lipid, some proteinaceous material, and some minerals and metals, in particular gadolinium, will be hyperintense (or "bright") on T1 weighted sequences. T2 weighted sequences (Figure 7.1B) are notable for showing water as bright; in the normal brain, cerebrospinal fluid within the ventricular system and in the subarachnoid space is well seen; however, increased water content due to edema or hypomyelinated white matter is also noted.

Fluid attenuated inversion recovery (FLAIR) (Figure 7.1C) is a technique that is typically applied to T2 weighted images whereby the hyperintense signal from pure water (plus or minus electrolytes) such as cerebrospinal fluid is negated. FLAIR sequences can increase the conspicuity of parenchymal edema or gliosis, and can help detect whether there are contaminants in the cerebrospinal fluid such as blood products in subarachnoid hemorrhage or proteinaceous material in meningitis.

Inversion recovery can be used in different ways, and in seizure patients inversion recovery sequences (Figure 7.1D) can offer excellent gray-white evaluation, which is important to detect subtle cortical dysplasia. A coronal inversion recovery sequence is often the best way to evaluate the morphology of the hippocampal formations. This is often paired with a coronal FLAIR image to look for hippocampal signal abnormalities.

Diffusion weighted imaging (DWI) is a technique that attempts to quantify the Brownian motion of water (Figure 7.2A). The more freely that water can move ("facilitated diffusion"), the less signal is seen. If there are limitations to water movement ("restricted diffusion"), a hyperintense signal is seen. The amount of signal seen is also related to the underlying water

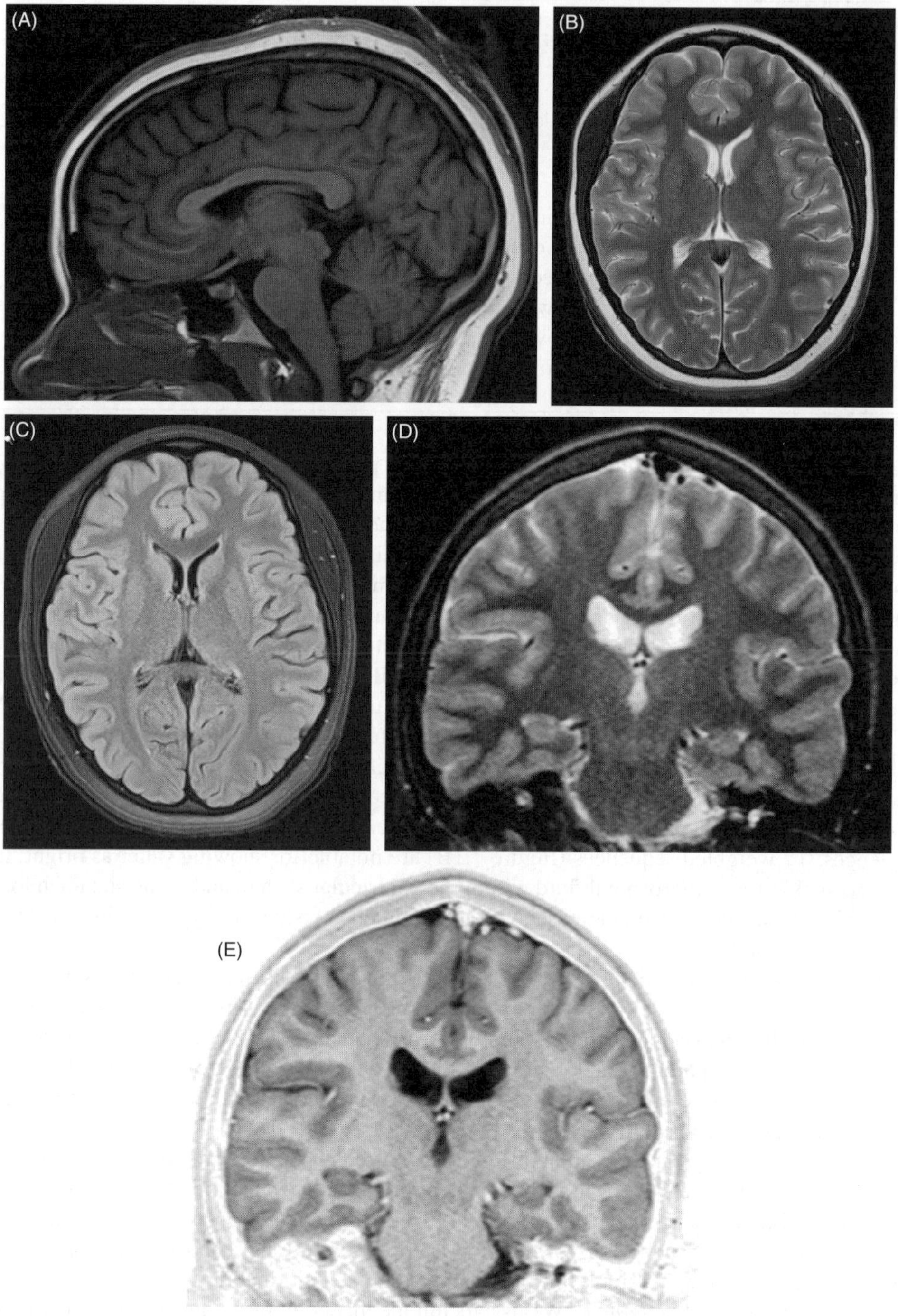

Figure 7.1 Imaging of a normal brain in multiple projections and sequences, including mid-sagittal T1 weighted image (A); axial T2 weighted image (B); axial fluid attenuated inversion recovery, or FLAIR (C); and a coronal short-tau inversion recovery sequence, or STIR (D). The STIR image can be post-processed by switching black and white to highlight the gray-white interface (E).

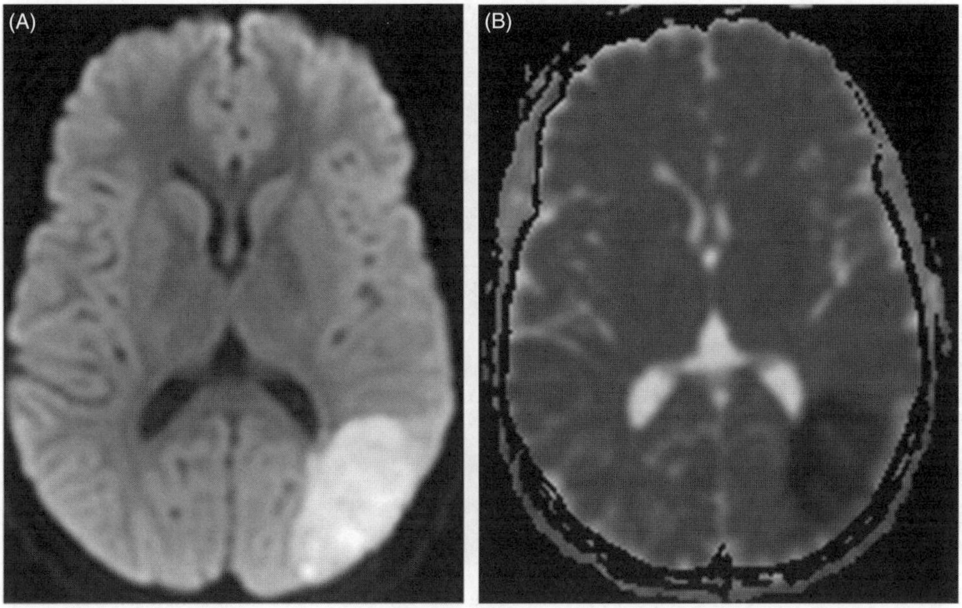

Figure 7.2 Axial diffusion weighted image (DWI, A) shows hyperintense signal in a confluent area at the junction of the left temporal and occipital lobes. The low values demonstrated on the apparent diffusion coefficient (ADC) map (B) confirm the DWI signal hyperintensity represents diffusion restriction in this patient with an acute infarction. Angiography confirmed the etiology of this stroke to be vasculitis.

concentration, so it is possible to mistake increased DWI signal in areas of increased water concentration for true diffusion restriction, a concept referred to as "T2 shine-through." It is possible to have a computer calculate the actual coefficient of diffusion for a given water molecule independent of the water concentration, which is graphically depicted as the apparent diffusion coefficient (ADC) map (Figure 7.2B). ADC values reflect the amount of diffusion that takes place, so restricted diffusion will have low ADC values and therefore appear hypointense on the graphical depiction.

DWI was once considered an advanced imaging technique used in very specific circumstances, in particular in suspected stroke (Figure 7.2A). Advances in technology have made this sequence very rapid, typically less than 1 minute, and it should be a part of all pediatric brain imaging protocols.

While CT traditionally has been considered the gold standard for detecting hemorrhage and mineral deposition, there are MR techniques that are very sensitive to the magnetic field alterations caused by areas of hemosiderin and mineral deposition. *Gradient recalled echo* (GRE) images, also referred to as T2-star (T2*), show areas of hemorrhage and mineral deposition as hypointense. *Susceptibility weighted imaging* (SWI) is a newer highly sensitive technique that can detect evidence of hemorrhage and mineral deposition (Figure 7.3).

Intravenous gadolinium chelates can result in a hyperintense T1 signal in areas where gadolinium is delivered. *Gadolinium-enhanced MR* scans are most commonly performed when there is concern for an active infectious/inflammatory process, or when there is

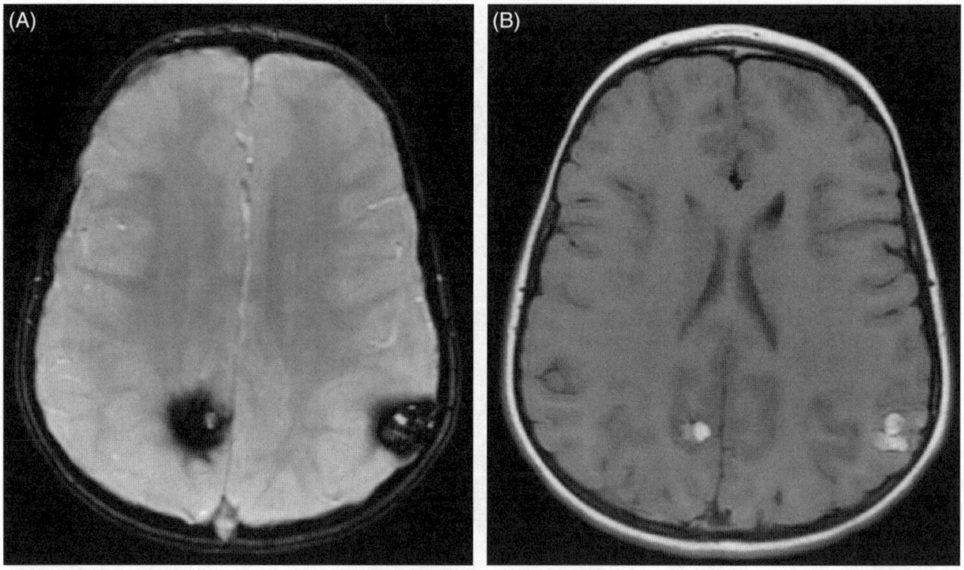

Figure 7.3 Axial susceptibility weighted imaging (SWI) (A) shows two hypointense lesions. Both are heterogeneous but predominantly hypointense with a continuous peripheral hypointense rim consistent with hemosiderin deposition surrounding two cavernomas. Axial T1W image (B) shows areas of T1 hyperintense signal within the lesions, consistent with areas of methemoglobin indicating subacute blood products.

suspicion for a neoplasm. These chelates do not cross an intact blood–brain barrier, so they are effective in finding areas of an active infectious/inflammatory process. Gadolinium-based contrast agents are also helpful in evaluating a neoplasm to look for signs of increased blood supply and loss of blood–brain barrier integrity. Enhancement in adult brain tumors typically indicates a higher grade; however, many low-grade pediatric neoplasms will enhance after gadolinium administration (Figure 7.4).

Advanced MR

Early MR neuroimaging was largely focused on structural evaluation of the brain. More recent advances have improved the ability to provide physiological characterization of the brain and of lesions.

Diffusion tensor imaging (DTI) is a specialized variant of DWI that can detect the freedom of water movement in different directions (Figure 7.5) [4]. If six or more directions are measured, it is possible to calculate whether the movement of water is the same in all directions ("isotropic"), or if it differs ("anisotropic"). The more unidirectional the movement the higher the degree of anisotropy, which is depicted in the fractional anisotropy (FA) maps (Figure 7.5A). These maps can be color-encoded to display the predominant direction of motion. DTI can be post-processed to calculate the likely course of white matter tracts, a technique known as diffusion-tensor fiber tracking, or "tractography" (Figure 7.5B).

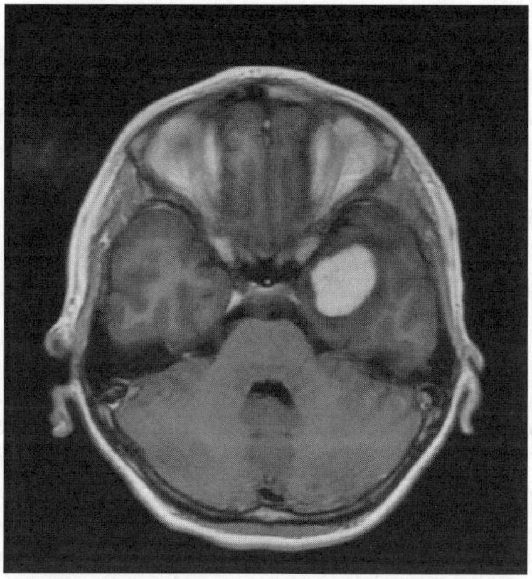

Figure 7.4 Axial T1W image after the intravenous administration of gadolinium shows a circumscribed enhancing mass in the left temporal lobe, centered approximately in the amygdala. This represented a ganglioglioma.

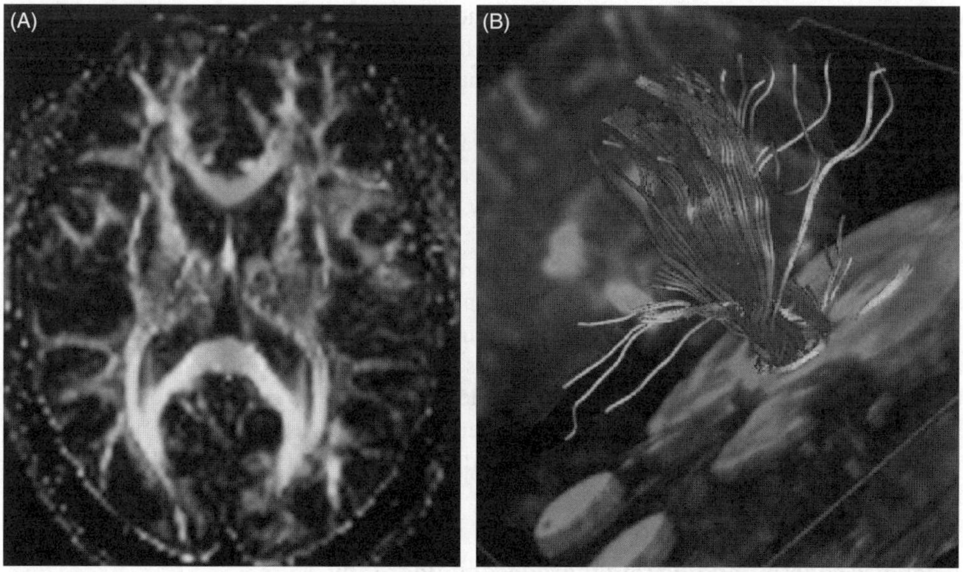

Figure 7.5 Axial directionally encoded fractional anisotropy map (A) from diffusion tensor imaging shows the predominant direction of water diffusion, encoded as red indicating movement in the left-right axis, green in the anterior-posterior axis, and blue in the cranio-caudal axis. The brightness of a given pixel indicates the degree of unidirectionality, or anisotropy, of the fibers in that region. Processed diffusion-tensor fiber tracking ("tractography") shows the fibers of the corticospinal tract (B).

Magnetic resonance spectroscopy (MRS) is a technique that is a clinical application of the chemistry principles of nuclear magnetic resonance spectra. Molecules such as choline, creatine, lactate, and *N*-acetyl-aspartate can be detected and the ratio of these substances can provide insight into disease processes. The main role in the pediatric population is in the evaluation of inborn errors of metabolism, as well as sometimes aiding in tumor characterization.

MR perfusion [4] is set of techniques to qualitatively and/or quantitatively assess the blood supply to different parts of the brain. This has traditionally been used in neurovascular evaluation, in particular in patients with strokes or vascular malformations, and for tumors.

Functional MRI

The greatest advance in physiological MRI has been the recent rapid evolution of functional MRI (fMRI) [4], which has been facilitated by advanced imaging processing techniques, improved MR scanning equipment, and higher field strength scanners. fMRI has been especially useful in localizing language and motor cortex in patients undergoing surgery. When an area of cortex is activated in a given task, there is increased metabolism resulting in increased oxygen extraction and therefore increased quantity of deoxyhemoglobin in the effluent venous blood. If there is intact cerebral autoregulation, there is regional arteriole vasodilation, which increases the total oxygen delivery to a greater extent than the increased oxygen extraction, so there is transiently decreased deoxyhemoglobin content in the effluent venous blood. This allows changes in deoxyhemoglobin concentration to be measured as an indirect marker of neuronal activity. Deoxyhemoglobin results in a greater T2* signal decrease than oxygenated hemoglobin, and therefore areas of neuronal activity that have regionally decreased deoxyhemoglobin will have a transient increase in signal on T2* images. Study paradigms can be set up to map cortex involved in various motor tasks, receptive language, and expressive language.

fMRI is a non-invasive technique that can evaluate the entire brain, which is an advantage over intraoperative cortical mapping. However, fMRI is a "positive activation" technique that only detects cortex involved in an activity, and does not depict cortex that is essential for that function.

Limitations of fMRI include the dependence upon intact cerebral autoregulation to accurately detect indirect evidence of neuronal activation. If cerebral autoregulation is disrupted, such as can occur with hyperemic tumors and vascular malformations, a concept referred to as neurovascular uncoupling occurs and activated cortex will not be detected as there is no significant measurable change in deoxyhemoglobin concentration, resulting in a false-negative result. While research is underway to use fMRI to measure memory, it is not clinically validated and an intracarotid sodium amobarbital test will still be needed in some patients.

Magnetic source imaging/magnetoencephalography

Electric currents moving through a wire generate a magnetic field, and action potentials within neurons are no different. Within a magnetically shielded environment, highly sensitive magnetic detectors coupled to a superconducting quantum interference device (SQUID) create a voltage proportional to the detected magnetic field [5,6]. The magnetic information can be overlayed upon structural brain imaging, typically MRI, to provide a visual depiction of the source of the field. Spontaneous interictal activity can be measured in an attempt to localize epileptogenic cortex (Figure 7.6A). Evoked dipoles can be measured after the patient has been presented with sensory stimuli (Figure 7.6B).

Nuclear medicine

Technetium (^{99m}Tc) exametazime is a radiotracer, also known by its chemical name HMPAO. HMPAO is lipophilic and can cross the intact blood–brain barrier. Neurons take up HMPAO, which is metabolized into a hydrophilic molecule that is trapped within the cell. The amount of HMPAO that is taken up by a given cell is proportional to mitochondrial metabolic activity. After an injection takes place and the tracer can distribute, a single-photon emission computed tomography (SPECT) can be performed by using rotating gamma cameras that detect and localize the source of the photons that are produced during the decay of ^{99m}Tc.

If injected shortly after onset of ictus (ictal study) (Figure 7.6C), there will be increased accumulation of tracer in hypermetabolic neurons. The earlier the injection, the greater the ability to identify the primary area of epileptogenic activity as opposed to areas involved by propagation. When injection is not shortly after a seizure, typically performed more than 24 hours after the most recent seizure activity (interictal study) (Figure 7.6D), epileptogenic areas tend to be hypometabolic due to underlying cellular dysfunction. Although the hypometabolism on interictal scans is more subtle than the hypermetabolism on ictal studies, ictal studies can be difficult to perform given that there must be tracer available to inject within seconds of seizure onset. If a successful ictal and interictal scan can be performed, subtraction imaging can be performed to further highlight the alterations in metabolic activity. This can further aid in distinguishing areas primarily involved from those secondarily involved in seizure propagation.

18F-deoxyglucose (FDG) is a modified glucose molecule that has been tagged with a positron-emitting fluorine isotope. FDG is thus an excellent marker for glucose metabolism, which can be localized within the body using positron emission tomography (PET). FDG-PET data can be superimposed upon CT datasets, which are often acquired simultaneously (PET-CT), and with advanced post-processing can be fused to MRI images. Due to the short half-life (109.8 minutes) of the expensive isotope, ictal injections are not practical. Interictal FDG-PET has a very high spatial resolution to detect hypometabolic areas within the brain, which gives indication of possible underlying dysfunction (Figure 7.6E). FDG-PET delivers a higher radiation dose than HMPAO-SPECT, and therefore the expected diagnostic yield must be weighed against the costs and radiation risks.

Angiography

Cerebral angiography has been less commonly performed in recent decades given the significant advances in non-invasive imaging techniques. However, the high spatial resolution and dynamic information provided about vascular flow makes angiography the gold standard for evaluation of arteriovenous malformations and dural arteriovenous fistulae. These intracranial vascular lesions can often be treated by endovascular techniques as well. Cerebral angiography is also the foundation for the intracarotid sodium amobarbital test, or Wada test, which is a well-established technique to confirm the lateralization of language and memory.

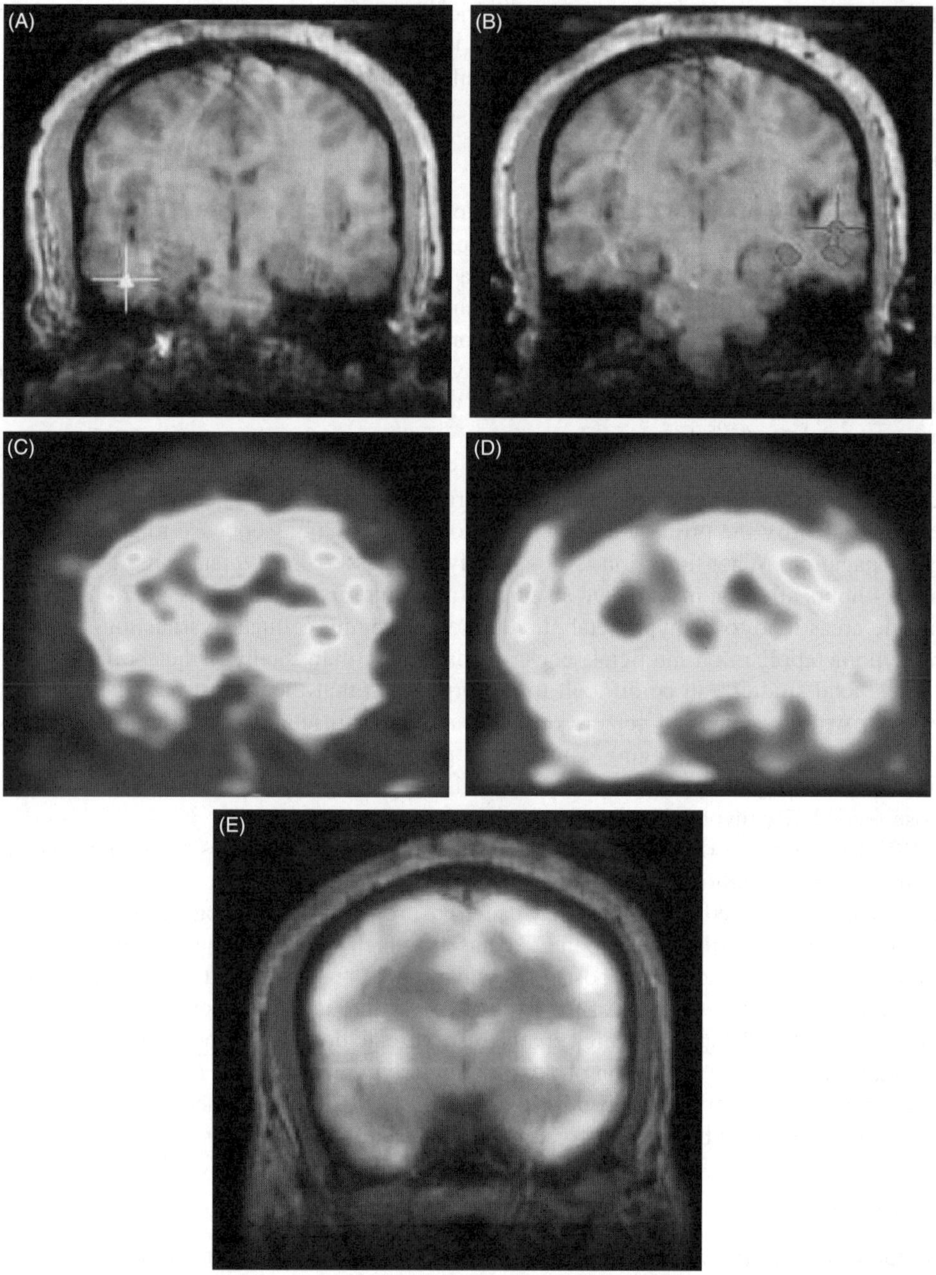

Figure 7.6 Magnetoencephalography (MEG) was fused with a coronal T1W magnetic resonance (MR) image to localize the epileptogenic source to the right temporal lobe (A) in a 17-year-old patient with seizures. MEG fused to a coronal T1W MR image also confirmed left-sided receptive language (B). Single-photon emission computed tomography (SPECT) perfusion imaging shows right temporal hypoperfusion on coronal interictal imaging (C) and increased perfusion on coronal ictal imaging (D). Interictal FDG-PET (18F-deoxyglucose-positron emission tomography) fused to a coronal T1W MR image (E) also confirmed right temporal hypometabolism. Pathology evaluation revealed right-sided hippocampal sclerosis.

Radiographs

Radiographs are primarily used in the evaluation of post-surgical patients, in particular the evaluation of shunt catheters, grid electrodes, and depth electrodes.

7.3 Congenital malformations

There is a vast array of malformations of cortical development, many of which are associated with seizure disorders. Appropriately recognizing the nature of the malformation can aid in determining whether optimal treatment may involve medical therapy, surgical resection, dietary modification, or some combination. As some malformations are sporadic and others have a syndromic or genetic association, proper identification of the type of malformation may allow appropriate triage of families to genetic counseling.

While many specific congenital malformations have extensive literature and even textbooks devoted to them, it is worth providing a survey of common abnormalities as well as some rarer malformations that have characteristic features.

Focal cortical dysplasia (FCD) [7] comprises areas of disorganized dysplastic neurons that typically represent an abnormality of neuronal proliferation. Cortical dysplasias are subdivided into three types. Type I FCDs are very subtle on imaging, and are typically detected as focal cortical thickening and/or blurring of the gray-white differentiation. Imaging sequences that highlight contrast between the gray and white matter are best for detecting FCD type I, in particular T1 weighted and inversion recovery sequences. FCD type II are commonly visible on T2 weighted and FLAIR sequences, with hyperintense signal in the white matter subjacent to the abnormal cortex. Differentiation between FCD and a low-grade glial neoplasm is often difficult on imaging as well as on biopsy. A subtype of FCD type II known as type IIb (also Taylor type FCD, or FCD with balloon cells) has a very characteristic imaging appearance with a conical transmantle T2/FLAIR signal abnormality that tapers as it extends from the cortex toward the superolateral margin of the lateral ventricles, reflecting the migration pathway of neurons from the germinal matrix to the cortex. The characteristic appearance of FCD IIb is radiographically indistinguishable from that of a cortical tuber in tuberous sclerosis (Figure 7.7A). FCD III is a dysplasia associated with another abnormality such as hippocampal sclerosis (IIIa), a tumor (IIIb), a vascular malformation (IIIc), or another structural abnormality (IIId). FCD should not exhibit enhancement after gadolinium administration, and enhancement should shift the differential diagnosis to a neoplastic or infectious/inflammatory process.

Hemimegaloencephaly is an abnormality with hamartomatous overgrowth of an entire cerebral hemisphere (Figure 7.8). The overgrowth can occur without involvement of the entire hemisphere (subhemispheric megaloencephaly), so the presence of normal-appearing parenchyma within a hemisphere does not exclude this class of malformation.

There is a complex collection of midline cleavage defects known as the *holoprosencephaly spectrum*. While textbooks often refer to specific subtypes known as (in decreasing order of severity) alobar, semilobar, and lobar holoprosencephaly, the clinical manifestations are a continuum. Two additional entities exist at the mildest end of the spectrum, syntelencephaly (also known as the middle interhemispheric variant) and septo-optic dysplasia.

Agenesis of the corpus callosum (ACC) is a midline developmental abnormality where the corpus callosum does not develop. As a result, there is a characteristic imaging appearance including colpocephaly, a high-riding third ventricle that communicates with the

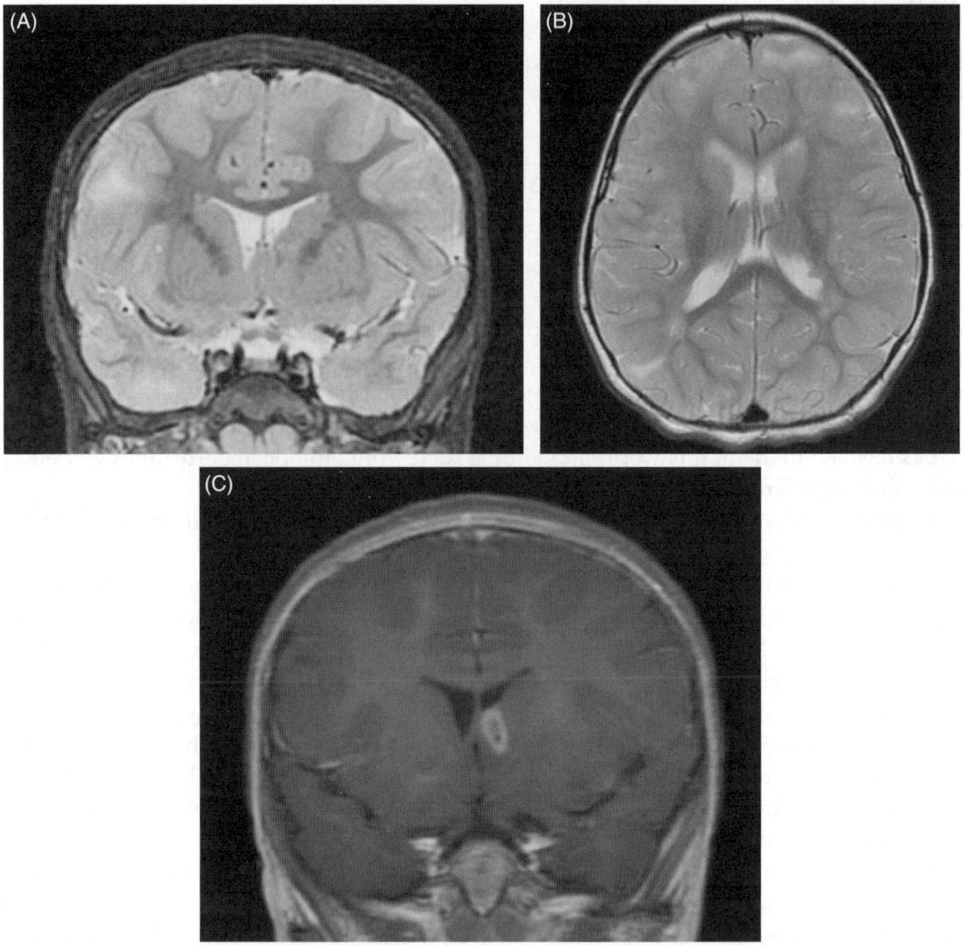

Figure 7.7 Coronal T2W-inversion recovery image (A) shows hyperintense signal in the juxtacortical white matter of a slightly expanded right inferior frontal gyrus, with signal abnormality that tapers as it reaches toward the superolateral margin of the right lateral ventricle; this is identical to the transmantle sign of focal cortical dysplasia (FCD) type IIb. Axial T2W image (B) shows multiple additional subcortical white matter signal abnormalities, representing cortical tubers in the setting of tuberous sclerosis complex. There is also a contour irregularity along the margin of the left lateral ventricle due to a subependymal nodule. Coronal T1W image after gadolinium administration (C) shows an enhancing subependymal lesion in the region of the left foramen of Monro, representing a subependymal giant cell astrocytoma (SEGA).

interhemispheric fissure, parallel lateral ventricles, a low course of the anterior cerebral and pericallosal arteries, and absence of the cingulate sulcus with parasagittal gyri radiating out from the third ventricle (Figure 7.9). ACC can be an isolated finding or be associated with a syndrome, such as Aicardi syndrome. Partial agenesis of the corpus callosum can also be present, typically with less pronounced phenotypes.

Polymicrogyria is not a specific entity or syndrome but a description of a malformation of cortical organization whereby there is absence of a normal sulcation pattern, which is

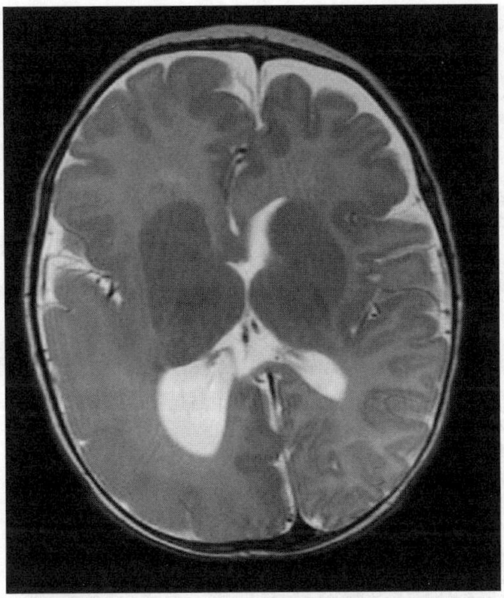

Figure 7.8 Axial T2W image shows asymmetric enlargement of the right cerebral hemisphere, with concomitant enlargement of the atrium of the right lateral ventricle and right temporo-occipital pachygyria. This represents hemimegaloencephaly, or hamartomatous dysplasia of the right cerebral hemisphere.

replaced by areas of multiple small, shallow gyri (Figure 7.10). Symmetric polymicrogyria patterns often have syndromic associations, while any parenchymal injury (such as a Toxoplasmosis, Otherinfections, Rubella, Cytomegalovirus, Herpes simplex virus-2 [TORCH] infection, all parinatal infections) in the second trimester, during cortical organization, can result in polymicrogyria.

Schizencephaly is a cleft in the cerebral hemisphere connecting the subarachnoid space overlying the convexities with the ventricular system (Figure 7.11). The cleft in schizencephaly is lined by gray matter, which differentiates this from a postnatal acquired abnormality such as a prior stroke or a surgical defect. The gray matter lining the cleft may have dysplastic cortex or areas of polymicrogyria. The cleft may have clearly demonstrable cerebrospinal fluid separating the margins ("open-lipped schizencephaly"), or may have direct apposition of the margins with a more subtle imaging appearance ("closed-lip schizencephaly").

An abnormality of neuronal migration during development can result in gray matter deposits that did not reach the intended location (Figure 7.12). Heterotopic gray matter can take many forms, including a periventricular nodular form, which is most common. The heterotopia can be a band of gray matter paralleling the cortex (band-heterotopia), and can also be a focal subcortical deposit.

Hamartomas of the hypothalamus, in particular the tuber cinereum, are non-enhancing lesions seen arising from the lateral walls or floor of the third ventricle (Figure 7.13). Due to the subtle nature of this lesion, there can be a delayed diagnosis despite multiple imaging studies. When patients present with gelastic seizures (ictal laughter), a characteristic clinical manifestation of these lesions, the morphology of the hypothalamus and third ventricle must be scrutinized.

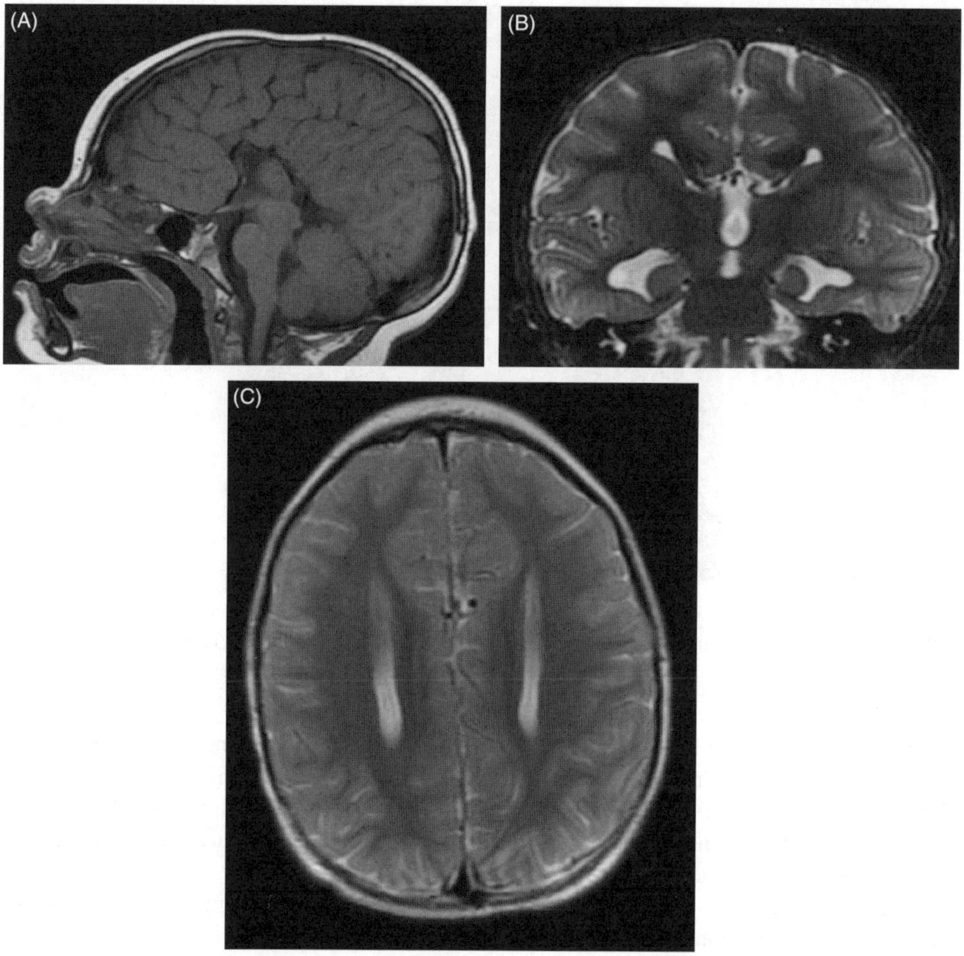

Figure 7.9 Sagittal T1W image (A) shows absence of the corpus callosum and a resultant low-riding anterior cerebral artery. There is also absence of the cingulate gyrus, with the parasagittal gyri radiating from the third ventricle. Coronal short-tau inversion recovery (STIR) image (B) shows continuity of the interhemispheric fissure with the third ventricle. Axial T2W image (C) shows a parallel orientation of the lateral ventricles.

Phakomatoses

There are numerous neurocutaneous syndromes (phakomatoses), each of which has characteristic imaging and clinical features. Familiarity with two phakomatoses in particular is important when dealing with childhood epilepsy – tuberous sclerosis complex and Sturge–Weber syndrome.

Tuberous sclerosis complex (TSC), also known as Bourneville disease, is a neurocutaneous syndrome that gets its name from the cortical "tubers" that are seen at autopsy (see Figure 7.7). These tubers are firm, earning the name tuberous sclerosis. The tubers represent areas of dysplastic cortex, which can serve as the origin of seizures. Previously

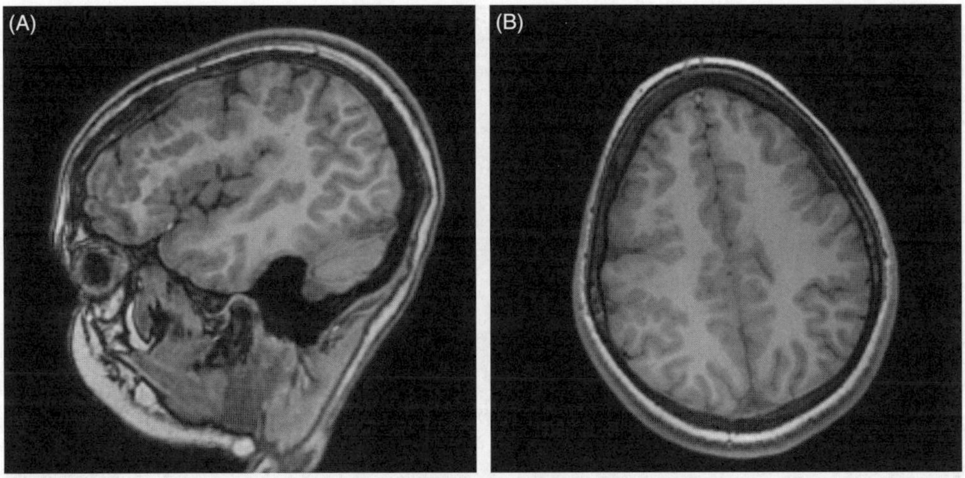

Figure 7.10 T1W images in the sagittal (A) and axial (B) planes show multiple areas of polymicrogyria in the right frontal and parietal lobes. Other images confirm additional areas of polymicrogyria in the left frontal and parietal lobes, as well as both temporal lobes.

patients with TS did not undergo resection of the epileptogenic tubers due to the difficulty in confirming which lesions were the true sources. Modern multimodality multispecialty evaluation has allowed successful localization of epileptogenic tubers with improved seizure control after lesionectomy. The other characteristic imaging feature in children with TS is the development of subependymal nodules along the margins of the lateral ventricles. These

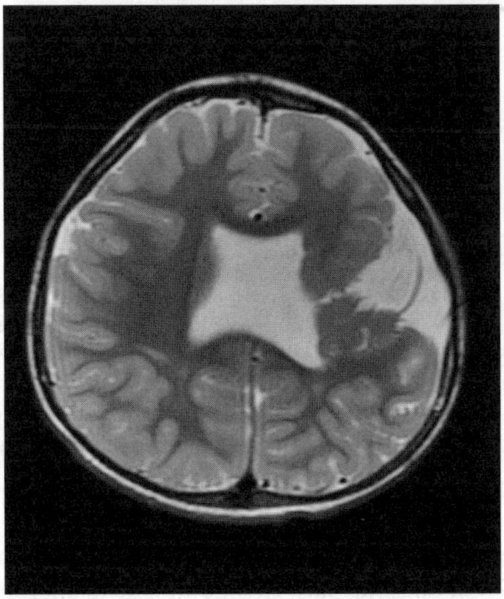

Figure 7.11 Axial T2W image shows continuity of the left lateral ventricle with the cerebrospinal fluid (CSF) space overlying the left frontal lobe, representing schizencephaly. The cleft is in an area of volume loss, and is lined with gray matter. There is also absence of the septum pellucidum.

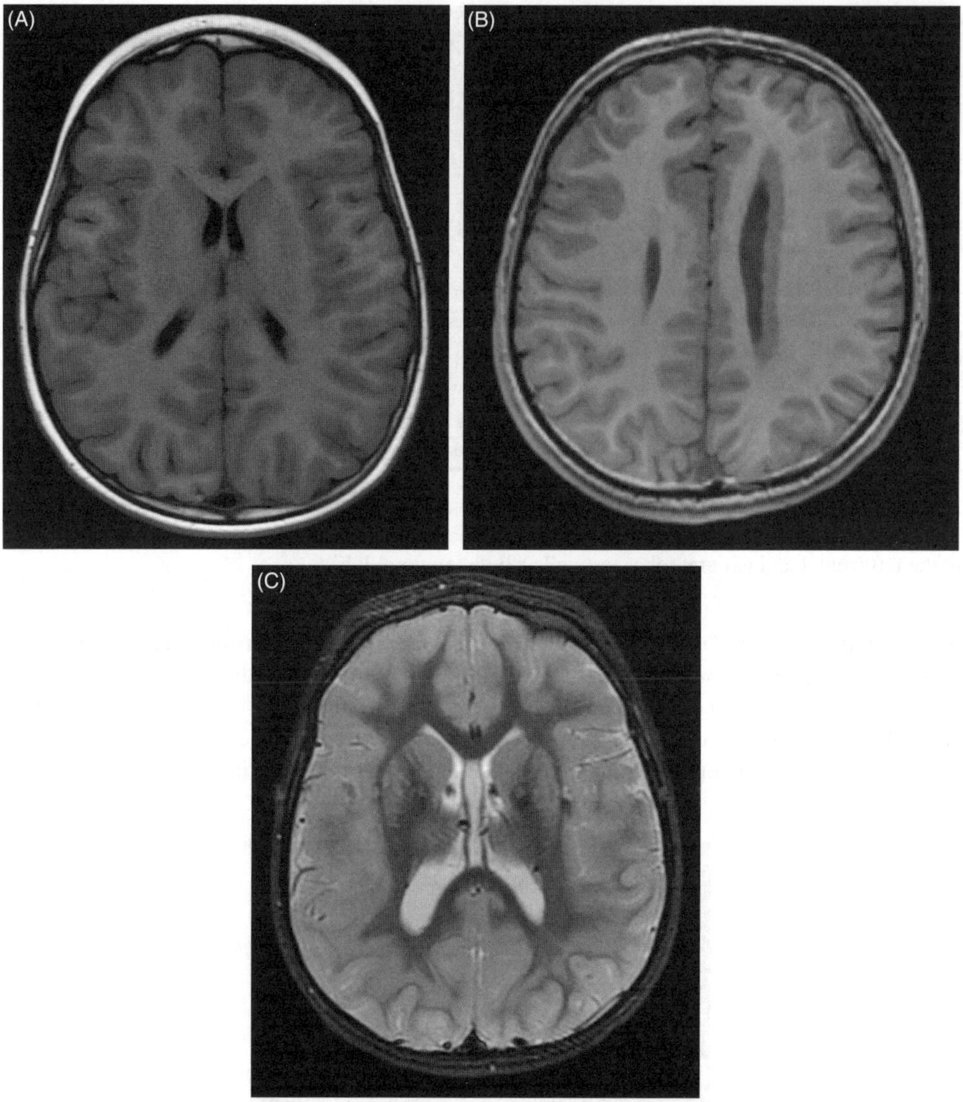

Figure 7.12 Axial T1W image shows a small focus of gray matter along the superolateral margin of the atrium of the left lateral ventricle (A), the most common location for isolated periventricular nodular heterotopia. An axial T1W image in another patient shows more extensive periventricular nodular heterotopia (B). An axial short-tau inversion recovery (STIR) image in a third patient demonstrates a band of gray matter paralleling the cortex but embedded in the white matter of both occipital and parietal lobes (C), representing band-type heterotopia.

nodules, which are often calcified, have the potential to develop into subependymal giant cell astrocytomas (SEGAs), and thus any change in size or morphology of these nodules warrants close follow-up. Subependymal nodules and SEGAs have been shown to stabilize and regress during treatment with inhibitors of the mammalian target of rapamycin (mTOR) pathway.

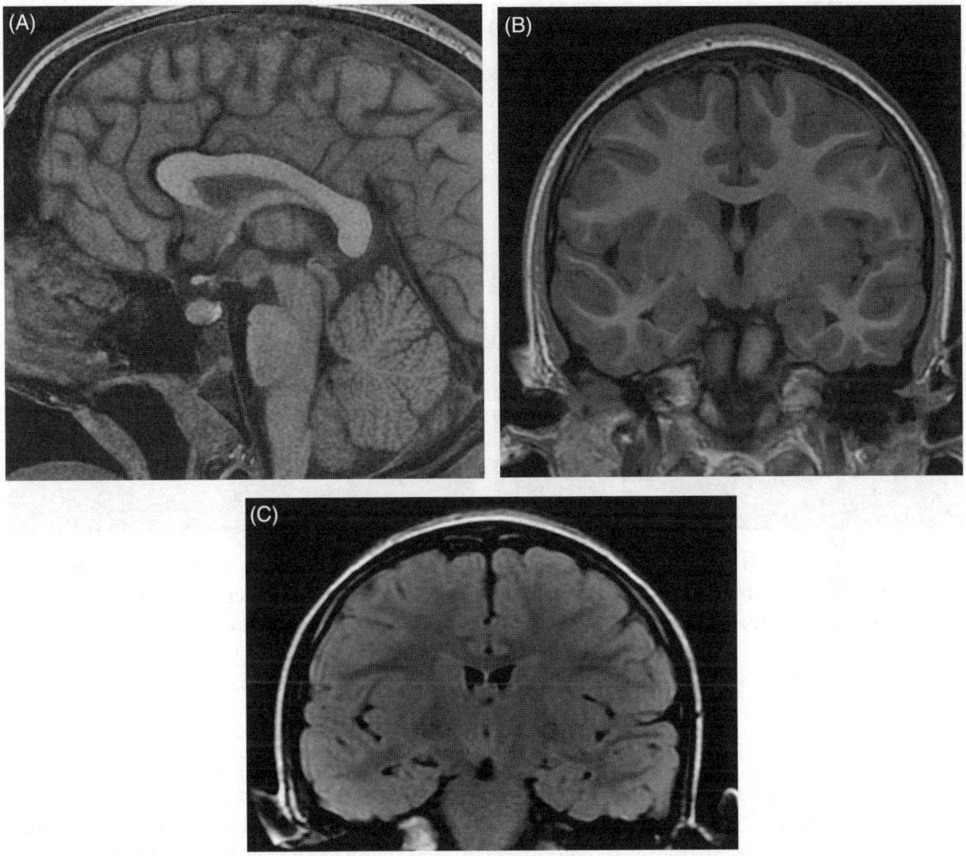

Figure 7.13 Sagittal T1W image (A) shows a soft tissue density within the body of the third ventricle, immediately above the mammillary bodies. A coronal T1W image (B) shows a hypointense appearance to the right hypothalamus, which is slightly expansile and effaces the right lateral aspect of the body of the third ventricle. Coronal fluid attenuated inversion recovery (FLAIR) image (C) shows this lesion has a higher signal intensity than the contralateral hypothalamus. This lesion did not enhance after gadolinium administration (not shown), and at resection was confirmed to be a hypothalamic hamartoma.

Sturge–Weber syndrome, also known as encephalotrigeminal angiomatosis, is a vascular phakomatosis in which there is maldevelopment of the superficial venous drainage system over portions of the brain, typically confined to a cerebral hemisphere (Figure 7.14). Patients have ipsilateral facial port-wine stains that conform to the dermatome of branches of the trigeminal nerve, in particular the maxillary division. The absent superficial drainage system results in rerouting of the venous drainage to the deep system through transmantle veins causing localized venous hypertension. The resulting chronic venous ischemia can lead to cortical mineralization, best depicted on CT or SWI, and volume loss.

Epilepsy related to a congenital disorder does not necessarily have to have an associated malformation. Many metabolic disorders have biochemical abnormalities that directly or indirectly involve the brain. Mitochondrial disorders such as Mitochondrial encephalopathy,

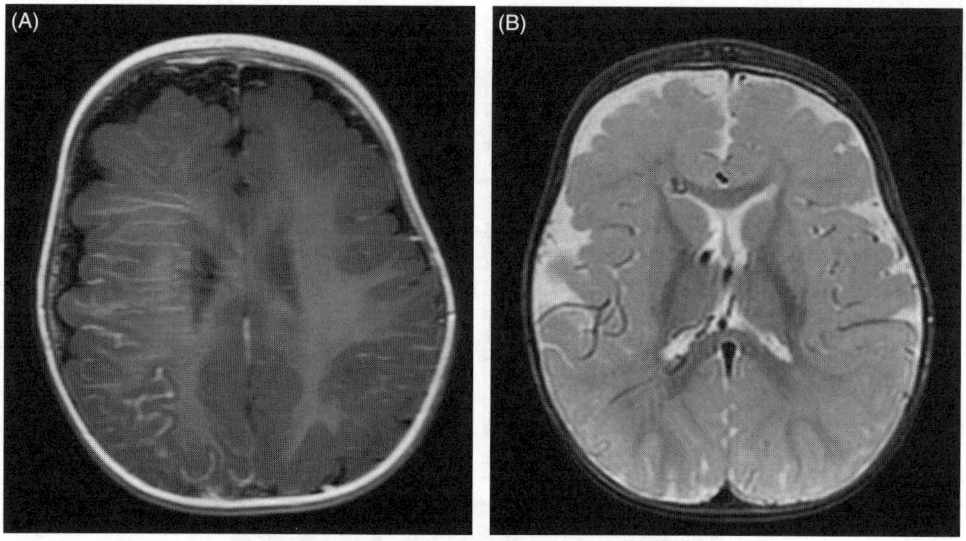

Figure 7.14 Axial T1W post-contrast image (A) in a child with Sturge–Weber syndrome shows transmantle veins draining the cortex of the right frontal lobe into the deep drainage system, and leptomeningeal enhancement overlying the right occipital lobe due to pial venous collaterals. There is also asymmetric prominence of the cerebrospinal fluid (CSF) space over the right cerebral hemisphere. Axial T2W image (B) shows a dilated right internal cerebral vein at the margin of the right lateral ventricle.

lactic acidosis and stroke like episodes (MELAS) will show multiple strokes due to energy deprivation. Organic acidurias and peroxisomal disorders can result in signal abnormalities in the cortex, the white matter, or the deep gray nuclei (such as the caudate, putamen, globus pallidus, and thalamus). If biochemical tests and conventional MR imaging do not yield a diagnosis, MRS may be of benefit.

Arteriovenous malformations are tangles of dysplastic vessels that result in shunting of arterial blood into the venous system. Seizures can occur in these patients for several reasons, including irritation from hemorrhage, ischemia due to steal phenomenon, direct mass effect, and a combination of etiologies.

7.4 Neoplasms

Low-grade glial neoplasms must be considered as a possibility in nearly all cases of seizures associated with a structural lesion, and this entity can be difficult to differentiate from cortical dysplasia on both imaging and histopathology. Although neoplasms that result in seizures are most commonly low grade, more aggressive tumors can result in seizures as well. It is noted that infratentorial tumors very rarely have a direct association with seizures; however, in the setting of metastases or post-treatment effects (such as radiation-induced cavernomas) seizures can occur.

It is worth reiterating that cortical dysplasia and low-grade glial neoplasms can be very difficult to differentiate on histopathology, and thus differentiation on imaging features is often not possible. As low-grade neoplasms will typically have a non-aggressive progression pattern, stability for several years may not be adequate to exclude a neoplasm.

While enhancement after gadolinium is typically a sign of high tumor grade in adult CNS neoplasms, low-grade pediatric neoplasms not uncommonly enhance.

While nearly any tumor has the potential to cause seizures, several specific lesions are important to be aware of, in particular *dysembryoplastic neuroepithelial tumor* (DNET) and *ganglioglioma*. Multiple additional neoplasms can be associated with seizures, including oligodendroglioma and pleomorphic xanthoastrocytoma.

DNET is a low-grade lesion that often occurs in the temporal lobes, commonly has cystic areas, and typically does not enhance after the administration of gadolinium (Figure 7.15). Gangliogliomas are mixed solid and cystic tumors that commonly have enhancing solid

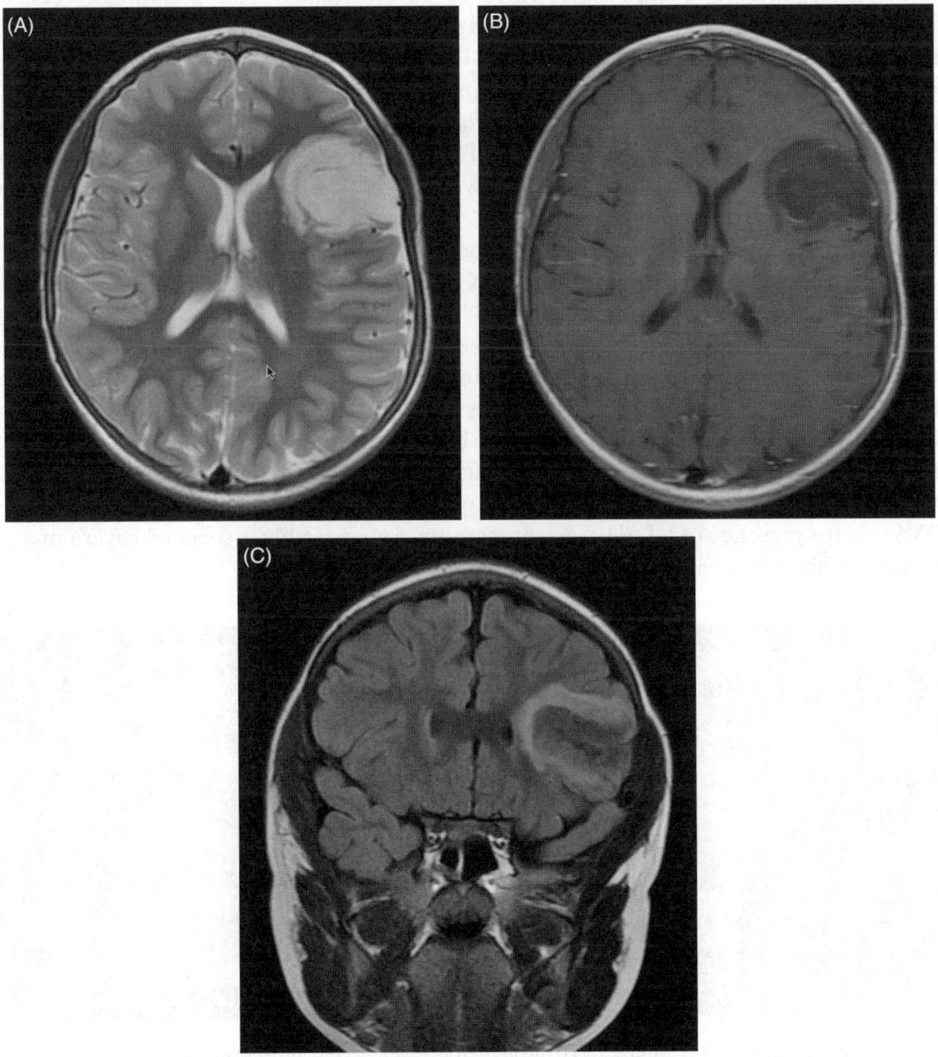

Figure 7.15 Axial T2W image (A) shows a hyperintense mass in the left frontal opercular region. Post-contrast T1W image (B) shows no solid enhancing component. Coronal fluid attenuated inversion recovery (FLAIR) (C) shows there is cortical thickening with a surrounding rim of vasogenic edema. At resection this was confirmed to be a dysembryoplastic neuroepithelial tumor (DNET).

tissue, often occur within the temporal lobes, and may have calcification on CT (see Figure 7.4).

7.5 Acquired/idiopathic abnormalities

Many brain abnormalities associated with seizures are acquired. Parenchymal injury after traumatic, ischemic, infectious, or inflammatory processes may induce epileptogenic activity.

Mesial temporal sclerosis (MTS), also known as hippocampal sclerosis, is a condition in which there is decreased hippocampal volume and abnormally increased signal intensity on T2/FLAIR images (Figure 7.16). In up to 20% of patients the abnormality can be bilateral, making it difficult to diagnose based upon asymmetry in the morphology or signal characteristics. The imaging findings of MTS do not indicate that this is the cause of the patient's seizures, and confirmation is imperative prior to any planned surgery. This can be especially tricky in patients with bilateral asymmetric MTS if the less atrophic hippocampus is the epileptogenic source. MTS typically is thought to be an etiology of seizures in adolescents and young adults; however, it is now known that this can be seen in children younger than 2 years of age.

Post-traumatic contusions can be the source of epilepsy, in particular if there are hemosiderin deposits within the cortex. SWI is very helpful in evaluating the brain in patients with a history of prior trauma.

SWI is also the optimal way to identify *cavernomas* (see Figure 7.3), which are focal areas of dysplastic blood vessels without intervening neuronal tissue. Cavernomas tend to have chronic microscopic hemorrhage. This gives a characteristic appearance of a peripheral continuous rim of hemosiderin, which will be hypointense on all sequences (best seen on SWI), with central mixed-age blood products giving a heterogeneous appearance on all imaging sequences. Cavernomas are often associated with a developmental venous anomaly (DVA), so the presence of a DVA warrants scrutiny for a possible associated cavernoma. A DVA in the absence of a cavernoma is felt to be a normal variant.

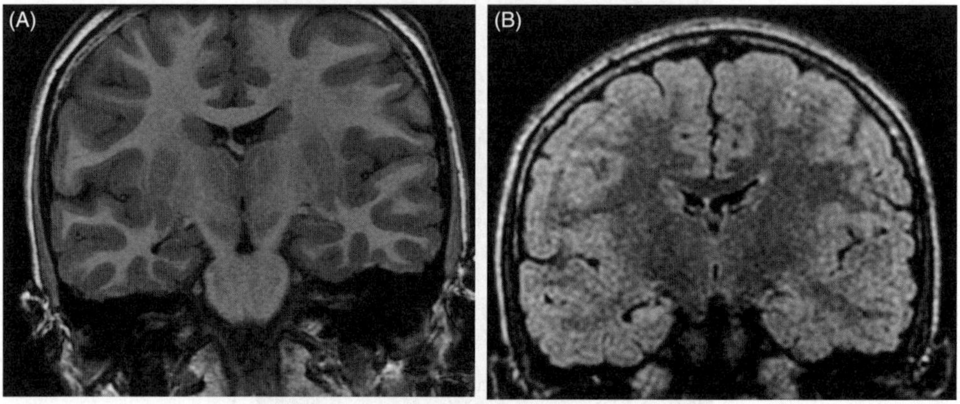

Figure 7.16 Coronal T1W image (A) through the level of the hippocampal formations shows asymmetric decreased gray matter volume in the right hippocampus and a corresponding subtle prominence of the temporal horn of the right lateral ventricle. Coronal fluid attenuated inversion recovery (FLAIR) image (B) shows asymmetrically increased signal in the right hippocampus.

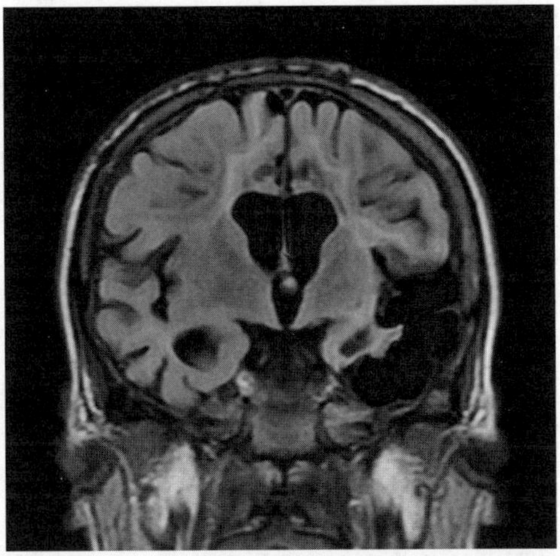

Figure 7.17 Coronal fluid attenuated inversion recovery (FLAIR) image in a child with a history of herpes simplex virus (HSV) encephalitis shows cystic encephalomalacia within the left temporal lobe, with additional areas of gliotic changes in both frontal lobes and volume loss in the right temporal lobe. The diploic space of the left parietal bone is noted to be thicker than that on the right, consistent with a Dyke–Davidoff–Masson phenomenon due to chronic left hemispheric volume loss.

Epileptogenic activity can be induced after *infectious/inflammatory injury* to the parenchyma. Congenital infections can predispose to seizures, in particular HSV encephalitis due to the propensity for hemorrhage (Figure 7.17).

Prior cerebral infarction is not uncommonly associated with seizure activity, in particular if there was a hemorrhagic component to the infarction. *In utero* or perinatal infarctions in the middle cerebral artery (MCA) territory can occur, presumably due to arterial dissection or an embolic event. This results in typical MCA territory encephalomalacia. Due to the loss of parenchymal volume during calvarial development, there will often be thickening of the diploic space in the ipsilateral parietal bone and squamosal portion of the temporal bone, which is known as the Dyke–Davidoff–Masson phenomenon.

Idiopathic inflammatory processes such as Rasmussen's encephalitis can result in hemispheric atrophy and profound seizure activity. Hemispheric asymmetry in the absence of signs of Sturge–Weber syndrome, hemimegaloencephaly, or discrete territorial infarction should raise suspicion for the sequelae of Rasmussen's encephalitis.

References

[1] Strain JD, Kushner DC, Babcock DS, *et al.* Imaging of the pediatric patient with seizures. American College of Radiology. ACR Appropriateness Criteria. *Radiology* 2000;**215**(Suppl.):787–800.

[2] Hirtz D, Ashwal S, Berg A, *et al.* Practice parameter: Evaluating a first nonfebrile seizure in children Report of the Quality Standards Subcommittee of the American Academy of Neurology, the Child Neurology Society, and the American Epilepsy Society. *Neurology* 2000;**55**:616–623.

[3] Goske MJ, Applegate KE, Boylan J, *et al.* The "Image Gently" campaign: increasing CT radiation dose awareness through a national education and awareness program. *Pediatr Radiol* 2008;**38**:265–269.

[4] Pillai JJ, Zaca D, Choudhri A. Clinical impact of integrated physiologic brain tumor imaging. *Technol Cancer Res Treat* 2010;**9**:359–380.
[5] Wheless JW, Castillo E, Maggio V, *et al.* Magnetoencephalography (MEG) and magnetic source imaging (MSI). *Neurologist* 2004;**10**:138–153.
[6] Schwartz ES, Edgar JC, Gaetz WC, Roberts TPL. Magnetoencephalography. *Pediatr Radiol* 2010;**40**:50–58.
[7] Blümcke I, Thom M, Aronica E, *et al.* The clinicopathologic spectrum of focal cortical dysplasias: a consensus classification proposed by an ad hoc Task Force of the ILAE Diagnostic Methods Commission. *Epilepsia* 2011;**52**:158–174.

8 Non-epileptic paroxysmal events of childhood

Sucheta M. Joshi

Pediatrics and Communicable Diseases, Division of Pediatric Neurology, University of Michigan, Ann Arbor, MI, USA

8.1 Introduction

A paroxysmal event is a set of clinical symptoms and signs that occur suddenly, either spontaneously or provoked, with changes in motor function, behavior, and/or consciousness. Seizures themselves manifest as episodic and sudden events, but they are not the only condition that occurs in a paroxysmal manner. Several other non-epileptic conditions can also have an episodic and paroxysmal presentation. The prospect of a paroxysmal event being a seizure is very concerning to parents and physicians alike, which usually prompts medical evaluation.

The prevalence of epilepsy in children is estimated to be around 1% [1]. The incidence of paroxysmal non-epileptic events (PNEs) is difficult to determine accurately, as there are few studies looking at their incidence. Kotagal *et al.* studied PNEs in a tertiary care epilepsy monitoring unit, and observed that they occurred in about 15% of their cohort [2]. Similar rates have been reported by others [3]. The range of PNEs reported varies, however, probably because the term "PNE" is broad and includes events of varied semiology and etiology, as well as varying with the population studied. In the National Child Development

Epilepsy in Children and Adolescents, First Edition. Edited by James W. Wheless.

Study in the United Kingdom (published in 1980), it was estimated that 6.7% of children had experienced at least one episode with loss of consciousness in the first decade of life [4]. Other studies have estimated the incidence of PNEs in the pediatric population to be 25% in the first 2 years of life [5].

Non-epileptic paroxysmal events occur across age groups in the pediatric population, including neonates. In children, PNEs occur as a result of several physiological or pathological processes, that may or may not primarily involve the central nervous system. Cardiac disease, respiratory processes, and behavioral spells can all present as PNEs. Some neurological conditions that are not epilepsy have an episodic presentation, and mimic seizures.

PNEs pose a particular diagnostic challenge in the pediatric population. Unlike adults, children are not always able to provide an accurate history, and the clinician must rely on a description from witnesses. Caregivers who often find the event frightening to witness, may not be the most accurate in their description. Differentiating epileptic from non-epileptic events can be difficult even for clinicians experienced in diagnosing seizures. Misdiagnosis of PNEs in children as epilepsy has been reported to be as high as 39% [6]. However, it is important that these non-epileptic paroxysmal events be accurately identified and differentiated from seizures. Accurate identification of PNEs will avoid unnecessary treatment of these events with antiepileptic drugs, which carry their own share of side effects and morbidity, including systemic and cognitive side effects. Misdiagnosis of PNEs as epileptic seizures can have consequences for lifestyle, such as unnecessary restriction of activities. Specific treatment for PNEs can also be instituted once an accurate diagnosis is established. Some PNEs such as cardiac arrhythmias mimicking seizures can be life threatening, further underscoring the need for accurate diagnosis.

Evaluation of paroxysmal events begins with a history, preferably from someone who has witnessed an event. Details regarding the event should be recorded including a description of the semiology of the event, time of the day when the event occurs, association with feeding, posture, awake or asleep states. While there isn't a sign or symptom that is characteristic for differentiating PNEs from epileptic seizures, certain simple observations of subtle clinical signs can be useful in steering the clinician toward the possibility of PNEs. In the paragraphs below, some of the PNEs occurring commonly in the pediatric population are discussed.

8.2 Breath-holding spells

Breath-holding spells (BHS) are common paroxysmal events that occur in early childhood, typically with onset in toddlerhood, usually between 12 and 18 months of age. Presentation at younger ages has been described [7]. There are reports of breath-holding spells occurring in neonates [8]. These typically occur in an otherwise neurologically normal child. Based on their semiology, the presence or absence of cyanosis, they are described as cyanotic or acyanotic (or pallid) breath-holding spells [9].

The more common, accounting for over 50% of cases, are cyanotic breath-holding spells. In the common scenario, breath-holding spells are provoked by crying. When the child is emotionally upset or fearful or angry, she/he starts crying relentlessly. The crying may or may not escalate, but after a variable period of crying, the child becomes quiet, accompanied by a pause in respiration. It is often perceived that the respiratory pause occurs during inspiration, and observers describe the child taking a deep breath and then not breathing. However, the pause occurs in the expiratory phase of the respiratory cycle. With milder cyanotic episodes, the spell ends at this point. DiMario describes these as simple breath-holding spell [7]. If the breath-holding spell progresses further, there is evolution to cyanosis, and often loss of consciousness as well as loss of tone. The child may become limp, but tonic stiffening can also occur. There may be associated myoclonic or clonic jerks. Usually the breath-holding spell ends with a deep inspiratory breath, and consciousness is regained. Following the episode the child is usually back to her/his pre-event baseline, but a period of fatigue after the spell can also occur.

A second, less commonly described breath-holding spell is the pallid breath-holding spell. Often this is provoked by seemingly minor trauma, such as a gentle bump to the head. This is followed by pallor and sudden loss of consciousness, often with loss of tone. Compared to a cyanotic breath-holding spell, the pathophysiology of a pallid breath-holding spell is different and thought to be secondary to a vagal reflex response to the minor trauma, similar to vasovagal syncope.

A breath-holding spell is a clinical diagnosis; EEGs are not needed for diagnosing, but are sometimes done, especially if the semiology of the event is unclear. The interictal EEG is normal. If a breath-holding spell is captured on EEG, initially there is slowing of the EEG background. As the child becomes bradycardiac, further slowing and suppression of the EEG background becomes apparent, at times with subsequent/concomitant asystole. As the child regains consciousness, there is rapid return of the EEG background to normal [9].

More commonly iron studies are recommended, which may show presence of iron deficiency anemia or iron deficiency in up to 56% of patients [10].

Breath-holding spells are benign paroxysmal events that tend to resolve over time. Parental education about their benign nature, and reassurance are key in managing breath-holding spells. Iron supplementation is often recommended as treatment, as iron supplementation has been shown to improve breath-holding spells [10]. Iron supplementation is most likely to be helpful in the presence of iron deficiency anemia, as suggested by several studies [11,12]. The mechanism of action of iron probably goes beyond simple correction of iron deficiency anemia. A low iron concentration has been implicated in serotonin metabolism, related to aldehyde oxidase, a serotonin-degrading enzyme, which shows reduced activity in iron deficiency. Piracetam has also been used for treating breath-holding spells [13]. In more severe cases, atropine has been used [14]. Severe breath-holding spells may require placement of a cardiac pacemaker [14,15].

In children with severe breath-holding spells, even those who have a convulsive component, treatment with antiepileptic drugs (AEDs) is not necessary. AEDs have their own share of undesirable side effects, and while AEDs may reduce the occurrence of the convulsive component of a breath-holding spell, they do not impact the frequency of breath-holding spells themselves. There may be a small subset of children with severe breath-holding spells, in whom the use of AEDs is considered; however, this determination must be made on a case-by-case basis, after careful consideration of various factors and extensive discussion with parents.

Breath-holding spells tend to improve over the course of time, and often resolve by 5–7 years of age.

8.3 Parasomnias

Parasomnias refer to unwanted, involuntary motor or sensory autonomic phenomena that occur in sleep. These can pose a particular diagnostic challenge to the clinician, and the dramatic symptoms that accompany them can be distressing to caregivers. Given the circumstances when these occur, an accurate description may be even more difficult to obtain, adding to the diagnostic dilemma. Some PNEs in sleep often have prominent motor activity that is dramatic and bizarre enough to arouse the suspicion of seizures such as frontal lobe seizures. An accurate diagnosis is important to avoid such misdiagnosis. Furthermore, parasomnias can be disruptive to the sleep of the child as well as for caregivers.

Parasomnias can occur in both non-rapid eye movement (NREM) and REM sleep. They can be primary or secondary (arising due to other conditions). This discussion will be limited to the primary parasomnias.

Parasomnias can be classified, based on their association with the sleep state that they occur in. The International Classification of Sleep Disorders classifies parasomnias into four categories: disorders of arousal, sleep-wake transition disorders, parasomnias associated with REM sleep, and other parasomnias [16]. The parasomnias that are commonly seen in children are: night terrors, periodic leg movements/restless legs syndrome (PLS/RLS), nightmares, sleep-walking, and sleep-talking.

Night terrors

Night terrors, also known as *pavor nocturnus*, occur in NREM sleep. It has been suggested that night terrors are better termed "sleep terrors," to differentiate them from nightmares [17]. These are most common in young children, with age of onset around 2–3 years. They commonly occur a few hours after the child falls asleep. The typical semiology is a sudden arousal from sleep, followed by inconsolable crying and screaming. There can be accompanying autonomic changes, including tachycardia, tachypnea, diaphoresis, and pupillary dilatation. Typically the child's eyes are open, but the child is seemingly unresponsive. The duration of the event is variable, commonly lasting for a few minutes, but prolonged spells have also been described. The event subsides on its own, and the child falls back asleep. Usually there is no recollection of the event the next morning. The frequency of night terrors is variable, and multiple events in one sleep period have been observed.

The etiology of night terrors is not known. They are not associated with emotional or psychological disturbances. They are a disorder of arousal, probably related to a child's maturational stage. Parasomnias usually resolve gradually over time, and do not require treatment other than parental reassurance. Low-dose benzodiazepines have been used to treat night terrors, but typically pharmacological treatment is not indicated.

Nightmares

Nightmares, or anxiety dreams as described by Sheldon [17], are parasomnias that occur out of REM sleep. The child suddenly arouses from REM sleep and is fully awake with recall of the contents of the dream. The theme of the dream can be scary, and there may be some minor autonomic symptoms accompanying the dream and arousal. Usually the child can be comforted, but takes time to return to sleep. Nightmares occur occasionally in almost all children, and the themes of the dreams as well as the child's recall and description are usually in keeping with her/his developmental stage. Usually no treatment is required.

Restless leg syndrome (RLS) and periodic limb movement disorder (PLMD)

These parasomnias are well described in adults with specific diagnostic criteria [18]. However, these parasomnias are only recently being recognized in children, as the awareness of this condition has increased. In the pediatric population, symptoms of RLS include an urge to move the legs, accompanied by dysasthesias, usually worse at night [19,20]. The symptoms are relieved by movement. On the other hand excessive periodic limb movements during sleep, with disturbed sleep, characterize PLMD. Objectively, more than five limb movements per hour (recorded during polysomnography) are needed to diagnose PLMD. Treatment with dopamine agonists has been used with relief of symptoms. Iron studies are also commonly done in children presenting with these symptoms, as low ferritin levels are often found in children with RLS/PLMD symptoms. Treatment with supplemental iron often alleviates symptoms [20].

Sleep-related rhythmic movement disorders

This is a distinct parasomnia characterized by stereotyped rhythmic movements during sleep. Some of the commonly observed symptoms include head banging or body rocking, and may be accompanied by humming or other vocalizations. Their stereotyped, repetitive nature arouses suspicion for seizures. Video telemetry as well as polysomnography is useful in differentiating these sleep-related movements as PNEs rather than epileptic seizures. Often having the parents videotape the event in question can also be helpful in diagnosis. These are benign conditions that occur in infancy and usually subside by the age of 5 years. Pharmacological treatment is usually not indicated, although treatment with benzodiazepines has been described for particularly severe symptoms [19]. Protective measures to prevent injury, such as padding the bed or installing guard rails for the bed, may also be considered in specific situations.

Benign sleep myoclonus of infancy

This PNE occurs in an otherwise normal infant, and is often seen in the first month of life [21]. The semiology consists of brief, repetitive synchronous or asynchronous jerks involving one or more extremities while the infant is asleep [22]. The jerks can sometimes be quite dramatic, and mistaken for multifocal clonic or myoclonic seizures. The association with sleep, and a normal neurodevelopmental assessment, should reassure about the benign nature of these movements, but not infrequently video telemetry with EEG monitoring is needed to make the diagnosis. EEG studies show a normal EEG, without electrographic seizures during the infant's symptoms. It has been postulated that an immature serotonergic system in the very young infant underlies these benign movements [23].

No treatment is required. These movements usually resolve on their own within a few months.

8.4 Benign paroxysmal positional vertigo of childhood

Benign paroxysmal positional vertigo in childhood (BPVC) is a disorder of peripheral vestibular dysfunction that can be mistaken for seizures. More commonly benign paroxysmal positional vertigo (BPPV) occurs in adults, but cases in children have been reported. BPVC can occur across age groups, occurring commonly in young children [24]. Typically children present with sudden onset of dizziness, loss of balance, and change in gait due to the dizziness. At times this can be accompanied by more systemic symptoms such as diaphoresis, nausea and vomiting, and pallor. The symptoms can be quite distressing to the child, and involve some behavioral manifestations such as crying or fearfulness. In young children articulation of symptoms can be difficult. Usually the spells are self-limited, and resolve spontaneously. The frequency can be quite variable. The episodic, sudden onset of the spells and the seemingly dramatic presentation usually brings up the question of seizures. However, with a thorough history, EEG studies are not mandated. BPVC has been reported in children as young as 4 years, and tend to improve or resolve by mid-childhood. There are several reports in the literature suggesting that BPVC is a precursor to or a variant of migraine [25,26,27]. It has been classified in the International Headache Classification under "migraines" (section 1.3.3) [28].

8.5 Syncope

Syncope is an episode of transient loss of consciousness, often associated with loss of tone, due to cerebral hypoperfusion, characterized by quick onset, short duration, and quick and complete recovery [29]. This paroxysmal event is common in children, particularly older children and adolescents. The most common pathophysiological mechanism underlying syncope is hypotension, which leads to transient cerebral hypoperfusion with resultant loss of consciousness. Often there is a prodrome of symptoms such as lightheadedness, altered vision, and diaphoresis, followed by rapid loss of consciousness and atonia. There may be associated tonic stiffening of extremities, and a brief period of convulsive jerking. All of this adds to the confusion of the diagnosis of a syncopal episode as a seizure.

Evaluation should include an electrocardiogram to measure the corrected QT interval, as long QT syndrome is associated with sudden cardiac death. When appropriate evaluation by a cardiologist should be considered. Electroencephalograms are normal, and are usually done when there is a convulsive element to the syncope.

Pharmacological treatment includes beta-adrenergic receptor blockers, fludrocortisone, and also specific serotonin reuptake inhibitors and midodrine. Ideally, therapy should be individualized based on clinical presentation [30].

8.6 Paroxymal non-epileptic events (PNEs) with a psychiatric or behavioral basis

PNEs with a psychiatric or behavioral basis have been described for centuries. Marsden provides an eloquent review of the history of functional disorders, and their relevance to neurology [31]. A variety of terms are used to describe paroxysmal events with a psychiatric or psychogenic basis: pseudoseizures, psychogenic seizures, hysterical spells, non-epileptic events or non-epileptic spells, and functional spells. Patel *et al.* suggested the use of the term non-epileptic seizures (NES), to convey a more neutral and unbiased tone [32], as the term "pseudo" often implies that a patient is putting on or faking clinical symptoms. These events are described more extensively and in greater detail in adults [33], but are known to occur in children and adolescents as well. The prevalence of NES in adults is estimated to be between 1/3000 and 1/50 000 [34]. Studies reporting the incidence of NES in pediatrics are limited. The etiology of NES in children and adolescents is likely to be different than in adults [32,35]. In the pediatric population, NES tend to occur in individuals with epilepsy, which can make the diagnosis that much more challenging. Up to 25% of children with epilepsy have been reported as having NES [35]. Another factor that influences the occurrence of NES is the presence of developmental, especially cognitive, delay.

NES should be considered as a possibility when a child is being treated for epilepsy, but does not respond to appropriately selected and adequately dosed antiepileptic medications, if clinical events are provoked by specific situations, and if repeated EEGs are normal. Symptoms of NES are also variable, and vary by age and gender. Patel and co-workers observed that in children under the age of 13, NES occurred equally in males and females, while in the older pediatric population (ages 13 and older), there was a female preponderance [32]. In the study by Kutluay *et al.*, gender differences were observed, with NES occurring more frequently in girls older than 12 years [35].

In younger children, NES tend to manifest as more subtle motor symptoms, and staring spells are the most common parent-reported sign. Other motor symptoms such as hand flapping and body rocking, are also described. In older children and in adolescents, motor manifestations are more prominent and more dramatic. Large-amplitude motor movements, non-rhythmic shaking, and left-to-right head-shaking movements are all common symptoms of NES. It can be somewhat difficult to distinguish NES from epileptic seizures, but there are features that can help in the distinction. There is no pathognomonic sign that differentiates epileptic from non-epileptic seizures. NES tend to occur during wakefulness. They can be of variable duration, some lasting seconds, some lasting for several minutes. If observed carefully, movements during a NES are not as stereotyped as in an epileptic seizure. They often occur when the patient is being observed, and seldom occur when the patient is alone. In certain individuals, they may be "provoked" by gentle suggestion during history-taking and physical examination.

Eye closure is a reliable sign that an event is non-epileptic in nature. In a study by Chung *et al.*, 50 out of 52 patients with NES had eyes closed during the event, while 152 out of 156 patients with epileptic seizures had their eyes open during the event [36]. Similar observations have been made in children. Korff and co-investigators observed, in a retrospective study [37], that persistent eye closure in infants presenting with paroxysmal events made it less likely that the events in question represented seizures.

It is thought that bladder incontinence and injuries are characteristic features of epileptic seizures. But this is not true solely for epilepsy, and these features are therefore not reliable in differentiating epilepsy from a non-epileptic event. Patterns of oral trauma may suggest that an event is a NES. DeToledo and colleagues reported that oral trauma involving the tip of the tongue or the lip was more likely to be from NES [38].

Risk factors for NES in children are similar to those in adults; psychosocial stressors are common risk factors in children, and particularly in adolescents with NES. The nature of the stressors can vary, however, from stressors in the house (parental divorce, abuse, etc.) to stressors outside the home (school, friends, etc.) [32,39].

In most children, NES occur as a manifestation of conversion disorder. In a cohort of 38 children with NES studied at the Cleveland Clinic Foundation, all were given a diagnosis of conversion disorder. However, in addition one-third of these children were given an additional diagnosis of a major mood disorder. In this group the incidence of abuse, particularly sexual abuse, was also notably high [40].

Diagnosing psychogenic NES involves a good history, with detailed description of the index event. When feasible, having parents videotape the event in question can be invaluable. Video EEG telemetry is also useful to assess the semiology of the event in question and to evaluate the EEG during an event.

Once a diagnosis of a NES is made, it is important to convey the diagnosis to the patient and family in a sensitive way, as often the diagnosis can be upsetting, especially if the patient and the family perceive that the physician is implying the events to be "fake" [41]. Psychological evaluation, and when appropriate psychiatric evaluation, should be considered.

Treatment of NES may include withdrawal of AEDs, counseling (individual or family), and pharmacological treatment of any underlying psychiatric disorder. Cognitive behavior therapy and group therapy focused on interpersonal issues have been described as useful tools in the management of NES in adolescents and adults [42,43], but data in the pediatric population are lacking.

The outcome of NES is also difficult to assess, and studies are lacking in children. Short duration of symptoms, no or mild psychiatric history, identifiable psychological trauma (or stressor), and absence of concomitant epilepsy are favorable factors for remission of NES [44].

8.7 Hyperekplexia

This is a rare disorder, with autosomal dominant inheritance. It occurs in neonates and young infants. The typical form is called hyperekplexia major [45]. The phenotype consists of a triad of clinical symptoms, which include stiffness in the newborn period, an exaggerated startle, and startle-induced stiffness. The stiffness observed in neonates with hyperekplexia underlies the term "stiff baby syndrome" used to describe this disorder. Paroxysmal onset of stiffness can be provoked by gentle stimulation such as tapping on the bridge of the nose, which induces a characteristic retraction of the head. In some of the pedigrees that have been studied, a defect in the gene encoding the alpha 1 subunit of the glycine receptor, *GLRA1*, on chromosome 5q33-35, has been identified. Another gene less commonly associated with this condition is the *GLYT2* gene [46] . Benzodiazepines such as clonazepam are usually effective in treating the symptoms of hyperekplexia. It is important to recognize the non-epileptic nature of this paroxysmal condition, as in severe cases sudden infant death has been described, presumably from the stiffness and complications such as aspiration pneumonia [47].

8.8 Alternating hemiplegia of childhood

Another rare condition, alternating hemiplegia of childhood (AHC), was first described by Verrett and Steele in 1971 [48]. As the name suggests, AHC is characterized by paroxysmal episodes of hemiplegia, involving alternating sides of the body. Other symptoms including episodes of dystonia, eye movement abnormalities such as nystagmus, or intermittent exotropia/esotropia have also been reported [49]. Onset of symptoms occurs in infancy or toddlerhood, usually before 18 months of age. Infants as young as 3 months can present with oculomotor symptoms. In the case series reported by Sweney and colleagues [49], episodes of hemiplegia occurred in 56% of a cohort of 103 subjects by 6 months of age. Other neurological symptoms include ataxia, and cognitive impairment has also been described as a common comorbidity. The duration of the hemiplegia is variable, lasting from hours to days. The symptoms abate during sleep, but may recur upon waking. Magnetic resonance imaging (MRI) scans done while symptoms are occurring are normal. Electroencephalograms recorded during a paroxysm of hemiplegia may show non-specific changes such as slowing of the background. Attacks can be provoked by triggers such as temperature extremes, stress or physical activity, foods, light sensitivity, or exposure to water.

The etiology of AHC is unclear. The episodic nature of the symptoms suggests a channelopathy, and there are reports suggesting AHC to be related to mutations in the ATP1A2 and the CACNA1A genes [50,51]. Several medications have been used for treatment of AHC. The most commonly used is flunarazine, a calcium channel blocker, which has been used to reduce the frequency and severity of attacks [52]. The use of other drugs such as beta-blockers, anticonvulsants, methysergide, amantadine, aripiprazole, and haloperidol has been described [52–54].

Outcome in AHC is often poor, with associated intellectual disability and deterioration after multiple severe attacks.

8.9 Movement disorders

Tics

Hyperkinetic movement disorders are common in childhood, occurring in about 5% of school-age children [55,56]. Motor tics are a common movement disorder presenting in childhood, usually in the early school-age years. Typically motor tics manifest as sudden-onset involuntary paroxysmal movements of short duration, occurring in a repetitive fashion. Some of the common semiologies of tics include eye blinking, facial grimacing, shrugging of shoulders, or extremity movements. They can be sudden and explosive in onset, but individual tics are short-lived, lasting of the order of seconds. They tend to be repetitive, occurring as clusters, and several times per day. They completely abate in sleep, and are often worse during periods of intercurrent illness, or physical or emotional stress. Associated comorbidities include attention-deficit/hyperactivity disorder and/or obsessive-compulsive disorder [57].

Diagnosis of motor tics is clinical. Electroencephalograms are normal, as are neuroimaging studies. If the nature of the movements is not clear based on clinical history, a video recording made by parents can be very helpful in diagnosis. Treatment of tics includes pharmacological treatment of motor symptoms if they are particularly severe or distressing to the child, and management of associated comorbidities. Behavior therapy for tics, such as cognitive behavior therapy and habit reversal therapy, can also be useful in some cases [58–60].

The long-term outcomes of tics are variable. In a study where subjects self-reported their tics, 26% reported almost complete disappearance of tics in young adulthood, 46% reported substantial reduction, and only 14% reported an increase in tics over time [61].

Paroxysmal dyskinesias

This refers to a group of movement disorders clinically characterized by sudden onset of involuntary movements that are brief and self-limited, and not accompanied by loss of consciousness. The movements may be dystonic, choreiform, or athetoid in nature. The neurological examination between episodes is completely normal. Paroxysmal dyskinesias can be primary or secondary. This review will be limited to the primary dyskinesias.

The paroxysmal dyskinesias can be classified as paroxysmal kinesigenic dyskinesias (PKD), and paroxysmal non-kinesigenic dyskinesias (PNKD), as suggested by Demirkiran and Jankovic [62].

In PKD, the dyskinesia is induced by a sudden movement, or sudden stimulation such as a loud sound. The movement itself is of short duration lasting several seconds. The average age at onset is around 11 years, but presentation at much younger ages has been described. Several patients achieve remission in their 20s [63]. The frequency is variable but several attacks per day are not uncommon. Over 50% of patients with PKD have a positive family history, suggesting autosomal dominant inheritance [64]. Diagnosis is clinical, based on typical history and a normal neurological examination. The locus of PKD has been mapped to chromosome 16p11.2-q12.1 [65]. PKD responds to anticonvulsants such as carbamazepine and phenytoin. Oxcarbazepine has also been used with good results [66–68].

In PNKD, the symptoms last longer, and as the name suggests are not induced by movement. They may be provoked by alcohol, emotion, or caffeine. Primary PNKD has its onset in childhood at around 8 years of age [69]. This disorder is inherited in an autosomal dominant mode [70]. The disease is associated with missense mutations in the *MR-1* gene [71–73]. Treatment with benzodiazepines may be useful in some cases. Other drugs that have been used include gabapentin, acetazolamide, and L-dopa. Avoiding triggers is also recommended.

8.10 Sandifer syndrome

This condition was first described in the 1960s [74]. It is a clinical syndrome consisting of dystonic posturing of the trunk and/or extremities or torticollis in association with gastroesophageal reflux. The age of presentation can vary, ranging from infancy to childhood. Adult cases have also been reported in the literature [75]. A history of gastroesophageal reflux may or may not be obvious. Typically the child presents with paroxysmal episodes of dystonic, or even opisthotonic posturing of the head, neck, and/or trunk. The range of symptoms can vary and can resemble infantile spasms in the semiology. This condition can be associated with hiatal hernia [76], but often occurs without it. It is thought that the dystonic posturing provides relief from the discomfort of the gastroesophageal reflux [74]. Gastroesophageal reflux occurs commonly in young children. The presentation of an infant with episodic tonic arm extension or arm, leg, and trunk flexion usually raises concern for infantile spasms. The diagnosis of infantile spasms needs to be made urgently, so that appropriate treatment can be instituted promptly. EEG studies in Sandifer syndrome are normal. Video EEG studies can be especially useful to view the semiology of the events and to exclude a diagnosis of infantile spasms. Specific gastroenterology testing such as a Ph-probe study, or endoscopy can further help confirm the diagnosis of gastroesophageal reflux.

Since this condition mimics a potentially devastating epilepsy in infancy and early childhood, prompt diagnostic evaluation is necessary. Further, identification of gastroesophageal reflux helps to institute specific and effective treatment.

8.11 Conclusion

Paroxysmal, episodic events are common in childhood and adolescence. They have a varied differential diagnosis ranging from physiological conditions to psychiatrically based phenomena. Video telemetry has made the diagnosis of these non-epileptic conditions much easier. Also, when feasible, having parents videotape the events in question can be a useful tool in diagnostic assessment. It is important to accurately identify the non-epileptic phenomena, not only to exclude a diagnosis of epilepsy and save the patient unnecessary treatment with antiepileptic drugs, but also to steer a patient toward appropriate treatments for the condition.

References

[1] Russ SA, Larson K, Halfon N. A National profile of childhood epilepsy and seizure disorder. *Pediatrics* 2012;**129**:256–264.
[2] Kotagal P, Costa M, Wyllie E, *et al*. Paroxysmal nonepileptic events in children and adolescents *Pediatrics* 2002;**110**:e46.
[3] Montenegro MA, Sproule D, Mandel A, *et al*. The frequency of non-epileptic spells in children: results of video-EEG monitoring in a tertiary care center. *Seizure* 2008;**17**:583–587.
[4] Ross EM, Peckham CS, West PB, *et al*. Epilepsy in childhood: findings from the National Child Development Study. *Br Med J* 1980;**280**:207–210.
[5] Hamiwka LD, Singh N, Niosi J, Wirrell EC. Diagnostic inaccuracy in children referred with "first seizure": role for a first seizure clinic. *Epilepsia* 2007;**48**:1062–1066.
[6] Uldall P, Alving J, Hansen LK, *et al*. The misdiagnosis of epilepsy in children admitted to a tertiary epilepsy centre with paroxysmal events. *Arch Dis Child* 2006;**91**:219–221.
[7] DiMario FJ Jr. Prospective study of children with cyanotic and pallid breath-holding spells. *Pediatrics* 2001;**107**:265–269.
[8] Breukels MA, Plötz FB, van Nieuwenhuizen O, *et al*. Breath holding spells in a 3-day-old neonate: an unusual early presentation in a family with a history of breath holding spells. *Neuropediatrics* 2002;**33**:41–42.
[9] Lombroso CT, Lerman P. Breathholding spells (cyanotic and pallid infantile syncope). *Pediatrics* 1967;**39**:563–581.
[10] Handan U, Sükrü C, Gülhis D, *et al*. Serum soluble transferrin receptor is a valuable diagnostic tool in iron deficiency of breath-holding spells. *Pediatr Hematol Oncol* 2005;**22**:711–716.
[11] Mocan H, Yildiran A, Orhan F, Erduran E. Breath holding spells in 91 children and response to treatment with iron. *Arch Dis Child* 1999;**81**:261–262.
[12] Colina KF, Abelson HT. Resolution of breath-holding spells with treatment of concomitant anemia. *J Pediatr* 1995;**126**:395–397.
[13] Azam M, Bhatti N, Shahab N. Piracetam in severe breath holding spells. *Int J Psychiatry Med* 2008;**38**:195–201.
[14] Legge LM, Kantoch MJ, Seshia SS, *et al*. A pacemaker for asystole in breath-holding spells. *Paediatr Child Health* 2002;**7**:251–254.
[15] Di Pino A, Calabrò MP, Gitto P, *et al*. Permanent cardiac pacing for severe pallid breath-holding spells. *Pacing Clin Electrophysiol* 2007;**30**:280–282.
[16] American Academy of Sleep Medicine. *International Classification of Sleep Disorders, Diagnostic and Coding Manual*, 2nd edn. Westchester, IL: American Academy of Sleep Medicine, 2005.
[17] Sheldon SH. Parasomnias in childhood. *Pediatr Clin N Am* 2004;**51**:69–88.
[18] Walters AS, The International Restless Legs Syndrome Study Group. Towards a better definition of the restless legs syndrome. *Mov Disord* 1995;**10**:634–642.
[19] Hoban TF, Chervin RD. Pediatric sleep-related breathing disorders and restless legs syndrome: how children are different. *Neurologist* 2005;**11**:325–337.
[20] Hoban TF. Sleep disorders in Children. *Ann N Y Acad Sci* 2010;**1184**:1–14.
[21] Cohen R, Shuper A, Straussberg R. Familial benign neonatal sleep myoclonus. *Pediatr Neurol* 2007;**36**:334–337.
[22] Maurer VO, Rizzi M, Bianchetti MG, Ramelli GP. Benign neonatal sleep myoclonus: a review of the literature. *Pediatrics* 2010;**125**:e919–924.
[23] Resnick TJ, Moshé SL, Perotta L. Benign neonatal sleep myoclonus. Relationship to sleep states. *Arch Neurol* 1986;**43**:266–268.
[24] Batson G. Benign paroxysmal vertigo of childhood: A review of the literature. *Paediatr Child Health* 2004;**9**:31–34.
[25] Goebel JA (ed). *Practical Management of the Dizzy Patient*. Philadelphia: Lippincott Williams & Wilkins, 2008.

[26] Fenichel GM. Migraine as a cause of benign paroxysmal vertigo of childhood. *J Pediatr* 1967;**71**:114–115.

[27] Parker C. Complicated migraine syndromes and migraine variants. *Pediatr Ann* 1997;**26**:417–421.

[28] Subcommittee of the International Headache Society. The International Classification of Headache Disorders, second edition. *Cephalalgia* 2004;**24**:9–160.

[29] Moya A, Sutton R, Ammirati F, *et al.* Guidelines for the diagnosis and management of syncope (version 2009). *Eur Heart J* 2009;**30**:2631–2671.

[30] Massin M. Neurocardiogenic syncope in children: current concepts in diagnosis and management. *Paediatr Drugs* 2003;**5**:327–334.

[31] Marsden CD. Hysteria – a neurologist's view. *Psychol Med* 1986;**16**:277–288.

[32] Patel H, Scott E, Dunn D, Garg B. Nonepileptic seizures in children. *Epilepsia* 2007;**48**:2086–2092.

[33] Ettinger AB, Devinsky O, Weisbrot DM, *et al.* A comprehensive profile of clinical, psychiatric, and psychosocial characteristics of patients with psychogenic nonepileptic seizures. *Epilepsia* 1999;**40**:1292–1298.

[34] Benbadis SR, Allen Hauser W. An estimate of the prevalence of psychogenic non-epileptic seizures. *Seizure* 2000;**9**:280–281.

[35] Kutluay E, Selwa L, Minecan D, *et al.* Nonepileptic paroxysmal events in a pediatric population. *Epilepsy Behav* 2010;**17**:272–275.

[36] Chung SS, Gerber P, Kirlin KA. Ictal eye closure is a reliable indicator for psychogenic nonepileptic seizures. *Neurology* 2006;**66**:1730–1731.

[37] Korff CM, Nordli DR Jr. Paroxysmal events in infants: persistent eye closure makes seizures unlikely. *Pediatrics* 2005;**116**:e485–486.

[38] DeToledo JC, Ramsay RE. Patterns of involvement of facial muscles during epileptic and nonepileptic events: review of 654 events. *Neurology* 1996;**47**:621–625.

[39] Bhatia MS, Sapra S. Pseudoseizures in children: A profile of 50 cases. *Clin Pediatr (Phila)* 2005;**44**:617–621.

[40] Wyllie E, Glazer JP, Benbadis S, Kotagal P, *et al.* Psychiatric features of children and adolescents with pseudoseizures. *Arch Pediatr Adolesc Med* 1999;**153**:244–248.

[41] Duncan R. Psychogenic nonepileptic seizures: diagnosis and initial management. *Expert Rev Neurother* 2010;**10**:1803–1809.

[42] LaFrance WC Jr, Miller IW, Ryan CE, *et al.* Cognitive behavioral therapy for psychogenic nonepileptic seizures. *Epilepsy Behav* 2009;**14**:591–596.

[43] Barry JJ, Wittenberg D, Bullock KD, *et al.* Group therapy for patients with psychogenic nonepileptic seizures: a pilot study. *Epilepsy Behav* 2008;**13**:624–629.

[44] Bodde NM, Brooks JL, Baker GA, *et al.* Psychogenic non-epileptic seizures – definition, etiology, treatment and prognostic issues: a critical review. *Seizure* 2009;**18**:543–553.

[45] Bakker MJ, van Dijk JG, van den Maagdenberg AM, *et al.* Startle syndromes. *Lancet Neurol* 2006;**5**:513–524.

[46] Rees MI, Harvey K, Pearce BR. Mutations in the gene encoding GlyT2 (SLC6A5) define a presynaptic component of human startle disease. *Nat Genet* 2006;**38**:801–806.

[47] Nigro MA, Lim HC. Hyperekplexia and sudden neonatal death. *Pediatr Neurol* 1992;**8**:221–225.

[48] Verrett S, Steele JC. Alternating hemiplegia in childhood: a report of eight patients with complicated migraine beginning in infancy. *Pediatrics* 1971;**47**:675–680.

[49] Sweney MT, Silver K, Gerard-Blanluet M, *et al.* Alternating hemiplegia of childhood: early characteristics and evolution of a neurodevelopmental syndrome. *Pediatrics* 2009;**123**:e534–541.

[50] Swoboda KJ, Kanavakis E, Xaidara A, *et al.* Alternating hemiplegia of childhood or familial hemiplegic migraine? A novel ATP1A2 mutation. *Ann Neurol* 2004;**55**:884–887.

[51] de Vries B, Stam AH, Beker F, *et al.* CACNA1A mutation linking hemiplegic migraine and alternating hemiplegia of childhood. *Cephalalgia* 2008;**28**:887–891.

[52] Tenney JR, Schapiro MB. Child neurology: alternating hemiplegia of childhood. *Neurology* 2010;**74**:e57–59.
[53] Haffejee S, Santosh PJ. Treatment of alternating hemiplegia of childhood with aripiprazole. *Dev Med Child Neurol* 2009;**51**:74–77.
[54] Aishworiya R, Low PS, Tay SK. Alternating hemiplegia of childhood: successful treatment with topiramate and flunarizine, a case report. *Ann Trop Paediatr* 2011;**31**:149–152.
[55] Dooley JM. Tic disorders in childhood. *Semin Pediatr Neurol* 2006;**13**:231–242.
[56] Scahill L, Tanner C, Dure L. The epidemiology of tics and Tourette syndrome in children and adolescents. *Adv Neurol* 2001;**85**:261–271.
[57] Mol Debes NM, Hjalgrim H, Skov L. Validation of the presence of comorbidities in a Danish clinical cohort of children with Tourette syndrome. *Child Neurol* 2008;**23**:1017–1027.
[58] Piacentini J, Woods DW, Scahill L, *et al.* Behavior therapy for children with Tourette disorder: a randomized controlled trial. *JAMA* 2010;**303**:1929–1937.
[59] Himle MB, Woods DW, Piacentini JC, *et al.* Brief review of habit reversal training for Tourette syndrome. *J Child Neurol* 2006;**21**:719–725.
[60] Singer HS. Treatment of tics and tourette syndrome. *Curr Treat Options Neurol* 2010;**12**:539–561.
[61] Erenberg G, Cruse RP, Rothner AD. The natural history of Tourette syndrome: a follow-up study. *Annala Neurol* 1987;**22**:383–385.
[62] Demirkiran M, Jankovic J. Paroxysmal dyskinesias: clinical features and classification. *Ann Neurol* 1995;**38**:571–579.
[63] Bruno MK, Hallett M, Gwinn-Hardy K, *et al.* Clinical evaluation of idiopathic paroxysmal kinesigenic dyskinesia: new diagnostic criteria. *Neurology* 2004;**28**:2280–2287.
[64] Nagamitsu S, Matsuishi T, Hashimoto K, *et al.* Multicenter study of paroxysmal dyskinesias in Japan – clinical and pedigree analysis. *Mov Disord* 1999;**14**:658–663.
[65] Tomita H, Nagamitsu S, Wakui K, *et al.* Paroxysmal kinesigenic choreoathetosis locus maps to chromosome 16p11.2–q12.1. *Am J Hum Genet* 1999;**165**:1688–1697.
[66] Chillag KL, Deroos ST. Oxcarbazepine use in paroxysmal kinesigenic dyskinesia: report on four patients. *Pediatr Neurol* 2009;**40**:295–297.
[67] Tsao CY. Effective treatment with oxcarbazepine in paroxysmal kinesigenic choreoathetosis. *J Child Neurol* 2004;**19**:300–301.
[68] Gökçay A, Gökçay F. Oxcarbazepine therapy in paroxysmal kinesigenic choreoathetosis. *Acta Neurol Scand* 2000;**101**:344–345.
[69] Bhatia KP. Paroxysmal dyskinesias. *Mov Disord* 2011;**6**:157–165.
[70] Zorzi G, Conti C, Erba A, *et al.* Paroxysmal dyskinesias in childhood. *Pediatr Neurol* 2003;**28**:168–172.
[71] Rainier S, Thomas D, Tokarz D, *et al.* Myofibrillogenesis regulator 1 gene mutations cause paroxysmal dystonic choreoathetosis. *Arch Neurol* 2004;**61**:1025–1029.
[72] Hempelmann A, Kumar S, Muralitharan S, *et al.* Myofibrillogenesis regulator 1 gene (MR-1) mutation in an Omani family with paroxysmal nonkinesigenic dyskinesia. *Neurosci Lett* 2006;**402**:118–120.
[73] Stefanova E, Djarmati A, Momcilović D, *et al.* Clinical characteristics of paroxysmal nonkinesigenic dyskinesia in Serbian family with myofibrillogenesis regulator 1 gene mutation. *Mov Disord* 2006;**21**:2010–2015.
[74] Lehwald N, Krausch M, Franke C, Assmann B, Adam R, Knoefel WT. Sandifer syndrome – a multidisciplinary diagnostic and therapeutic challenge. *Eur J Pediatr Surg* 2007;**17**:203–206.
[75] Somjit S, Lee Y, Berkovic SF, *et al.* Sandifer syndrome misdiagnosed as refactory partial seizures in an adult. *Epileptic Disord* 2004;**6**:49–50.
[76] Senocak ME, Arda IS, Büyükpamukçu N. Torticollis with hiatus hernia in children. Sandifer syndrome. *Turk J Pediatr* 1993;**35**:209–213.

Section 3
Principles of treatment

James W. Wheless

9 Pharmacology of antiepileptic drugs

James W. Wheless

Department of Pediatric Neurology, University of Tennessee Health Science Center; Le Bonheur Comprehensive Epilepsy Program and Neuroscience Institute, Le Bonheur Children's Hospital, Memphis, TN, USA

Pharmacokinetics is the study of the movement of drugs through the body, whereas pharmacodynamics is the discipline examining the relationship between a drug's concentration and its physiological effect (e.g., pharmacokinetics is how the body affects the drug, pharmacodynamics is how the drug affects the body) [1,2]. Pharmacokinetics is a discipline that describes the absorption, distribution, metabolism, and excretion of a given substance. A basic understanding of its principles can contribute to better patient care by improving anticonvulsant dosing and monitoring, and in some cases ameliorate dose-dependent adverse effects. Clinicians can greatly benefit from recognizing variables that alter the pharmacokinetics of given anticonvulsants. It is well established that age, certain disease states, food, and concurrent medications (including other anticonvulsants) affect the pharmacokinetics of anticonvulsants. This chapter will review basic anticonvulsant pharmacokinetics with emphasis on clinical aspects. It will also provide an overview of pharmacogenomics and its potential application to care of epilepsy patients.

Epilepsy in Children and Adolescents, First Edition. Edited by James W. Wheless.

9.1 Pharmacokinetics

Absorption

Absorption describes the entrance of an anticonvulsant into the intravascular space, typically from the gastrointestinal tract, skin, or muscle. Both the rate and extent of absorption are important. The rate of absorption is described by the absorption rate constant (k_a, units 1/unit time) or the time to maximal plasma concentration (T_{max}). For intravenously (i.v.) administered anticonvulsants the absorptive phase is minimal, the T_{max} is most rapid and coincides with the end of bolus. Typically the rate of absorption, from slowest to fastest, is: intramuscular, rectal, sustained-release capsules/tablets, subcutaneous, immediate release oral capsules/tablets, and solutions. For most of the currently available anticonvulsants the k_a is a first-order process meaning that a constant percentage of drug is absorbed per unit of time. Gabapentin is the exception, in that its intestinal absorption is saturable (k_a becomes zero order above doses >1200 mg) making the k_a dependent on dose. Regardless of the route of administration, the more rapid the absorption (shorter T_{max}), the higher the peak concentration (C_{max}). It seems that both the rate at which concentrations increase and the actual peak in the concentration affect the probability of acute central nervous system side effects. Extended-release dosage formulations attempt to blunt these acute side effects by slowing the rate of drug absorption, by lowering the C_{max} below the minimally toxic concentration (MTC) (Figure 9.1). Optimally, these dosage forms maintain plasma concentrations above the minimally effective concentration (MEC) for 12–24 hours so that once-daily dosing may be possible. It is hoped that by manipulating the pharmacokinetics through these dosage forms toxicity will be reduced and adherence will be maximized.

Two terms that are commonly mistaken are bioavailability (F) and bioequivalence. Absolute bioavailability refers to the proportion of an active drug that reaches the systemic circulation (and to the site of action) following non-parenteral administration. The values of F range from 0 to 1 with $F = 0.0$ when no drug is absorbed to $F = 1.0$ when all a drug dose is absorbed. Since all of a parenterally administered drug reaches the systemic circulation, i.v. administered drugs by definition have an F of 1.0. When medications are administered by extravascular routes, the absolute bioavailability generally decreases. This can be because of incomplete dissolution-absorption of a dosage form or because of extensive first-pass hepatic metabolism following oral administration. Relative bioavailability is the term describing the relative proportion of the same drug when given in two different products (tablet a and tablet b) or formulations (liquid, tablet, capsule) that reaches the systemic circulation. An understanding of bioavailability can be important when converting a patient from differing dosage forms (e.g., i.v. dosage to tablet and vice versa) or products (e.g., from brand to a generic). Non-equivalent conversion of a dose and interval can lead to changes in efficacy or toxicity.

Other medications (prokinetics – e.g., metoclopramide; cation-containing antacids; sequestrants – e.g., cholestyramine) and food can affect the bioavailability of some anticonvulsants. For example, the bioavailability of gabapentin and phenytoin is decreased by concurrent administration of antacids and gastric-tube feedings, respectively. Carbamazepine and phenytoin have poor oral absorption, especially in the first 2 years of life, limiting their use in this age group. Clinically these factors are important; if absorption is decreased this increases the risk of subtherapeutic plasma concentrations resulting in an increased likelihood of seizures. For most anticonvulsants food does not affect their bioavailability, although it may delay absorption (e.g., increased T_{max}).

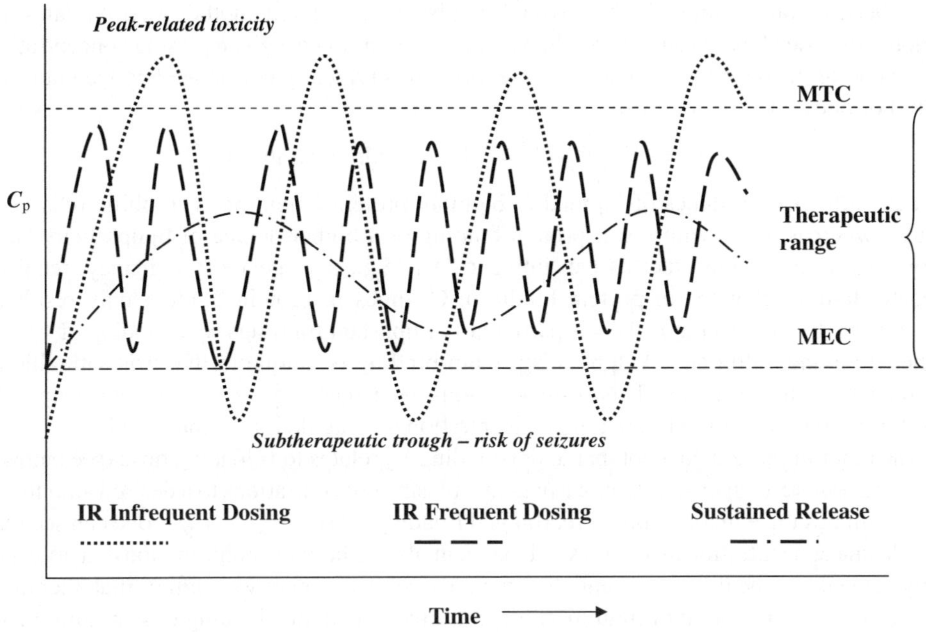

Figure 9.1 Immediate-release versus sustained-release pharmacokinetic profiles. In the figure, three different dosage forms of the same medication are shown. The immediate-release (IR) dosage form results in large variations in peak-trough concentrations. Concentrations above the minimum toxic concentration (MTC) can result in peak-related side effects (nausea, vomiting, dizziness), whereas concentrations below the minimum effective concentration (MEC) may result in subtherapeutic anticonvulsant concentration and seizures. In clinical practice we try to maintain drugs within the therapeutic range (below the MTC and above the MEC) to maximize the potential benefits of the anticonvulsant. To minimize the larger variations that occur with anticonvulsants with short half-lives, two approaches may be used. The first is to give the IR dosage form more frequently (lower C_{max}, higher C_{min}). The second is to give a sustained-release dosage form that releases drug slowly such that the peak trough fluctuations are small. This also has the advantage of less frequent dosing, which may improve patient adherence. C_p, plasma concentration.

Bioequivalence is an important consideration in epilepsy, particularly since many of the currently available anticonvulsants have a narrow therapeutic index. Bioequivalence can be thought of as the interchangeability of two dosage forms (immediate vs sustained release) or products (e.g., brand vs generic). Therapeutic equivalence is another term associated with the use of generics. In order to be therapeutically equivalent two products/forms must be expected to exert the same clinical effect when given to the same treatment population. This definition includes two products or dosage forms being bioequivalent.

Distribution

Distribution describes the extent to which a drug transfers into various parts of the body. The extent of a drug's distribution is determined by its lipid-water solubility and affinity for plasma proteins (e.g., albumin or α_1-acid glycoprotein) or tissues. The term volume of distribution (V_d) is used to characterize or quantify these properties. V_d is refers to a hypothetical volume into which a given drug distributes. Stated another way, it relates the amount of dose (D) of drug that would be required to produce a given plasma concentration at the end of the dose (C_{p0}). When V_d is reported it is typically normalized by weight (e.g., L/kg) or body surface area (L/m^2).

$$V_d = FD/C_{p0} (F = 1 \text{ for i.v. administration})$$

Drugs with smaller values of V_d tend to be more protein bound or hydrophilic (charged) drugs, whereas drugs with lower protein binding or a higher degree of lipophilicity have larger V_d values. Many factors can influence V_d (e.g., age, gender, pregnancy, renal or hepatic failure, changes in protein binding). Changes in protein binding may result in changes in drug distribution. This is particularly important for drugs with binding of $\geq$90% (phenytoin and valproate). Valproate's protein binding is unique in that it is saturable at therapeutic concentrations. This results in non-linear increases in free (active) valproate concentrations compared to the total concentration as drug doses are increased.

The other important concept that understanding V_d relates to is loading dose (see below). Loading doses are given to increase a patient's plasma concentrations to a desired amount. If one examines the equation above (rearranged Loading Dose = $V_d \times C_{p0}$), one can see that the plasma concentration of a drug is independent of metabolism or elimination of a drug and only depends on the dose given and the drug's V_d. Stated another way, things that alter drug clearance (e.g., induction or inhibition) do not affect a patient's loading dose requirement.

Metabolism

The liver is the organ responsible for the majority of metabolism. Hepatic metabolic pathways are typically divided into phase I and phase II reactions, with the outcome of making the drug more polar and therefore more readily excreted. During phase I reactions, drugs undergo oxidation, reduction, or hydrolysis to a more polar or hydrophilic product. These reactions are non-synthetic and either unmask or add a functional group, so that the resultant product can be active. Major enzymes involved in phase I biotransformation of anticonvulsants include: the cytochrome P450 system (CYP450), alcohol and aldehyde dehydrogenases, epoxide hydroxylase, and non-specific amidases and esterases (Table 9.1). Phase II reactions are synthetic and result in the conjugation of a drug or drug product to either glucuronic acid (via UDP-glucuronosyltransferases, UGTs), sulfonates (via sulfonotransferases), acetylation (via *N*-acetyltransferase), or an amino acid (via glutathione *S*-transferase, amino acid *N*-acyltransferases). In contrast, to phase I reactions the end product is always inactive. Orally administered drugs are first circulated to the liver where they may undergo biotransformation before reaching the site of action (i.e., *first-pass effect*). When the metabolism is extensive, there can be a significant difference in the bioavailability and ultimately dosing requirements depending upon whether a medication is given orally or intravenously.

Most anticonvulsants undergo linear pharmacokinetics, meaning that the dose and resulting total and free plasma concentrations increase in direct proportion with each other (Figure 9.2). The exceptions to this are gabapentin (saturable absorption), carbamazepine, phenytoin, and valproate (saturable protein binding). Carbamazepine and phenytoin undergo non-linear metabolism. Carbamazepine induces its own metabolism (autoinduction or time-dependent metabolism). The increase in metabolism occurs during the first month of therapy, often at the point of dose titration. Because dosage increases may not result in

Table 9.1 Antiepileptic drug metabolism and excretion.

Medication	Metabolizing pathway	Induction	Inhibition	Renal elimination	Protein binding
Carbamazepine	CYP3A4 Minor: 1A2, 2C8, 2C9	1A2/2C/3A4, UGT, epoxide hydoxylase	None	<1%	75%
Clobazam	CYP3A4, 2C19 (NDM)	None	None	Yes	85%
Ethosuximide	CYP3A4 Minor: CYP2B/2C/2E1	None	None	20%	0%
Felbamate	C3A4, 2E1, UGT	3A4	2C19, β-oxidation	50%	25%
Gabapentin	None	None	None	100%	0%
Lacosamide	CYP2C19	None	None	40%	<15%
Levetiracetam	Cellular amidases	None	None	66%	<10%
Lamotrigine	UGT	Weak UGT	None	10%	55%
Oxcarbazepine	Cellular enzymes, UGT	3A4/5 (weak)	2C19*	95%	40% (MHD)
Phenobarbital	2C9 Minor: 2C19, 2E1	1A2, 2C, C3A Families, UGT	Rare 2C†	25–30%	50%
Phenytoin	2C9, 2C19	1A2, 2C, C3A Families, UGT	Rare 2C†	<5%	90%
Pregabalin	None	None	None	90%	0%
Primidone	2C9	2C, C3A Families, UGT	Rare 2C†	15–65%	10%
Rufinamide	Carboxylesterases	None	None	85%	27%
Tiagabine	3A4	None	None	<2%	98%
Topiramate	Unknown	CYP3A4 (weak)	2C19*	70%	13–17%
Valproate	2C9, 2C19, β-oxidation	None	2C9, UGT, epoxide hyroxylase	<5%	93%‡
Vigabatrin	None	None	None	100%	100%
Zonisamide	CYP3A4	None	None	62%	40%

*May increase phenytoin concentrations.
†Coadministration of phenobarbital and phenytoin can result in inhibition of 2C family metabolic pathways.
‡Saturable protein binding, proportion free increases with increasing total concentration.
MHD, monohydroxy derivative; UGT, UDP-glucuronosyltransferase.

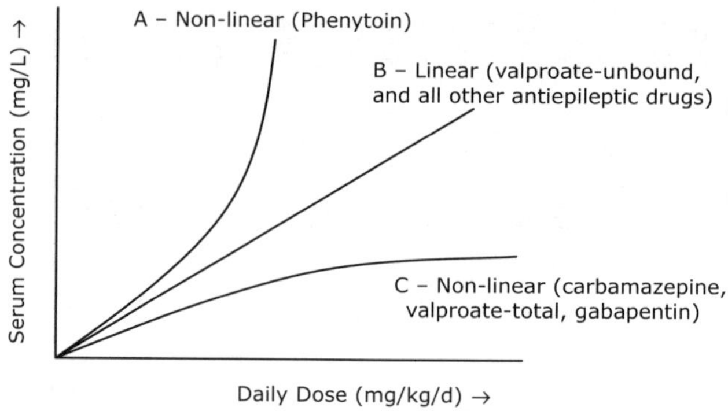

Figure 9.2 Pharmacokinetics.

linear increases in carbamazepine plasma concentrations, it can be misconstrued as medication non-adherence. Phenytoin has saturable metabolism that results in disproportionately larger increases in plasma concentrations with increasing dose.

Elimination

Elimination is the irreversible loss of a drug from the site of measurement. It occurs by both excretion and metabolism (see Table 9.1). Excretion is the irreversible loss of chemically unchanged drug. The kidney is responsible for the excretion of most drugs; however, some undergo biliary or fecal excretion. The majority of anticonvulsants available today undergo some degree of metabolism before renal elimination. The exceptions are vigabatrin, gabapentin, and pregabalin, which are not metabolized (and levetiracetam, which has minimal non-hepatic metabolism). Net renal elimination is governed by the processes of glomerular filtration, tubular secretion, and reabsorption. Pharmacological properties that affect renal excretion include the degree of protein binding, acid-base properties (pK_a), and lipophilicity. Patient factors that affect the elimination of drugs include hepatic or renal disease, age, and gender.

Pharmacokinetic parameters

Anticonvulsants have different pharmacokinetic properties that define them (reviewed in Tables 9.1 and 9.2) [1–8]. Drugs with linear elimination have proportional increases of plasma concentrations (C_p) with increasing dose (D). Adjusting doses based upon a known plasma-concentration dose is done simply by cross-multiplying and solving for the new dose. For example, if you have a phenobarbital concentration of 20 mg/L on a dose of 300 mg/day, what dose would be needed to maintain a concentration of 30 mg/L?

$$\frac{D1}{C_p1} = \frac{D2}{C_p2}$$

Solving for the example:

$$\text{Dose 2} = \frac{D1 \times C_p2}{C_p1} = \frac{300\text{ mg} \times 30\text{ mg/L}}{20\text{ mg/L}} = 450\text{ mg/day}$$

Table 9.2 Antiepileptic medication pharmacokinetic parameters.

Medication	Reference range (mcg/ml)	Volume of distribution, V_d (L/kg)		Elimination half-life (h)		Time to steady state, C_{pss} (days)		Time AED Levels*
		Adult	Pediatric	Adult	Pediatric	Adult	Pediatric	
Carbamazepine	CBZ 4–12 (10,11-epoxide 0.4–4)	0.59–2	Neo: 1.5 Child: 1.9	Init: 18–55 Chronic: 8–20	Init: 3–32 Chronic: 8–14	Init: 4–9 Chronic: 3–4	Init: 4–6 Chronic: 2–3	Init: 1 wk, 3 wks Chronic: 3–4 days
Clobazam	0.03–0.3 (0.3–3 desmethyl/ metabolite)	1	1	10–30 (36–46 NDM)	10–30 (36–46 NDM)	7–10	7–10	10 days
Ethosuximide	50–100	0.69	0.65–0.75	40–60	24–41	8–13	5–9	1.5–2 wks
Felbamate	40–100	0.75	0.54–0.73	14–22	14	3–7	3	3–7 days
Gabapentin	2–20	0.65–1.04	0.65–1.04	5–9	4–5	1–2	1	2–5 days
Lacosamide	2–12	0.6	0.6	13	10–12	3	3	3 days
Lamotrigine	2–20	0.9–1.3	1.3–2.4	MTX 15–32 VPA 48–71 EIA 8–15	MTX 13–27 VPA 45–66 EIA 6–12	MTX 5–7 VPA 10–15 EIA 3–4	MTX 3–6 VPA 9–14 EIA 2–3	MTX 1 wk VPA 2 wks EIA 4 days
Levetiracetam	15–45	0.5–0.7	0.67	6–8	5–7	1–2	1–2	2 days
Oxcarbazepine (MHD)	(MHD) 5–35	0.65	0.75	7–12	7–12	2–3	2–3	3 days
Phenobarbital (PB)	10–40	0.54–0.73	N: 0.8–1.1 I/C: 0.6–0.8	53–140	N: 45–150 I/C: 20–133	11–30	N: 10–42 I/C: 4–28	1 wk then 1 mo. 1–24 h post-LD

(continued)

Table 9.2 (*Continued*)

Medication	Reference range (mcg/ml)	Volume of distribution, V_d (L/kg)		Elimination half-life (h)		Time to steady state, C_{pss} (days)		Time AED Levels*
		Adult	Pediatric	Adult	Pediatric	Adult	Pediatric	
Phenytoin (PHT), fosphenytoin (FPHT)	10–20	0.7	P: 1–1.2 N: 0.8–1 I/C: 0.7	30–100	<10	7–28	7	7 days PHT 1–24 h post-LD FPHT 2–24 h post-LD
Pregabalin	2–12	0.4	0.4	6	4.6–6.8	2	2	2 days
Primidone (PRM)	PRM 5–12 (PEMA 1.5–10, PB 15–40)	0.86–2	0.86	PRM 10–22 PEMA 16	PRM 4.5–11 PEMA N/A	2–4	1–3	1 wk, then 1 mo.
Rufinamide	10–40	0.7	0.7	6–10	6–10	3	3	3
Tiagabine	20–200 ng/ml	1.3–1.6	2.4	4–9	3.2–5.7	1–2	1–2	2 days
Topiramate	2–20	0.6–0.8	0.56–0.72	20–22	4.2–13.5	4–5	1–3	5 days
Valproate (VPA)	50–100	0.12	02.–0.25	14	7.5–15	3–4	2–4	4 days 30 min post-LD
Vigabatrin	0.8–36	0.8	0.8	5–8	5–8	1–2	1–2	2 days
Zonisamide	10–40	1.45	1.5	56–78	25–35	12–17	10	2 wks

*Time in which anticonvulsant concentrations are indicated based upon time to steady state or for post-loading dose confirmation of reaching a therapeutic concentration.
AED, antiepileptic drug; EIA, enzyme-inducing agent; MTX, monotherapy; N, neonate; I/C, infant/children; PEMA, phenylethyl malonamide; Init, initiation of therapy; LD, loading dose; NDM, *N*-desmethylclobazam; MHD, monohydroxy derivative, active metabolite.

In this example, the phenobarbital dose would need to be increased to 450 mg/day to achieve a steady-state concentration of 30 mg/L. Because phenobarbital's half-life and time to steady state are so long, the resulting effect from a change in dose may take 2 weeks. Therefore, one may consider giving a loading dose in this patient. Given an estimated population $V_d = 1$ mg/kg (Table 9.3), a loading dose can be calculated by rearranging the equation from above:

$$\text{Loading dose} = \frac{C_{\text{target}} - C_{\text{observed}}}{V_d}$$

$$= \frac{30 \text{ mg/L} - 20 \text{ mg/L}}{1 \text{ L/kg}} = 10 \text{ mg/kg}$$

The patient in the example would require a 10 mg/kg dose to achieve a phenobarbital plasma concentration of 30 mg/L. The patient's new maintenance dose (450 mg/day) could then be started. In general, assessment of the adequacy of the phenobarbital loading dose is between 1 and 24 hours after infusion. Maintenance doses typically are assessed at steady state (see Table 9.3). A general principle for drugs with first-order kinetics is that the approximate time required to achieve a steady state is five times the half-life.

Half-life ($t_{1/2}$ in 1/time) is the time it takes for the plasma concentration for a given drug to reach half of its previous concentration. Stated another way, over one half-life, the concentration decreases by 50%; following another half-life, one-quarter ($^1/_2 \times {}^1/_2$) of the original concentration remains, and so on. An understanding of half-life is important because it determines both dosing frequency and time to steady state (see Table 9.2). As a general rule, the shorter the half-life the more frequent the dosing needs to be. For anticonvulsants with half-life values in the range of 1–8 hours, usually doses need to be given every 1–3 half-lives; for those with half-lives greater than 8–24 hours, doses are typically given every half-life; and for those with half-lives greater than 24 hours, doses can be given once daily for convenience. This is why a medication such as carbamazepine (immediate-release tablet or liquid) needs to be given many times per day, whereas phenobarbital can be given once daily. At a constant rate of drug input, drugs reach a steady state, in which the peak-trough fluctuation remains constant or plateaus. The time for this is roughly 4–5 times a drug's half-life. This is important in evaluating the efficacy of a maintenance dose. Assessments before steady state can under- or overestimate the overall efficacy of a dose and mistakenly motivate an unnecessary dose adjustment.

Therapeutic drug monitoring

Therapeutic drug monitoring (TDM) is generally aligned with pharmacokinetics and is usually applied to drugs with a narrow therapeutic index. TDM is based upon the concepts that in order for a drug to be effective it must usually be above a minimum effective concentration (MEC), and to be free of side effects it typically needs to be below a minimum toxic concentration (MTC). The concentration difference in the MEC and MTC is the therapeutic range, and the ratio of MTC/MEC is the therapeutic index. As the ratio gets closer to 1, the index is narrower. Many of the older anticonvulsants possess a narrow therapeutic index and therefore TDM is advocated to improve response. The new anticonvulsants have a greater difference in MEC and MTC and they seem to possess a larger therapeutic index. One thing that makes anticonvulsant therapy complex, particularly in cases of anticonvulsant

Table 9.3 Antiepileptic drug-drug interactions.

	Medication <u>added</u> to therapy																	
Existing-affected drug	CBZ	CLB	ETX	FLB	GPB/PGB	LEV	LCS	LTG	OXC	PB	PHT	PRM	RFM	TGB	TPM	VPA	VGB	ZNS
Carbamazepine (CBZ)	A	0	0	$\downarrow^{CBZ}\uparrow^{E}$	0	0	0	$\uparrow^{PD}$	$\downarrow^{ns}$	↓	↓	↓	0	$\uparrow^{PD}$	0	$\uparrow^{E}$	0	$\downarrow^{ns}$
Clobazam (CLB)	↓	—	0	↑	0	0	0	0	0	↓	↓	↓	0	NI	0	0	0	0
Ethosuximide (ETX)	↓	0	—	NI	0	0	0	NI	NI	↓	↓	↓	0	0	0	↑↓	0	0
Felbamate (FLB)	↓	0	0	—	0	0	0	0	NI	↓	↓	↓	0	NI	0	↑	0	NI
Gabapentin/pregabalin (GPB/PGB)	0	0	0	0	—	0	0	0	0	0	0	0	0	0	0	0	0	0
Levetiracetam (LEV)	0	0	0	0	0	—	0	0	0	0	0	0	0	0	0	0	0	0
Lacosamide (LCS)	↓	0	0	0	0	0	—	0	0	↓	↓	↓	0	0	0	0	0	0
Lamotrigine (LTG)	↓	0	0	0	0	0	0	A	$\downarrow^{ns}$	↓	↓	↓	0	0	0	↑	0	0
Oxcarbazepine (OXC)	↓	0	0	0	0	0	0	0	—	↓	↓	↓	0	NI	0	0	0	NI
Phenobarbital (PB)	0	0	0	↑	0	0	0	0	$\uparrow^{ns}$	—	↑	—	0	0	0	↑	0	NI
Phenytoin (PHT)	$\downarrow\uparrow^{R}$	0	0	↑	0	0	0	0	$\uparrow^{R}$	↑↓	—	↑↓	0	0	$\uparrow^{R}$	↑	0	0
Primidone (PRM)	$\downarrow^{PRM}\uparrow^{PB}$	↑	0	NI	0	0	0	0	$\uparrow^{ns}$	—	$\downarrow^{PRM}\uparrow^{PB}$	—	0	0	0	↑	0	NI
Rufinamide (RFM)	↓	0	0	0	0	0	0	0	0	↓	↓	↓	—	0	0	↑	0	0
Tiagabine (TGB)	↓	0	0	NI	0	0	0	NI	NI	↓	↓	↓	0	—	0	$\uparrow^{IV}$	0	NI
Topiramae (TPM)	↓	0	0	NI	0	0	0	NI	NI	↓	↓	↓	0	0	—	$\downarrow^{ns}$	0	NI
Valproate (VPA)	↓	↑	$\downarrow^{R}$	↑	0	0	0	$\downarrow^{ns}$	0	↓	↓	↓	0	0	$\downarrow^{ns}$	—	0	0
Vigabatrin (VGB)	0	0	0	0	0	0	0	0	0	0	0	0	0	0	0	0	—	0
Zonisamide (ZNS)	↓	0	0	NI	0	0	0	$\uparrow^{R}$	NI	↓	↓	↓	0	NI	NI	0	0	—
Oral contraceptives	↓	$\downarrow^{ns}$	0	↓	0	0	0	↓LTG	↓	↓	↓	↓	0	0	↓	0	0	0

A, autoinduction, induces its own metabolism; E, increases the formation of 10,11-epoxide; IV, *in vitro* drug interaction, not definitively found in humans; NI, no information; NS, not a clinically significant increase/decrease in the affected drug's concentration; PD, pharmacodynamic reaction, AED concentrations do not change; R, rare, but possible interaction.

NDM, *N*-desmethylclobazam.

Oral contraceptives decrease serum LTG levels.

Table 9.4 Indications for anticonvulsant therapeutic drug monitoring.

Time point	Rationale
Following a loading dose	To confirm therapeutic concentrations are achieved before starting the maintenance dose If drawn as peak (C_{p0}), can be used to calculated V_d
At steady state on a maintenance dose	To establish individual therapeutic concentration, when desired clinical outcome achieved Once an effective dose is achieved, to record that concentration relationship for future dosage adjustment needs
In cases of seizures	To determine the need for a loading dose or maintenance dose adjustment, or adherence to therapy
Suspected acute toxicity	As an aid in the diagnosis of clinical toxicity
Suspected non-adherence	To confirm daily doses are being taken, especially in patients with uncontrolled seizures
Addition or removal of a drug known to alter the pharmacokinetics of the patient's anticonvulsant	To ensure a compromise in efficacy or toxicity does not occur secondary to drug-drug interactions (displacement, elimination changes)
In cases of a clinically significant change in the physiological function that results in a change in the absorption, binding, metabolism, or elimination of an anticonvulsant (e.g., pregnancy, ↓ protein binding, change in renal or hepatic function, change in drug formulation)	To ensure a compromise in efficacy or toxicity does not occur secondary to changes in pharmacokinetics, or in a situation with known pharmacokinetic variability

polytherapy, is the extent of drug-drug interactions (Table 9.3) [9–14]. The therapeutic ranges of the anticonvulsants are listed in Table 9.2, and suggested indications for TDM in Table 9.4 [15,16]. Serum drug concentrations should be measured with a clear indication, and are interpreted clinically, taking into account the whole clinical context.

9.2 Pharmacogenomics

The terms pharmacogenetics and pharmacogenomics are often used interchangeably. Although both attempt to correlate a given individual's genetic background with how it predicts the effects of a drug, there is a slight difference in their scope. Pharmacogenetics evaluates the relationship between individual or small numbers of gene variations and drug disposition (pharmacokinetics), response, and toxicity (pharmacodynamics) [17–19]. Pharmacogenomics takes a much broader focus and examines the genome and how it relates to the pharmacokinetics and/or pharmacodynamics of a given drug. Both fields attempt to maximize a given patient's therapy by using genetic data to guide the selection of the optimal drug and dose. It is well known that individuals with the same condition respond differently to the same drug and same dose, and this variation currently is difficult to predict *a priori*. It is hoped in the future that pharmacogenetic data will facilitate individualization of drug therapy. In theory, patients with a diagnosis would come to clinic and have pharmacogenomic testing performed. Results from this testing would aid in the selection of the most efficacious medication with the least side effects for that patient. It is hoped this more logical prescreening method would minimize the need for the trial-and-error approach that is practiced today, in which medications with similar indications are selected generically for an affected patient population rather than an individual genotype.

Pharmacogenetics focuses on single nucleotide polymorphisms (SNPs, or "snips"). For SNPs located in coding regions there is a potential for the actual transcribed protein to be different between two patients. In this case, the altered amino acid sequence of the protein has the potential to alter the activity of the protein, be it a metabolic enzyme or receptor. It is also important to remember that only those SNPs that produce a change in a protein's amino acid sequence have the potential to produce a clinical effect (non-synonymous SNPs).

Approximately half of patients with epilepsy fail their first anticonvulsant due to incomplete response or intolerability or both. With further therapy, one-third will ultimately be refractory to anticonvulsant therapy. There can be many reasons for this variation of response, some with a pharmacogenomic basis. Pharmacogenomics in the field of epilepsy has focused largely on genes producing differences in the pharmacokinetics of anticonvulsants. The remaining portion of this chapter will review available information regarding the pharmacogenomics of anticonvulsants.

Metabolizing pathways

Logically, alterations in the rate at and/or extent to which an anticonvulsant is metabolized or eliminated from the body will ultimately affect the dose requirements [20–23]. Clinically relevant differences in oxidative metabolism have been identified for the CYP2C9 and CYP2C19 isoenzymes. Several studies support the role of polymorphisms affecting the functioning of these enzymes in patients with epilepsy receiving either phenytoin, phenobarbital, or diazepam. CYP2C19 has been shown to have more than 10 different alleles. These alleles lead to the translation of a non-functional protein. Before genetic testing was available, two clinical populations were described based upon the ability to *p*-hydroxylate mephenytoin (a measure of 2C19 activity). Poor metabolizers (PM) were later found to have both alleles of this locus affected. There is significant variation in the incidence of the PM phenotype. In Caucasians and Blacks the frequency is lowest (2–5% of the population), whereas in Japanese and Chinese populations the frequency rises to 18–23%. The clearance of medications can be impaired in 2C19 PMs but the extent is variable based upon the relative contribution of 2C19 to the overall metabolism of the anticonvulsant. For example, approximately 60% of diazepam undergoes biotransformation through 2C19 (via two separate steps), whereas 40% of a given dose of phenobarbital is metabolized through this pathway. This results in many patients of Asian ancestry having toxic side effects when given standard doses of diazepam.

Other metabolic enzymes have SNPs identified and have been considered for possible pharmacogenomic significance (CYP1A2, 2A6, 3A4, 2B1, UGT1A4, 1A6); however, none has proven to be of clinical relevance in predicting anticonvulsant dosage requirements or adverse effects.

The genetic contribution to anticonvulsant drug hypersensitivity reactions – Stevens–Johnson syndrome (SJS), toxic epidermal necrolysis (TEN) – has also been examined. The literature has examined a relationship between the human leukocyte antigen (HLA) and carbamazepine. Specifically, in Chinese patients the HLA-B∗1502 allele has been associated with a significantly higher risk of SJS; however, these findings have not been replicated in Caucasians. In Caucasians, the HLA-B*0702 allele is thought to be protective against carbamazepine-associated hypersensitivity.

Anticonvulsant pharmacogenomics is still in its infancy, particularly when it comes to the consideration of pharmacodynamics. There are many receptors relevant to anticonvulsants' mechanism of action for which SNPs have been identified but have yet to be explored. Likewise, there are epilepsies with defined mutations in drug targets – e.g., generalized epilepsy with febrile seizures plus additional symptoms (GEFS +) or juvenile myoclonic epilepsy – for which pharmacogenomic studies would be a logical pursuit. Future studies need to address limitations in study populations, confounding variables, and possible linkage disequilibrium.

References

[1] Anderson GD. Pharmacokinetic, pharmacodynamic and pharmacogenetic targeted therapy of anti-epileptic drugs. *Ther Drug Monit* 2008;**30**:173–180.

[2] Bourgeois B. Pharmacokinetic properties of current anti-epileptic drugs: what improvements are needed? *Neurology* 2000;**55**(11, Suppl. 3):S11–S16.

[3] Perucca E. Clinical pharmacokinetics of new generation anti-epileptic drugs at the extremes of age. *Clin Pharmacokinet* 2006;**45**:351–363.

[4] Perucca E. Pharmacological problems in the management of epilepsy in children. *Seizure* 1995;**4**:139–143.

[5] Gilman JT. Developmental principles of anti-epileptic drug therapy. *J Child Neurol* 1994;**9**(Suppl. 1):S20–S25.

[6] Bartelink IH, Rademaker CMA, Schobben AFAM, vandenAnker JN. Guidelines on pediatric dosing on the basis of developmental physiology and pharmacokinetics considerations. *Clin Pharmacokinet* 2006;**45**:1077–1097.

[7] Anderson GD, Lynn AM. Optimizing pediatric dosing. A developmental pharmacologic approach. *Pharmacotherapy* 2009;**29**:600–690.

[8] Bialer M. The pharmacokinetics and interactions of new anti-epileptic drugs. *Ther Drug Monit* 2005;**27**:722–726.

[9] Spina E, Perucca E. Clinical significance of pharmacokinetic interactions between anti-epileptic and psychotropic drugs. *Epilepsia* 2002;**43**(Suppl. 2):37–44.

[10] Patsalos PN, Perucca E. Clinically important drug interactions in epilepsy: general features and interactions between anti-epileptic drugs. *Lancet Neurol* 2003;**2**:347–356.

[11] Johannessen LC, Patsalos PN. Drug interactions involving the new second- and third-generation anti-epileptic drugs. *Expert Rev Neurother* 2010;**10**:119–140.

[12] French JA, Gidal BE. Anti-epileptic drug interactions. *Epilepsia* 2000;**41**(Suppl. 8):S30–S36.

[13] Perucca E. Clinically relevant drug interactions with anti-epileptic drugs. *Br J Clin Pharmacol* 2005;**61**:246–255.

[14] Patsalos PN, Perucca E. Clinically important drug interactions in epilepsy: general features and interactions between antiepileptic drugs. *Lancet Neurology* 2003;**2**:347–356.

[15] Patsalos PN, Berry DJ, Bourgeois BFD, *et al.* Anti-epileptic drugs best practice guidelines for therapeutic drug monitoring: A position paper by the subcommission on therapeutic drug monitoring, ILAE Commission on Therapeutic Strategies. *Epilepsia* 2008;**49**:1239–1276.

[16] Glauser TA, Pippenger CE. Controversies in blood-level monitoring: Re-examining its role in the treatment of epilepsy. *Epilepsia* 2000;**41**(Suppl. 8):S6–S15.
[17] Klotz U. The role of pharmacogenetics in the metabolism of anti-epileptic drugs. *Clin Pharmacokinet* 2007;**46**:271–279.
[18] Ferraro TN, Buono TN. The relationship between the drugs and human gene variation: An overview. *Epilepsy Behav* 2005;**7**:18–36.
[19] Hung CC, Tai JJ, Lin CJ, Lee MJ, Lio HH. Complex haplotypic effects of the ABCB1 gene on epilepsy treatment response. *Pharmacogenomics* 2005;**6**:411–417.
[20] Seo T, Ishitsu T, Ueda N, *et al.* ABCB1 polymorphisms influence the response to antiepileptic drugs in Japanese epilepsy patients. *Pharmacogenomics* 2006;**7**:551–561.
[21] Nakajima Y, Saito Shiseki K, Fukushima-Uesaka H, *et al.* Haplotype structures of EPHX1 and their effects on the metabolism of carbamazepine-10,11-epoxide in Japanese epileptic patients. *Eur J Clin Pharmacol* 2005;**61**:25–34.
[22] Hung CC, Lin CJ, Chen CC, Chang CJ, Liou HH. Dosage recommendation of phenytoin for patients with epilepsy with different CYP2C9/CYP2C19 polymorphisms. *Ther Drug Monit* 2004;**26**:534–540.
[23] Tate SK, Depondt C, Sisodiya SM, *et al.* Genetic predictors of the maximum doses patients receive during clinical use of the anti-epileptic drugs carbamazepine and phenytoin. *Proc Natl Acad Sci* 2005;**102**:5507–5512.

10 Therapeutic efficacy of antiepileptic drugs

James W. Wheless

Department of Pediatric Neurology, University of Tennessee Health Science Center; Le Bonheur Comprehensive Epilepsy Program and Neuroscience Institute, Le Bonheur Children's Hospital, Memphis, TN, USA

The choice of an antiepileptic drug (AED) for the treatment of seizure disorders in infants and children must be made not only on the basis of efficacy but also taking into account a number of other considerations (Table 10.1). The first step is determining the seizure type and epilepsy syndrome. While there are many different seizure types and epilepsy syndromes that occur in children, knowing the age of the child, their neurological examination, seizure etiology, and EEG characteristics will help guide the clinician to the appropriate seizure type and epilepsy syndrome [1]. The importance of the correct diagnosis cannot be overstated.

The challenge the clinician then faces is selecting the antiepileptic drug that is efficacious for a given seizure type or epilepsy syndrome, and applying the results of large population-based studies to their individual patient. For example, the clinician may be confronted with a patient with Lennox–Gastaut syndrome, and needs to know not only which drugs are effective in treating the syndrome, but what medications are effective for the different seizure types associated with this syndrome. In this chapter, I will primarily focus on the efficacy of antiepileptic drugs, while realizing that many other factors are critical in drug selection (adverse effect profile, pharmacology, etc.; these topics are covered in other chapters).

Epilepsy in Children and Adolescents, First Edition. Edited by James W. Wheless.

Table 10.1 Selection of antiepileptic drug therapy: general considerations.

• Efficacy for seizure type, epilepsy syndrome	• Pharmacokinetics, pharmacogenomics
• Etiology	• Need for laboratory monitoring
• Side-effect profile	• Dosing requirements/ drug formulations
• Safety (acute, long-term)	• Speed, ease of initiation
• Teratogenicity	• Comorbidities
• Mechanism of action	• Cost
• Drug interactions	• Regulatory status, national approval
• Route of elimination	

10.1 Efficacy-based treatment guidelines

In 2004, the Therapeutics and Technology Assessment Subcommittee and Quality Standard Subcommittee of the American Academy of Neurology and the American Epilepsy Society published practice parameters for the use of new antiepileptic drugs [2]. They examined the relevant medical literature from 1987 to the spring of 2003 for evidence pertaining to the efficacy, tolerability, and safety of the new generation of antiepileptic drugs, applying the American Academy of Neurology guidelines for the assessment of the quality of the available data (Table 10.2). On the basis of the available evidence that met their criteria, they were able to endorse only gabapentin, lamotrigine, topiramate, and oxcarbazepine for initial use as monotherapy for partial and secondary generalized seizures in adolescents and adults. Additionally, they did not address situations that are commonly encountered by pediatric neurologists (i.e., younger patients and the multitude of pediatric epilepsy syndromes). However, they were able to endorse the use of lamotrigine as additional therapy for the treatment of absence seizures in children. In 2006, the International League Against Epilepsy (ILAE) published evidence-based treatment guidelines [3]. These were based on a review of the literature of all antiepileptic drugs available. The document was under development from 1999 until 2005. This comprehensive review noted an especially alarming lack of well-designed, properly conducted, randomized controlled trials for patients with generalized seizures/epilepsies and for children in general. While these guidelines comprehensively reviewed the literature, it was clear there was not a substantial source of evidence-based medicine to guide the pediatric neurologist in selection of antiepileptic drug therapy.

Parents clearly expect the drug chosen to be efficacious for the seizure type, desire the medication to have no serious side effects and minimal nuisance or other side effects, and be available in a pediatric formulation. The pediatric neurologist must balance the epilepsy syndrome and its expected outcome and ability to be controlled with the risks and

Table 10.2 Evidence-based medicine: American Academy of Neurology (AAN) guidelines.

- Class I: prospective, random, controlled trial
- Class II: prospective, matched group cohort study
- Class III: all other controlled trials (natural history controls, patient serving as own control)
- Class IV: expert opinion, case series, uncontrolled studies

Source: Neurology, 2003;**60**:166–175.

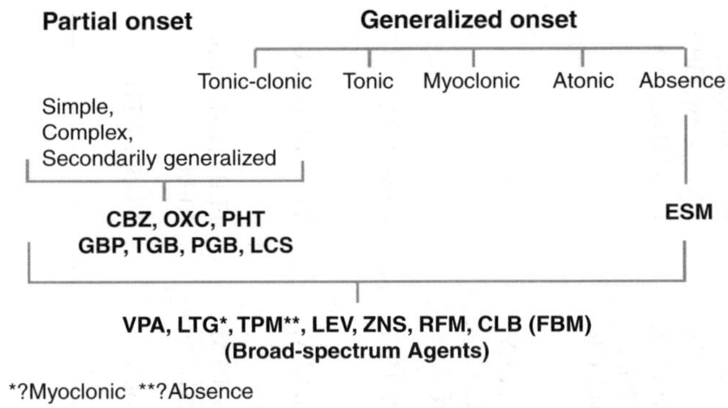

Figure 10.1 Antiepileptic drug treatment options by seizure type.

benefits of each medicine. There are some epilepsy conditions that tend to be more benign and easily controlled, such as childhood absence epilepsy and the primary generalized tonic-clonic seizures. For these conditions, a drug with minimal side effects would be preferable. However, there are also epilepsy syndromes seen in childhood that are often chronic and progressive with adverse neurological outcomes such as infantile spasms, Lennox–Gastaut syndrome, and some partial-onset seizures. For these epilepsy syndromes, and their associated intractable seizures, a drug with a higher risk-to-benefit ratio may be acceptable, given the difficulty in controlling the seizure. Risk assessment is critical in determining the best therapy for each child based on their epilepsy syndrome and seizure type. Knowing the efficacy of each antiepileptic drug in each pediatric epilepsy syndrome is critical to treatment selection [5–8].

Given the lack of evidence-based controlled trials in children, algorithms have been proposed that divide the world of epilepsy into partial-onset or generalized seizures (Figure 10.1). This model proposes that there is a group of compounds that are primarily niche medications or narrow-spectrum agents that are effective against partial-onset seizures. On the other hand, there are broad-spectrum agents that are effective against partial seizures, primary generalized tonic-clonic seizures, and one or more of the other generalized seizure types. Additionally, these broad-spectrum agents carry a lower risk than the narrow-spectrum agents of aggravating generalized seizures. In contrast, the narrow-spectrum agents are typically effective against partial seizures and secondary generalized tonic-clonic seizures (and some primary generalized tonic-clonic seizures). However, these agents have a greater risk of aggravating non-convulsive seizures such as absence or myoclonic seizures.

Ideally, the physician faced with treating a specific seizure type or epilepsy syndrome in a given child would like to have well-conducted, randomized controlled trials with available data to make decisions about the care of individual patients. This degree of evidence-based medicine is often lacking in pediatric epilepsy. When there is an absence of controlled trials, the clinician must rely on other levels of evidence, either the expert consensus method, which focuses on specific clinical questions, or empirical therapy that is based on practical experience but is scientifically unproven (uncontrolled case series or historical controls). Tables 10.3, 10.4, and 10.5 list the drug therapies that have regulatory approval in children, whether they have regulatory approval in children or adults, and if they are

Table 10.3 Comparison of recommendations for the treatment of pediatric epilepsy.

Type of epilepsy	Japan approved*	ILAE[†]	SIGN[‡]	NICE[§]	USA FDA approved**
Partial onset	CBZ, VPA, ZNS, PHT, CLB, LTG	A: OXC B: None C: CBZ, PB, PHT, TPM, VPA	PHT, VPA, CBZ, LTG, TPM, OXC, VGB, CLB, LEV	LTG, CBZ-ER, LEV, OXC, VPA, TPM, GBP, CLB, LCS, PB, PHT, PGB, TGB,VGB, ZNS	PB, PHT, CBZ, OXC, TPM, GBP, LTG, TGB, LEV
BECT	CBZ	A,B: None C: CBZ, VPA	Not mentioned	CBZ, LTG, LEV, VPA, OXC, CLB, GBP, TPM	None
CAE	VPA	A,B: None C: ESM, LTG, VPA	VPA, ESM, LTG	ESM, VPA, LTG	ESM, VPA
JME	VPA	A, B, C: None	VPA, LTG, TPM	VPA, LTG, LEV, TPM	TPM, LEV, LTG
LGS	LTG	Not reviewed	VPA, LTG, TPM, CLB, FBM, RFM	VPA, LTG, RFM, TPM, (FBM)	FLB, TPM, LTG, RFM
IS	ZNS	Not reviewed	VGB, hormonal therapy	VGB, steroids	VGB, ACTH

Sources: *Accessed 1 March 2012, Pharmaceutical and Medical Devices Agency, Japan, 2011. www.pmda.go.jp.
[†]International League Against Epilepsy: Glauser T, *et al. Epilepsia* 2006;**47**(7):1094–1120.
[‡]Scottish Intercollegiate Guidelines Network: www.sign.ac.uk/pdf/sign81.pdf (March 2005).
[§]National Institute for Health and Clinical Excellence: www.nice.org.uk/cg137 (January 2012).
**US Food and Drug Administration: www.pdr.net.
BECT, benign epilepsy of childhood with centrotemporal spikes; CAE, childhood absence epilepsy; JME, juvenile myoclonic epilepsy; LGS, Lennox–Gastaut syndrome; IS, infantile spasms.

Table 10.4 Treatment of partial seizures in children, adolescents, and adults (USA).

	1–24 months		2–16 years		Adults	
AED*	Add on	Mono	Add on	Mono	Add on	Mono
Gabapentin	N	N	Y(>3)	N	Y	N
Topiramate	N	N	Y(>2)	Y(>10)	Y	Y
Lamotrigine	N	N	Y(>2)	N	Y	Y*
Tiagabine	N	N	Y(>12)	N	Y	N
Oxcarbazepine	N	N	Y(>2)	Y(>4)	Y	Y
Zonisamide	N	N	N	N	Y	N
Levetiracetam	N	N	Y(>4)	N	Y	N
Pregabalin	N	N	N	N	Y	N
Lacosamide	N	N	N	N	Y	N
Vigabatrin	N	N	N	N	Y	N
Rufinamide	N	N	N	N	N	N

*AED, antiepileptic drug; Add on, adjunctive therapy approval; Mono, monotherapy approval by the FDA, USA; Y, yes; N, no.

Table 10.5 National Institute for Health and Clinical Excellence (NICE) Clinical Guidelines (GC137) (January 2012).

Seizure type/ epilepsy syndrome	First-line	Second-line	Adjunctive
Partial-onset seizures	LTG, CBZ-ER	LEV, OXC, VPA	CLB, GBP, TPM; then LCS, PB, PHT, PGB, TGB, VGB, ZNS
BECT/BOEC	CBZ, LTG	LEV, OXC, VPA	CBZ, CLB, GBP, LTG, LEV, OXC, VPA, TPM; then LCS, PB, PHT, PGB, TCB, VGB, ZNS
Generalized tonic-clonic	VPA, LTG, CBZ, OXC		CLB, LTG, LEV, VPA, TPM
Absence	ESM, VPA	LTG	Combine (2 of these 3): LTG, ESM, VPA; OR CLB, CNZ, LEV, TPM, ZNS
Myoclonic	VPA	LEV, TPM	CLB, CNZ, ZNS
Tonic/atonic	VPA		LTG, TPM, RFM
Infantile spasms	VGB, steroid (VGB is TSC)		
Dravet syndrome	VPA, TPM		CLB, Stiripentol
Lennox–Gastaut syndrome	VPA		LTG, RFM, TPM, (FLB)
Idiopathic generalized epilepsy	VPA	LTG, TPM	LTG, LEV, VPA, TPM; then CLB, CNZ, ZNS
Juvenile myoclonic epilepsy	VPA	LTG, LEV, TPM	CLB, CNZ, ZNS
Childhood or juvenile absence epilepsy	ESM, VPA	LTG	Combine (2 of these 3): ESM, VPA, LTG; then CLB, CNZ, LEV, TPM, ZNS

Source: www.nice.org.uk/cg137.

BECT, benign epilepsy of childhood with centrotemporal spikes; BOEC, benign occipital epilepsies of childhood; TSC, tuberous selerosis complex.

Box 10.1 Drug abbreviations

ACTH – adrenocorticotropic harmone
CBZ – carbamazepine
CBZ-ER – carbamazepine extended release
CLB – clobazam
CZP – clonazapam
ESM – ethosuximide
FBM – felbamate
GBP – gabapentin
LCS – lacosamide
LEV – levetiracetam
LTG – lamotrigine
NTZ – nitrazepam
OXC – oxcarbazepine
PB – phenobarbital
PGB – pregabalin
PHT – phenytoin
RFM – rufinamide
Steroid (Hormonal Therapy) = Prednisolone or Tetracosactide
TGB – tiagabine
TPM – topiramate
VPA – valproate
VGB – vigabatrin
ZNS – zonisamide

approved as monotherapy or adjunctive therapy [3,9,10]. Additionally, Table 10.6 lists, by epilepsy syndrome, which antiepileptic drug has undergone randomized controlled trials (and the rare negative ones that are reported) in a given epilepsy syndrome and which other medications have been reported in the literature, but not in controlled trials. Finally, Table 10.7 lists, by epilepsy syndrome and seizure types, recommendations for treatment using the expert consensus method (studies performed in the United States, Europe, Japan, and India) [11–14]. (Medication abbreviations used in these tables are listed in Box 10.1.)

10.2 Antiepileptic drug selection based on specific pediatric epilepsy syndromes

Only a few comparative trials have been conducted in newly diagnosed childhood epilepsy with multiple antiepileptic drugs (Table 10.8) [15–22]. These have been typically conducted in children with partial-onset seizures or secondary generalized seizures that are cryptogenic or symptomatic in etiology. Almost all of these studies have shown equivalence for the medications as pertains to efficacy, with the primary differences noted being related to their side-effect profiles.

Neonatal seizures

Neonatal seizures can present as focal seizures, migrating events, or multifocal seizures. Various etiologies are found, but the most common are hypoxic ischemic encephalopathy, brain malformations, general infections, and metabolic disturbances. The treatment of neonatal seizure remains unsatisfactory. Most situations require intravenously administered antiepileptic drug therapy. Phenobarbital and fosphenytoin (or phenytoin) are commonly used but are less than satisfactory and only control seizures in less than half of the neonates when used alone [23]. On the other hand, antiepileptic drugs such as topiramate appear to have anticonvulsant and neuroprotective properties in animal models of neonatal seizures.

Table 10.6 Epilepsies and epilepsy syndromes: current antiepileptic drug therapy.

Type of seizure/epilepsy	Controlled trials	Uncontrolled series
I. Neonatal seizures	Fosphenytoin (phenytoin), phenobarbital	Benzodiazepines (diazepam lorazepam), valproate, primidone, levetiracetam
II. Febrile seizures	Phenobarbital, diazepam (PO) valproate	Diazepam (PR, PO), clobazam
III. Idiopathic generalized epilepsies		
A. Benign myoclonic epilepsy in infancy		Valproate, topiramate, lamotrigine, levetiracetam, zonisamide, clonazepam, ethosuximide
B. Childhood absence epilepsy	Ethosuximide and valproate > lamotrigine*	Clonazepam, zonisamide, topiramate
C. Juvenile absence epilepsy		Valproate, lamotrigine, topiramate, zonisamide, clonazepam (felbamate)
D. Generalized tonic-clonic seizures upon awakening	Levetiracetam	
E. Juvenile myoclonic epilepsy	Topiramate, lamotrigine, levetiracetam	Valproate, lamotrigine, clonazepam, zonisamide (felbamate)
IV. Symptomatic generalized epilepsies		
A. Severe myoclonic epilepsy of infancy (Dravet syndrome)	Stiripentol	Valproate, clobazam, topiramate, clonazepam, methsuximide, zonisamide, i.v. immunoglobin, bromide, levetiracetam
B. Early myoclonic encephalopathy		ACTH, prednisone, vitamin B6, valproate, lamotrigine, topiramate, zonisamide
C. Early infantile epileptic encephalopathy (Ohtahara syndrome)		
V. Cryptogenic or symptomatic generalized epilepsies		
A. Infantile spasms	ACTH, prednisone, vigabatrin, nitrazepam, sultiame	Vitamin B6, topiramate, valproate, lamotrigine, zonisamide, sultiame, levetiracetam, (felbamate)
B. Lennox–Gastaut syndrome	Topiramate, lamotrigine, felbamate, rufinamide, clobazam	Valproate, clonazepam, zonisamide, vigabatrin, levetiracetam
C. Doose syndrome (myoclonic-astatic seizures)		Valproate, topiramate, lamotrigine, ACTH, clonazepam, ethosuximide, levetiracetam, zonisamide, (felbamate)

(*continued*)

Table 10.6 (*Continued*)

Type of seizure/epilepsy	Controlled trials	Uncontrolled series
D. Tassinari syndrome (epilepsy with myoclonic absences)		Valproate, lamotrigine, ethosuximide, clonazepam, topiramate, (felbamate)
E. Jeavons syndrome (eyelid myoclonia with absences)		Valproate, lamotrigine, ethosuximide, levetiracetam, clonazepam, (felbamate)
VI. Undetermined epilepsies		
A. Acquired epileptic aphasia (Landau–Kleffner syndrome)	None	Valproate, lamotrigine, prednisone, immunoglobins, benzodiazepines
B. Epilepsy with continuous spike waves during slow-wave sleep	None	
VII. Idiopathic localization-related epilepsies		
A. Benign rolandic epilepsy	Gabapentin, sultiame	Carbamazepine, phenobarbital, phenytoin, valproate, oxcarbazepine, levetiracetam, lamotrigine, topiramate, zonisamide, clonazepam, clobazam
B. Benign occipital epilepsy		Carbamazepine, phenytoin, valproate, clobazam, levetiracetam
VIII. Cryptogenic, symptomatic, localization-related epilepsies†		
	Carbamazepine, phenytoin, valproate, oxcarbazepine, gabapentin, lamotrigine, topiramate, tiagabine, clobazam, vigabatrin, felbamate, levetiracetam, zonisamide, pregabalin, rufinamide, lacosamide	

*Controlled trial negative results for levetiracetam (Fattore C, *et al. Epilepsia* 2011;**52**(4):802–809) and gabapentin (Trudeau V, *et al. J Child Neurol* 1996;**11**(6):470–475).
†Adjunctive therapy or monotherapy.

Table 10.7 Comparison of recommendations for the treatment of pediatric epilepsy.

Type of seizure/epilepsy	USA expert opinion*	European expert opinion†	Indian Academy of Pediatrics‡	Japanese expert consensus§
Partial-onset	OXC, CBZ	CBZ, OXC, VPA	CBZ, VPA, PB, PHT, OXC, LTG	CBZ, ZNS
BECT	OXC, CBZ	VPA	CBZ, VPA	CBZ, VPA, ZNS
CAE	ESM	ESM, VPA, LTG	VPA, ESM**, LTG, benzodiazepine	VPA, ESM
JME	VPA, LTG	VPA, LTG (LEV)	VPA, LTG, PB	VPA, CZP
LGS	VPA, TPM, LTG	VPA, LTG, TPM	VPA, CLB, LTG, TPM (LEV)	VPA, CZP, CLB
IS	VGB, ACTH	VGB, ACTH, prednisone	ACTH, VGB, VPA, TPM, NTZ	VPA, ACTH, CZP, ZNS

*Wheless JW, *et al. J Child Neurol* 2005;**20**(Suppl. 1):S1–S60 [12].
†Wheless JW, *et al. Epilept. Disord* 2007;**9**:353–412 [11].
‡Naik N, *et al. Indian Pediatr* 2009;**46**:681–698 [14].
SSOguni H, *et al. No To Hattatsu* 2010;**42**:262–266 [13].
‖ESM not currently available.
BECT, benign epilepsy of childhood with centrotemporal spikes; CAE, childhood absence epilepsy; JME, juvenile myoclonic epilepsy; LGS, Lennox–Gastaut syndrome; IS, infantile spasms.

Table 10.8 Comparative trials in newly diagnosed childhood epilepsy.

Year	Antiepileptic drugs	Citation
1987	Phenobarbital, carbamazepine	Mitchell WG *et al. Epilepsia.*[1]
1995	Carbamazepine, valproate	Verity CM *et al. Dev Med Child Neurol.*[2]
1996	Phenobarbital, phenytoin, carbamazepine, valproate	de Silva M *et al. Lancer.*[3]
1997	Oxcarbazepine, phenytoin	Guerreiro MM *et al. Epilepsy Res.*[4]
1998	Clobazam, carbamazepine, phenytoin	Canadian Study Group. *Epilepsia.*[5]
1999	Carbamazepine, vigabatrin	Zamponi N *et al. Arch Neurol.*[6]
2004	Topiramate, valproate, carbamazepine	Wheless JW *et al. J Child Neurol.*[7]
2005	Carbamazepine, lamotrigine, valproate	Steinhoff BJ *et al. Seizure.*[8]

[1]Mitchell WG, Chavez JM. *Epilepsia* 1987;**28**:56–60; [2]Verity CM, *et al. Dev Med Child Neurol* 1995;**37**:97–108; [3]de Silva M, *et al. Lancet* 1996;**347**:709–713; [4]Guerreiro MM, *et al. Epilepsy Res* 1997;**27**:205–213; [5]Canadian Study Group for Childhood Epilepsy. *Epilepsia* 1998;**39**:952–959; [6]Zamponi N, Cardinall C. *Arch Neurol* 1999;**56**:605–607; [7]Wheless JW, *et al. J Child Neurol* 2004;**19**:135–141; [8]Steinhoff BJ. *et al. Seizure* 2005;**148**:597–605.

Unfortunately, there are only anecdotal reports of nasal, gastric, or oral use of topiramate and currently no intravenous formulation is available. As such, fosphenytoin and phenobarbital remain the drugs of choice in treating neonatal seizures, and if seizures are not controlled with one of the agents, the addition of the second agent can be helpful in some children.

Febrile seizures

Most febrile seizures are self-limiting, terminating in a few minutes, and the recurrence risk does not warrant daily preventive treatment with antiepileptic drugs. The American Academy of Pediatrics does not advocate the use of long-term therapy after febrile seizures [24]. No medication introduced in the United States in the last 30 years has undergone an efficacy trial for the prevention of febrile seizures. If the child has a complex febrile seizure that is prolonged, they are at high risk of recurrence of a prolonged seizure. It has become common practice to advise families to have rectal diazepam available for use in the event of a recurrent prolonged febrile seizure. While this is the current practice, there are no controlled trials that have investigated this use, only uncontrolled studies.

Infantile spasms (West syndrome)

The American Academy of Neurology and the Child Neurology Society published a practice parameter for the treatment of infantile spasms in 2004 [25]. This was based on an extensive review of literature dating back to 1966; the authors concluded that adrenocorticotropic hormone (ACTH) was probably effective in the short-term treatment of infantile spasms, and vigabatrin was possiblye effective. Since that time, both drugs have undergone controlled trials and have been approved by the US Food and Drug Administration (FDA) as treatments for infantile spasms. These two are currently considered the drugs of choice for treating this condition. Other controlled studies have been performed with other hormonal therapies (primarily prednisone) and there have been limited studies performed with valproic acid and sulthiame. In patients who do not respond to ACTH or vigabatrin there are anecdotal reports of the use of valproic acid, topiramate, zonisamide, and other agents [26–28]. An ongoing study is evaluating the efficacy of combination therapy using ACTH and vigabatrin versus hormonal therapy alone. The goal in treating infantile spasms is different to that for many other seizure types. Here the goal is not only to control the seizure but to change the EEG so that the characteristic signature of infantile spasms, hypsarrthymia, is no longer present. This condition should be treated aggressively with close follow-up and EEG monitoring to see if this has occurred; if it has not, therapy should be changed to alternative effective agents.

Lennox–Gastaut syndrome

Many children with infantile spasms go on to develop multiple seizure types associated with Lennox–Gastaut syndrome [8]. Historically, valproic acid has been a first choice for the treatment of this condition, but it has never undergone a controlled blinded trial specifically for this syndrome [29]. Felbamate was the first drug to show efficacy in treating this condition in randomized controlled trials, but potential side effects and organ toxicities have limited its use in Lennox–Gastaut syndrome. However, other options, including topiramate, lamotrigine, rufinamide, and clobazam are available in the modern era, giving the clinician more treatment options than ever for this refractory epilepsy syndrome.

Dravet syndrome

Mutations in the alpha subunit of the voltage-gated sodium channel (NaV1.1) have been frequently implicated in severe myoclonic epilepsy of infancy (SMEI, or Dravet syndrome) and other related infantile epileptic encephalopathies (including Lennox–Gastaut syndrome and Doose syndrome). The use of antiepileptic drugs targeting voltage-gated sodium channels is discouraged in the treatment of *SCN1A*-related epilepsy syndromes. Indeed, exacerbation of seizures in SMEI has been observed with lamotrigine and carbamazepine. Stiripentol, a direct modulator of the $GABA_A$ receptor, resulted in dramatic reduction in seizure frequency when evaluated in two placebo-controlled trials as adjunct to therapy with clobazam and valproate in children with Dravet syndrome [8]. Open label studies have suggested topiramate is also refractory in the treatment of the convulsive seizures. For the treatment of Dravet syndrome, valproate is used as first-line therapy, and then typically clobazam is added to this. Topiramate is also frequently used. Stiripentol is not available in the United States, and when obtained from international sources, this can cost 7000–8000 US dollars per year. A ketogenic diet is also effective in treating these conditions (see Chapter 13).

Landau–Kleffner Syndrome/Syndrome of Continuous Spikes and Waves in Sleep (CSWS)

Electrical status epilepticus in slow-wave sleep (ESES) is the electroencephalographic signature shared by Landau–Kleffner syndrome and the syndrome of continuous spike waves in sleep [30]. In these two syndromes, ESES is associated with profound language disturbances and neurodevelopmental impairment. An overnight electroencephalogram (EEG) is usually required for diagnosis, and there are no reliable data regarding the incidence and prevalence. The vast majority of children with ESES have comorbid epilepsy, and treatment with antiepileptic drugs is commonplace. Unfortunately, no controlled trials have been performed in these conditions. High-dose oral diazepam (1 mg/kg at bedtime on the first day and then 0.5–1 mg/kg for several weeks to months) is the preferred initial treatment for ESES; with divalproex, corticosteroids (prednisone, ACTH), or intravenous immunoglobulin used in benzodiazepine-refractory cases. Small, uncontrolled case series report favorable clinical or electroencephalographic responses to clobazam, ethosuximide, and levetiracetam.

Benign epilepsy of childhood with centrotemporal spikes (BECTS)

This syndrome is considered benign, with a high likelihood of remission, and as such has not been subject to many randomized controlled antiepileptic drug trials [31]. Only two have been performed, one in the United States using gabapentin and one in Europe with sulthiame. Historically, almost every drug that has shown efficacy in the treatment of partial seizures or secondary generalized tonic-clonic seizures has been used in the treatment of this benign condition. If the clinician uses one of these medications and the parents report a deterioration in behavior, cognitive function, and possible worsening of seizures, the clinician needs to be aware that these medications rarely can exacerbate this condition. If this occurs, the clinical approach would be to discontinue the offending agent rather than increasing the dose to treat the ongoing seizures.

Childhood and juvenile absence epilepsy

In the late 1950s, ethosuximide was the first medication to be reported effective in this condition, and it still is the drug of choice. Valproate and lamotrigine have also showed efficacy in this condition, and recently a National Institutes of Health (NIH)-sponsored trial was performed, which was multicentered and evaluated over 400 children with new-onset childhood absence epilepsy [32]. In this study both ethosuximide and valproate were shown to be equally efficacious, and more efficacious than lamotrigine. Additionally, ethosuximide was slightly better tolerated. As such, ethosuximide is commonly used as first choice in children who only have absence epilepsy. If they have had any associated generalized tonic-clonic seizures (e.g., juvenile absence epilepsy), there is concern that this medication will not treat their convulsive seizures and the preference may be to begin therapy with valproate or lamotrigine. Additional studies have established that if a child does not respond to one of these agents used in monotherapy, after trials of appropriate monotherapy agents, they should pursue a combination of two of these three agents. Some children who have not had a satisfactory response to two of these agents when used as monotherapy, will have complete seizure control when they are used together in combination therapy.

Several antiepileptic drugs (phenytoin, carbamazepine, gabapentin, vigabatrin, tiagabine, and oxcarbazepine) can exacerbate epilepsy syndromes associated with generalized spike wave discharges on EEG, such as the absence epilepsies.

Juvenile myoclonic epilepsy (JME)

The treatments for generalized tonic-clonic seizures upon awakening, and juvenile myoclonic epilepsy are very similar, with both representing genetic epilepsies. Few studies have been performed in either of these, but most have been associated with juvenile myoclonic epilepsy. The overlap among these idiopathic generalized epilepsies may have as its basis a common susceptibility gene. The agent used in the treatment of juvenile myoclonic epilepsy requires efficacy against multiple seizure types. Historically, valproic acid has been the drug of choice for this syndrome [33]. While this may be one of the more effective agents, concerns about toxicity, especially in females of child-bearing age, limit its use in this population (as it is common for this epilepsy syndrome to show up in adolescence). Other broad-spectrum antiepileptic drugs, including lamotrigine, topiramate, and levetiracetam, have been evaluated. The selection of these agents will depend on the associated seizure types that are occurring in the given patient with juvenile myoclonic epilepsy (e.g., frequency of absence seizures, myoclonic seizures, and generalized tonic-clonic seizures), the age of the patient, and other treatment factors. Valproate is of well-known teratogenic potential in women of child-bearing age. If this medication needs to be used, it should be given in an extended-release formulation, dosed twice daily, to minimize peak levels, and at the lowest possible effective dose.

Partial-onset seizures

Partial-onset seizures, or localization-related epilepsies, represent the majority of seizure types seen in both children and adults. As such, this is a seizure type for which almost every new drug is tested in randomized controlled trials. Some of the medications listed in Table 10.6 have been tested in monotherapy, but most have been tested as adjunctive

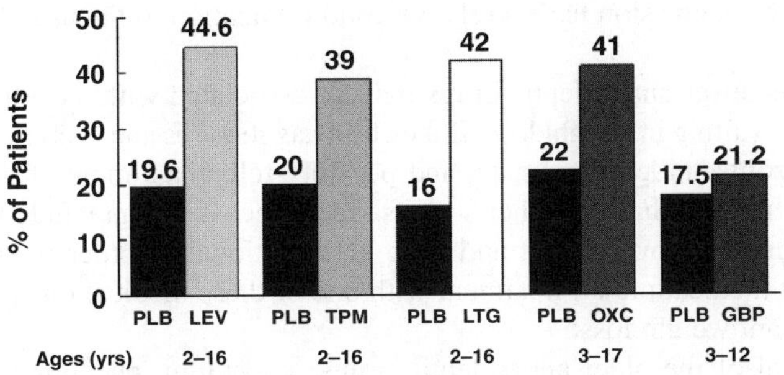

Figure 10.2 Responder rates across pediatric antiepileptic drug partial seizure trials: adjunctive therapy vs placebo (PLB). Glauser TA. *Neurology* 2006;**66**(11):1654–1660, Elterman RD, *Neurology* 1999;**52**(7):1338–1344, Duchowny M. *Neurology* 1999;**53**(8):1724–1731, Glauser TA. *Neurology* 2000;**54**(12):2237–2244, Appleton R. *Epilepsia* 1999;**40**(8):1147–1154.

treatment for partial onset seizures. Figure 10.2 illustrates the efficacy rates for newer antiepileptic drugs as adjunctive therapy in children [34–38]. While they are tested as adjunctive therapy, in order to gain regulatory approval, every medication that has ever shown efficacy for treatment of partial-onset seizures as adjunctive therapy, has been effective when used as monotherapy. A few studies have compared relative efficacy of these medications, and they typically show equal efficacy with the primary difference being side-effect profile and tolerability. As such, when the clinician is making a decision regarding drug selection for partial-onset epilepsy, he or she is guided more by the other selection factors than the efficacy of the medication.

10.3 Influence of comorbidities in children with epilepsy

After determining the seizure type and epilepsy syndrome, the clinician is typically faced with three or four medications that may be efficacious. After weighing the other factors involved in drug selection (see Table 10.1), especially the side-effect profile, the other consideration that may heavily influence the treatment selection is the comorbidity the child has. In the modern era, this has become more and more important as there is increased recognition that children with epilepsy often have other comorbidities, and these may be improved or exacerbated according to the antiepileptic drug chosen. As many as 20% of children with epilepsy have migraine headaches, and there may be a frequent temporal association with headaches and seizures. In children with epilepsy and migraines, the use of a single drug to treat both disorders is appealing. Valproate, topiramate, and gabapentin have all been found to be useful in the preventive treatment of migraines in children.

Affective disorders are common in children with epilepsy. Many antiepileptic drugs have mood stabilization properties, and some have a psychiatry indication in light of this. Positive behavioral effects and mood regulation have been noted with valproate, lamotrigine, oxcarbazepine, topiramate, carbamazepine, pregabalin, and tiagabine. If a child is taking one of these medications, and has been seizure free long enough for the medication to be discontinued, an indicator that it was also having a positive effect on mood may be worsening behavior when this medication is discontinued. If this occurs, the clinician should have a discussion with the child's family about reinitiating the medication at a dose to treat the mood or affective disorder (rather than the epilepsy). Children with significant mood disorders or depression have a relative contraindication to the use of barbiturates or benzodiazepines.

Several of the newer antiepileptic drugs may be associated with a central appetite suppressant effect, resulting in weight loss. If the child has seizures and is obese, this may make treatment with zonisamide, topiramate, and possibly felbamate more attractive treatment options (however, for felbamate other serious side effects often preclude this use). Additionally, if children are overweight and have an attentional disorder requiring treatment with a stimulant medication, co-treatment with one of these medications for epilepsy may result in significant weight loss.

Finally, several of the older antiepileptic drugs (phenytoin, phenobarbital, and carbamazepine) have significant broad spectrum inducing effects in the liver. This potent enzyme induction renders drugs that are metabolized by the liver less available and dramatically lowers their serum levels and shortens their half-life. This is especially important in children who are being treated for epilepsy and have an oncology illness (where chemotherapy regimens cannot be altered without life-threatening side effects), children on immunotherapy (organ transplantation or disease maintenance), children being treated for HIV infection, and children with elevated cholesterol (as these medications may cause further elevations, and interfere with the effects of the cholesterol-lowering medications).

10.4 Conclusions

The choice of an antiepileptic drug for the treatment of epilepsy in a child must begin with an accurate identification of the seizure type and epilepsy syndrome. Individualized assessment of risk factors and consideration of comorbidities is essential to optimization of therapy. In most epilepsy syndromes and seizure types, the newer antiepileptic drugs seem to offer at least equivalent efficacy and often far superior tolerability and fewer long-term side effects. The available options for treating children, especially those with certain refractory conditions, have increased substantially. In spite of all the progress made in recent years, epilepsy in many children remains refractory to antiepileptic drug therapy, and some children have difficulty adapting to the antiepileptic drugs. This fact should provide a strong stimulus for the continuing development of new antiepileptic drugs, especially agents targeting the developing brain. These challenges also highlight the importance of dietary and non-pharmacological therapies, discussed elsewhere in this textbook (see Chapters 12 and 13). All of these therapies are critically important in the armamentarium of the physician treating childhood epilepsy.

References

[1] Nordli DR Jr. Diagnostic difficulty in infants and children. *J Child Neurol* 2002,**17** (Suppl. 1):S28–S35.

[2] French JA, Kanner AM, Bautista J. *et al.* Efficacy and tolerability of the new anti-epileptic drugs, I: Treatment of new-onset epilepsy: report of the TTA and QSS Subcommittees of the American Academy of Neurology and the American Epilepsy Society. *Epilepsia* 2004;**45**:401–409.

[3] Glauser T, Ben-Menachem E, Bourgeios B, *et al.* ILAE Treatment Guidelines: evidence-based analysis of antiepileptic drug efficacy and effectiveness as initial monotherapy for epileptic seizures and syndromes. *Epilepsia* 2006;**47**:1094–1120.

[4] Asconape J. The selection of antiepileptic drugs for the treatment of epilepsy in children and adults. *Neurol Clin* 2010;**28**:843–852.

[5] Sankar R. Initial treatment of epilepsy with antiepileptic drugs. *Neurology* 2004;**63** (Suppl. 4):S30–S39.

[6] Hussain S, Sankar R. Pharmacologic treatment of intractable epilepsy in children: a syndrome based approach. *Semin Pediatr Neurol* 2011;**18**:171–178.

[7] Patsalos PN. Properties of antiepileptic drugs in the treatment of idiopathic generalized epilepsies. *Epilepsia* 2005;**46**(Suppl. 9):140–148.

[8] Wheless JW. Managing severe epilepsy syndromes of early childhood. *J Child Neurology* 2009;**24**:8S, 24S–32S.

[9] National Institute for Health and Clinical Excellence. The epilepsies: the diagnosis and management of the epilepsies in adults and children in primary and secondary care. *NICE,* 2012. Available at: www.nice.org.uk/cg137.

[10] Scottish Intercollegiate Guidelines Network. Diagnosis and management of epilepsies in children and young people. Available at: awww.sign.ac.uk/guidelines/fulltext/81/index.html.

[11] Wheless JW, Clarke DF, Arzimanoglou A, Carpenter D. Treatment of pediatric epilepsy: European expert opinion. *Epileptic Disord* 2007;**9**:353–412.

[12] Wheless JW, Clarke DF, Carpenter D. Treatment of pediatric epilepsy: expert opinion. *J Child Neurol* 2005;**20**(Suppl. 1):S1–S56.

[13] Oguni H, Hirano Y, Katoh I. Treatment of childhood epilepsies: Japanese Expert Consensus study and a comparison of the results with those of the USA and EU. *No To Hattatsu* 2010;**42**:262–266.

[14] Expert Committee on Pediatric Epilepsy, Indian Academy of Pediatrics. Guideline for diagnosis and management of childhood epilepsy. *Indian Pediatr* 2009;**46**:681–698.

[15] Mitchell WG. Carbamazepine versus phenobarbital for partial onset seizures in children. *Epilepsia* 1987;**28**:56–60.

[16] de Silva M, MacArdie B, McGowan M, *et al.* Randomised comparative monotherapy trial of phenobarbitone, phenytoin, carbamazepine, or sodium valproate for newly diagnosed childhood epilepsy. *Lancet* 1996;**347**:709–713.

[17] Verity CM, Hosking G, Easter DJ. A multicentre comparative trial of sodium valproate and carbamazepine in paediatric epilepsy. The Paediatric EPITEG Collaborative Group. *Dev Med Child Neurol* 1995;**37**:97–108.

[18] Guerreiro MM, Vigonius U, Pohlmann H, *et al.* A double-blind controlled clinical trial of oxcarbazepine versus phenytoin in children and adolescents with epilepsy. *Epilepsy Res* 1997;**27**:205–213.

[19] Canadian Study Group for Childhood Epilepsy. Clobazam has equivalent efficacy to carbamazepine and phenytoin as monotherapy for childhood epilepsy. *Epilepsia* 1998;**39**:952–959.

[20] Zamponi N, Cardinali C. Open comparative long-term study of vigabatrin vs carbamazepine in newly diagnosed partial seizures in children. *Arch Neurol* 1999;**56**:605–607.

[21] Wheless JW, Neto W, Wang S, EPMN-105 Study Group. Topiramate, carbamazepine, and valproate monotherapy: double-blind comparison in children with newly diagnosed epilepsy. *J Child Neurol* 2004;**19**:135–141.

[22] Steinhoff BJ, Ueberall MA, Siemes H, *et al.* The LAM-SAFE Study: lamotrigine versus carbamazepine or valproic acid in newly diagnosed focal and generalized epilepsies in adolescents and adults. *Seizure* 2005;**148**:597–605.

[23] Painter MJ, Scher MS, Stein AD. Phenobarbital compared with phenytoin for the treatment of neonatal seizures. *N Engl J Med* 1999;**341**:485–489.

[24] Steering Committee on Quality Improvement and Management, Subcommittee on Febrile Seizures American Academy of Pediatrics. Febrile seizures: clinical practice guideline for the long-term management of the child with simple febrile seizures. *Pediatrics* 2008;**121**:1281–1286.

[25] Mackay MT, Weiss SK, Adams-Webber T, *et al.* Practice parameter: medical treatment of infantile spasms: report of the American Academy of Neurology and the Child Neurology Society. *Neurology* 2004;**62**:1668–1681.

[26] Pellock JM, Hrachovy R, Shinnar S, *et al.* Infantile spasms: a U.S. consensus report. *Epilepsia* 2010;**51**:2175–2189.

[27] Lux AL, Edwards SW, Hancock E, *et al.* The United Kingdom Infantile Spasms Study comparing vigabatrin with prednisolone or tetracosactide at 14 days: a multicentre, randomized controlled trial. *Lancet* 2004;**364**:1773–1778.

[28] Elterman RD, Shields WD, Bittman RM, *et al.* Vigabatrin for the treatment of infantile spasms: final report of a randomized trial. *J Child Neurol* 2010;**25**:1340–1347.

[29] Arzimanoglou A, French J, Blume WT, *et al.* Lennox–Gastaut syndrome: a consensus approach on diagnosis, assessment, management, and trial methodology. *Lancet Neurol* 2009;**8**:82–93.

[30] Wheless JW, Simos PF, Butler IJ. Language dysfunction in epileptic conditions. *Semin Pediatr Neurol* 2002;**9**:218–228.

[31] Oguni H. Treatment of benign focal epilepsies in children: when and how should be treated? *Brain Dev* 2011;**33**:207–212.

[32] Glauser TA, Cnaan A, Shinnar S, *et al.* Ethosuximide, valproic acid, and lamotrigine in childhood absence epilepsy. *N Engl J Med* 2010;**362**:790–799.

[33] Mantoan L, Walker M. Treatment options in juvenile myoclonic epilepsy. *Curr Treat Options Neurol* 2011;**13**:355–370.

[34] Appleton R, Fichtner K, LaMoreaux L, *et al.* Gabapentin as add-on therapy in children with refractory partial seizures: a 12-week, multicentre, double-blind, placebo-controlled study. Gabapentin Paediatric Study Group. *Epilepsia* 1999;**40**:1147–1154.

[35] Glauser TA, Nigro, Sachdeo R, *et al.* Adjunctive therapy with oxcarbazepine in children with partial seizures. The Oxcarbazepine Pediatric Study Group. *Neurology* 2000;**54**:2237–2244.

[36] Duchowny M, Pollock JM, Graf WD, *et al.* A placebo-controlled trial of lamotrigine add-on therapy for partial seizures in children. Lamictal Pediatric Partial Seizures Study Group. *Neurology* 1999;**53**:1724–31.

[37] Elterman RD, Glauser TA, Wylie E, *et al.* A double-blind, randomized trial of topiramate as adjunctive therapy for partial-onset seizures in children. Topiramate YP Study Group. *Neurology* 1999;**52**:1338–1344.

[38] Glauser TA, Avala R, Elterman RD, *et al.* Double-blind placebo-controlled trial of adjunctive levetiracetam in pediatric partial seizures. *Neurology* 2006;**66**:1654–1660.

11 Adverse effects of antiepileptic drugs

James W. Wheless

Department of Pediatric Neurology, University of Tennessee Health Science Center; Le Bonheur Comprehensive Epilepsy Program and Neuroscience Institute, Le Bonheur Children's Hospital, Memphis, TN, USA

11.1 Introduction

Antiepileptic drugs constitute the mainstay of treatment for children with epilepsy. Efficacy for the specific seizure or epilepsy syndrome drives drug selection, but the side-effect profile of the medication and the potential for toxicity are also important considerations [1,2]. Adverse events in children related to antiepileptic drugs and reported to the US Food and Drug Administration's (FDA's) adverse event reporting system rank in the top reported categories, something not observed in adults. Drug reactions that lead to hospital admission are more common among certain drug classes, including antiepileptic drugs [3]. Treatment of children with epilepsy strives for complete seizure control without medication side effects. An antiepileptic drug's retention rate is mainly determined by its side-effect profile. Parents and patients must have adequate participation in treatment decisions and provide informed consent. Treatment must balance the goal of complete seizure control with potential drug toxicity during both the acute and chronic stages of treatment. Antiepileptic drugs can cause non-specific dose-related responses, unique

Epilepsy in Children and Adolescents, First Edition. Edited by James W. Wheless.

effects specific to a given drug, or rare but potentially dangerous idiosyncratic reactions [4–6]. Drug treatment, in the absence of a specific history of allergy, is a matter of trial and error. However, specific cellular mechanisms or metabolic abnormalities may account for some adverse drug effects. In addition, the potential for adverse effects in young children is greater than in adults, because young children have immature detoxification mechanisms and because doses must be individually adjusted for a much wider range of body sizes and weights.

Treatment requires accurate diagnosis followed by knowledgeable use of drugs based on pharmacokinetics and pharmacodynamics. Although commonly used antiepileptic drugs are effective in many patients, the efficacy of any selected drug for a specific patient cannot be predicted. Therefore, sequencing of treatment using several drugs is often required. Plasma levels, determined by therapeutic drug monitoring, guide treatment in some cases, but titration of dose, using development of dose-related symptoms as an end point, should be completed before a drug is declared ineffective.

Common problems can be anticipated, but dangerous, unexpected, and rare individual responses and reactions require physicians to provide detailed information during the process of informed consent. Thus, the parents and any other people involved in the care of the child must be informed in explicit terms about the potential for serious or even fatal reactions to drugs and how to appropriately monitor for these. Adverse drug reactions are noxious effects occurring at doses of drugs used appropriately in children for prevention, diagnosis, or therapy. Some of these reactions depend on pharmacokinetic effects, with dose-dependent responses that correlate with plasma concentrations of a drug.

Pharmacodynamic effects occur when target organ responses are altered in a way that is independent of plasma concentrations: such effects may be unique to a drug or to an individual patient. Serious non-dose-related adverse drug reactions cause drug-induced disease, which may be acute or may occur following chronic treatment (potentially fatal idiosyncratic reactions are listed in Table 11.1) [4,6]. Neurotoxicity, either dependent on dose or pharmacodynamic in nature, may occur at the time of drug initiation, during dose escalation, or at the time of peak plasma levels. These mild and reversible effects include sedation, changes in behavior, tremor, vertigo, diplopia, nystagmus, ataxia, or even dysarthria.

Dose-related neurotoxicity becomes more common when two or more antiepileptic drugs are used in combinations. Monotherapy improves patient adherence, reduces total costs of medication, and may eliminate interactions that could cause additive adverse effects. Monotherapy use of commonly available antiepileptics results in seizure control in 50–70% of patients with epilepsy.

Almost all antiepileptic drugs have caused idiosyncratic reactions or drug allergies. Such reactions may be severe, unpredictable, and although rare, may be life threatening. Idiosyncratic responses to antiepileptic drugs in a given patient are associated with cellular, immunological, or enzymatic characteristics that are unique to that patient [6]. Drug clearance by oxidation requires catalyzed effects of microsomal membrane-bound mixed function oxidases that contain cytochrome P450. The P450 terminal oxidases receive electrons from reduced nicotinamide adenine dinucleotide phosphate (NADPH) and reduced nicotinamide adenine dinucleotide (NADH). Heterogeneity of the P450 system causes apparent specificity, with isozyme families produced by the same gene family. Some antiepileptic drugs are metabolized through such mixed function oxidases, yielding stable, unstable, or

Table 11.1 Idiosyncratic reactions to antiepileptic drugs

	Drug															
Reaction	CBZ	ETS	FBM	GBP	LCS	LEV	LTG	OXC	PB	PHT	PGB	RFM	TPM	TGB	VPA	ZNS
Agranulocytosis	x	x	x						x	x					x	
Allergic dermatitis	x	x	x				x	x	x	x		x	x	x	x	x
Aplastic anemia	x	x	x							x					x	
Bone metabolism	x								x	x						
Hepatic failure	x		x						x	x					x	
Nephrolithiasis													x			x
Pancreatitis	x														x	
Serum sickness	x	x							x	x					x	
Stevens–Johnson syndrome	x	x					x		x	x					x	

CBZ, carbamazepine; ETS, ethosuximide; FBM, felbamate; GBP, gabapentin; LCS, lacosamide; LEV, levetiracetam; LTG, lamotrigine; OXC, oxcarbazepine; PB, phenobarbital; PHT, phenytoin; PGB, pregabalin; RFM,rufinamide; TPM, topiramate; TGB, tiagabine; VPA, valproate; ZNS, zonisamide.

potentially reactive molecular species. Accumulation of reactive and toxic intermediates as a result of drug treatment and metabolism is determined by genetically derived enzyme activity. Thus, the metabolism of ring compounds via arene oxidase with impairment of metabolism of the arene oxide product could occur with deficiency of the enzyme epoxide hydrolase. The arene form of phenytoin has been implicated as the cause of hepatotoxicity, teratogenicity, bone marrow toxicity, and allergic skin reactions.

Antiepileptic drug hypersensitivity reaction – the DRESS syndrome (**d**rug **r**eaction (or **r**ash) with **e**osinophilia and **s**ystemic **s**ymptoms) – occurs early in the treatment with aromatic antiepileptic medications [7–9]. Components include rash, fever, and eosinophilia and may include lymphadenopathy and life-threatening hepatic necrosis. Skin rash may or may not be pruritic and in the form of an exanthema. More severe reactions include exfoliative dermatitis, erythema multiforme, Stevens–Johnson syndrome, or even toxic epidermal necrolysis. Adverse reactions of the idiosyncratic type tend to be immune-mediated effects in a susceptible individual.

The mechanisms are not completely understood, but most rash and hypersensitivity syndromes probably are related to pharmacogenetic variation and drug biotransformation. Immune involvement is suggested by the occurrence of a sensitization interval of 7–10 days after first exposure to a drug. In fact, T lymphocytes have been found in the perivascular infiltrate and epidermis (CD8C, CD4C) of patients with carbamazepine-induced toxic epidermal necrolysis. Reactive metabolites produced by bioactivation are cytotoxic by binding to microsomal proteins. Such covalent adducts are formed in hepatic cytochrome P450-mediated reactions.

Antibodies to P450 enzymes, with epitopes such as anti-CYP2D6 and anti-CYP3A, have amino acid sequences similar to those of viral or fungal origin that suggest prior host-dependent immune responses to infections that are unique to a person's human lymphocyte antigen (HLA) genotype. With exposure to a bioactivated antiepileptic drug, a chemical modification of the P450 enzyme occurs. These effects may be from formation of reactive drug metabolites, free radical species, or impairment of the detoxification enzyme. These changes in enzyme function yield altered peptide structures that result in the immune response.

The impact of enzyme-inducing drugs on bone health must be considered in all children. Although most institutionalized patients in the modern era are given calcium and vitamin D supplementation, these simple interventions and the need for assessment of bone density in children on long-term antiepileptic drugs (especially if non-ambulatory) must be kept in mind and monitored. Fracture rates in children with epilepsy, although not clearly defined, are higher than the general population. Seizure-related falls, trauma, osteopenia and osteoporosis, and incoordination secondary to a comorbid condition or antiepileptic drug exposure likely all contribute [5,10]. Osteoporosis or low mineral density occurs in children with epilepsy, particularly in association with chronic exposure to certain antiepileptic drugs including enzyme-inducing antiepileptics (e.g., phenobarbital, phenytoin, and carbamazepine) and valproate. Children with epilepsy who are not fully ambulatory or have decreased exposure to sunlight and are on chronic antiepileptic therapy are at increased risk of osteoporosis. Screening with dual-emission X-ray absorptiometry (DXA) scanning and serological testing of vitamin D levels should be routinely considered. When a child with epilepsy treated with antiepileptic drugs shows evidence of a pathological fracture or osteoporosis, treatment options are available and changing the antiepileptic drug may be necessary.

11.2 Specific drugs [11]

Adrenocorticotropic hormone (ACTH)

Although ACTH is used as a first-line treatment of infantile spasms, its well-documented side effects act as a deterrent to its general use in this context. This drug carries a class warning for common side effects related to glucocorticoids. Older case reports describe the development of *Pneumocystis carinii* pneumonia, bacteremia, meningitis, and disseminated intravascular coagulopathy in patients being treated with ACTH for infantile spasms. However, the dose and duration of therapy in those cases would be considered prolonged and unconventional by more contemporary standards. A more recent retrospective review of side effects in the modern era using a high-dose ACTH protocol (starting at 150 U/m^2/day then tapered over 5–6 weeks) reported an improved side-effect profile [12]. This study showed increased weight gain in the first 2 months on ACTH, and transient increases in systolic and diastolic blood pressure seen over the same time interval, with typical normalization by 3 months. Rarely did a patient require short-term therapy with an antihypertensive agent. All patients were able to continue with ACTH. Other side effects noted were minor and included psychomotor agitation, sleep disturbance, minor infections, and electrolyte abnormalities, all of which were readily reversible as the dose was reduced. There was no increased rate of emergency or primary visits, hospitalizations, or infections requiring intravenous therapy.

Carbamazepine

Carbamazepine (CBZ) is catalyzed by the hepatic mono-oxygenases, forming an epoxide at the 10-11-double bond of the azepine ring (CBZ-10,11-epoxide). This new compound is associated with toxic symptoms. Hydration of the epoxide occurs through the microsomal epoxide hydrolase. Inhibition of that enzyme, as occurs with concomitant valproate administration, increases the quantity of the epoxide.

Severe reactions to carbamazepine can cause hematopoietic, skin, hepatic, and cardiovascular changes. Rash occurs in 5–8% of patients, and rarely may progress to exfoliative dermatitis or to bullous reaction, such as Stevens–Johnson syndrome, especially in patients of Oriental descent. Transient leukopenia is observed in 10–12% of patients; however, fatal reactions such as aplastic anemia are rare. Both parents and patients must be reassured that frequent monitoring of blood counts and liver values is unnecessary.

Presymptomatic blood test abnormalities have not been reported in patients who develop systemic hypersensitivity reactions to carbamazepine. Genetic susceptibility among patients who of Oriental ethnicity means that pretreatment screening is critically important for patient care [13].

Clobazam

Pivotal US trials with clobazam were performed in the treatment of the Lennox–Gastaut syndrome [14]. At the doses studied (0.25–1.0 mg/kg/day) adverse events were generally mild or moderate and were similar between dose groups. Adverse events experienced by more than 5% of patients include somnolence, lethargy, sedation, salivary hypersecretion, constipation, aggression, hypomania, and insomnia. Patients discontinue medication because of aggression, reduced oral intake as a consequence of sedation and drooling, or ongoing seizures, somnolence, chorea, defiant behavior, and encephalopathy. All of the events resolve with discontinuation of clobazam. General laboratory abnormalities were not detected.

Ethosuximide

Ethosuximide has a half-life that would allow single daily dosing, but such large doses of the drug can cause nausea, gastric distress, and abdominal pain unless the drug is given with meals and in divided doses. Rash and headaches, and on rare occasion leukopenia, pancytopenia, and aplastic anemia have occurred. Neurological effects include headache (which may be severe), lethargy, agitation, aggressiveness, depression, and memory problems. Psychiatric disorders and drug-induced lupus have been reported to occur in children.

Ezogabine (retigabine)

Ezogabine (ezogabine is US, retigabine in rest of world) is a unique antiepileptic chemical entity with broad-spectrum anticonvulsant properties; it enhances the potassium current mediated by human KCNQ2 and KCNQ3 potassium channels, as well as potentiating gamma-aminobutyric acid (GABA)-evoked currents [15]. The most common adverse events were central nervous system related. These included dizziness, somnolence, fatigue, confusion, asthenia, ataxia, blurred vision, and tremor. In addition, nausea and urinary tract infections were seen. Bladder epithelium contains voltage-gated potassium channel isoforms, and ezogabine causes urodynamic effects in animals. Ezogabine can cause a reddish-orangish discoloration of urine, which is harmless and is unrelated to bladder function. ECGs were performed in human trials due to concerns about possible cardiac effects of the potassium channel action. No abnormalities were noted. No changes in hematological parameters or hepatic enzymes were noted and there have been no significant rashes reported.

Felbamate

Felbamate can cause headaches, insomnia, and weight loss. Drug interactions with felbamate are significant and may cause clinical toxicity or seizure exacerbation. When felbamate is added to carbamazepine, levels of the parent compound decline by 20–25%, but the metabolite carbamazepine-10,11-epoxide increases by as much as 50%. These effects suggest induction of cytochrome P450, along with partial inhibition of epoxide hydrolase. This interaction induces carbamazepine's side effects; the combination also causes headaches.

Serious idiosyncratic reactions to felbamate, including aplastic anemia and hepatoxicity, have occurred, and clinical risk profiles for felbamate suggest the need for a screening strategy [16]. Importantly, no cases of aplastic anemia have been reported in children younger than 13 years of age. The mean time for presentation is 154 days, with very few cases being reported after 6 months of exposure. Similarly, severe hepatoxicity associated with felbamate has been reported, but this risk seems to be similar to that reported for valproate. Although felbamate has no predilection for age, children have been affected by severe, life-threatening hepatoxicity associated with the drug. The clinical risk profile for the idiosyncratic reactions includes some features such as Caucasian race, female gender, and adulthood that are not specific. However, more worrisome clinical risk factors were: a previous antiepileptic drug allergic reaction; cytopenia; an immune disorder, especially lupus erythematosus; and less than 1 year of treatment.

Guidelines for the use of felbamate emphasize that this drug should be used for severe epilepsy that is refractory to other therapies, for example in patients with Lennox–Gastaut syndrome. Treatment should be preceded by a careful history to uncover past indications of hematological toxicity, hepatoxicity, and autoimmune diseases. Women with autoimmune disease account for the largest proportion of those who develop aplastic anemia. Baseline routine hematological and liver function tests should be performed and the parents and child should be fully informed of the potential risk. Parents should be educated about symptoms that may signify either hematological change or hepatotoxicity. Dose escalations should be made slowly, and dosages of adjunctive medication must be corrected for known drug interactions.

Gabapentin

Gabapentin, 1-(aminomethyl)-cyclohexane acetic acid, is structurally related to gamma-aminobutyric acid (GABA). Uniquely for an antiepileptic drug, gabapentin is not bound to plasma proteins nor is it metabolized. Its bland pharmacokinetic properties include no hepatic enzyme induction and little effect on plasma levels of other antiepileptic drugs. Adverse effects detected in treated patients were typically neurotoxic, but withdrawal from studies was infrequent. Children and adults have similar adverse effect profiles. Patients may experience weight gain. Peripheral edema with normal plasma protein and albumin is rare. Use in children who have cognitive impairment may be accompanied by an increased incidence of hyperactivity and aggressive behavior.

Lacosamide

Lacosamide is a functionalized amino acid that selectively enhances slow activation of voltage-gated sodium channels [17]. In controlled clinical trials, the adverse effects most commonly leading to discontinuation were dizziness, ataxia, vomiting, diplopia, nausea, vertigo, and blurred vision.

The majority of adverse events in patients were reported as mild or moderate. Many of the adverse events were dose related. Those events occurring in more than 5% of patients were diplopia, nausea, vomiting, and central nervous system disorders (dizziness, headache, ataxia, and somnolence).

Dose-dependent prolongations in the PR interval with lacosamide were observed in clinical studies in patients and healthy volunteers. First-degree atrioventricular (AV) block and second-degree or higher AV block have been reported as rare incidents. Lacosamide should be used with caution in patients with known conduction problems or with severe cardiac disease. In such patients, obtaining an ECG before beginning lacosamide and after lacosamide is titrated to steady state is recommended. Patients should be made aware of the symptoms of second-degree or higher AV block (e.g., slow or irregular pulse, feeling light-headed and fainting) and told to contact their physician should any of these occur.

Lamotrigine [18]

Central nervous system-related side effects of lamotrigine include lethargy, fatigue, and mental confusion. Serious rashes have occurred and appear to be correlated with the rate of dose increase and are more common in children, especially if they are taking valproate concomitantly. Current guidelines in the United States require that lamotrigine be discontinued if a rash develops.

An erythematous rash with a morbilliform pattern or urticaria, or patterns with a maculopapular component are most common; however, some patients can develop erythema multiforme and blistering skin reactions such as Stevens–Johnson syndrome or toxic epidermal necrolysis. Simple rashes require careful assessment to ensure that hypersensitivity syndrome is not developing. Such sensitivity reactions often include fever, lymphadenopathy, elevated liver enzyme values, and altered numbers of circulating cellular elements of blood.

In drug trials conducted in the United States, rash was observed in about 10% of patients, 3.8% had to discontinue the drug, and 0.3% were hospitalized. Most serious rashes developed within 6 weeks of beginning treatment with lamotrigine. In children treated in drug trials, rash was observed in 12.9%, and was serious in 1.1%, with half of that group having Stevens–Johnson syndrome. Of note, more than 80% who experienced a serious rash were being treated with valproate or had been given higher than recommended doses. Rash was suspected to be a drug interaction with valproate, which inhibits the metabolism of lamotrigine, causing diminished clearance and resulting in higher blood levels. When treatment guidelines are followed, the incidence of serious rash is reduced. In the United States, if a rash develops, it is advised that the drugs be discontinued.

Table 11.2 provides the suggested drug initiation treatment plan for lamotrigine in children, and strict adherence to this results in dramatic lowering of the rate of rash and serious rash.

Levetiracetam [19]

Levetiracetam is effective against partial-onset seizures, primary generalized tonic-clonic seizures, juvenile myoclonic epilepsy, and photosensitivity-related epilepsy syndromes. Treatment-emergent side effects typical for a CNS-active drug have been reported from the clinical trials, including somnolence, asthenia, dizziness, nervousness, and anorexia. Behavioral changes reported in children include aggression, emotional lability, oppositional behavior, and psychosis. A possible mechanism for these side effects may be exacerbation of a pre-existing tendency. Rarely, significant thrombocytopenia may occur.

Oxcarbazepine [20]

Oxcarbazepine is a keto analog of carbamazepine that is rapidly converted to 10,11-dihydro-10-hydroxycarbamazepine by cytosol arylketone reductase. Renal clearance of the metabolites correlates with measured creatine clearance. Dizziness, sedation, and fatigue, possibly

Table 11.2 Guidelines for use of lamotrigine

	For patients taking valproate	For patients NOT taking carbamazepine, phenytoin, phenobarbital, primidone, or valproate	For patients taking carbamazepine, phenytoin, phenobarbital, primidone, and NOT taking valproate
A. Escalation regimen for children 2–12 years of age			
Weeks 1 & 2	0.15 mg/kg/day in one or two divided doses	0.3 mg/kg/day in one or two divided doses	0.6 mg/kg/day in two divided doses
Weeks 3 & 4	0.3 mg/kg/day in one or two divided doses	0.6 mg/kg/day in one or two divided doses	1.2 mg/kg/day in two divided doses
Weeks 5 onward to maintenance	Increase 0.3 mg/kg/day every 1 to 2 weeks	Increase 0.6 mg/kg/day every 1 to 2 weeks	Increase 1.2 mg/kg/day every 1 to 2 weeks
Usual maintenance dose	1–5 mg/kg/day in one or two divided doses (maximum 200 mg/day)	4.5–7.5 mg/kg/day in one or two divided doses (maximum 300 mg/day)	5–15 mg/kg/day in one or two divided doses (maximum 400 mg/day)
B. Escalation regimen for children over 12 years of age			
Weeks 1 & 2	25 mg every other day	25 mg every day	50 mg every day
Weeks 3 & 4	25 mg every day	50 mg every day	100 mg every day in two divided doses
Weeks 5 onward to maintenance	Increase by 25–50 mg/day every 1–2 weeks	Increase by 50 mg/d every 1–2 weeks	Increase by 100 mg/day every 1–2 weeks
Usual maintenance dose	100–200 mg/day with valproate alone	225–375 mg/day in two divided doses	300–500 mg/day in two divided doses

dose related, were reported in clinical trials. Hyponatremia has occurred with this drug, and may be more common with children taking other medication that may affect sodium balance (diuretics, selective serotonin reuptake inhibitors, etc.). Rash occurs infrequently, and Stevens–Johnson syndrome and toxic epidermal necrolysis are rare. Cross-reactivity in patients allergic to carbamazepine has been reported.

Phenobarbital

Phenobarbital has been in continual use for almost 100 years. Common side effects in children include behavioral changes with hyperactivity and irritability; adults experience drowsiness. Altered attention, effects on cognition, and even depression may be dose related or occur in specific patients unrelated to plasma levels. Dose-related neurotoxic effects include nystagmus, ataxia, altered coordination, cognitive changes, dyskinesia, and altered sleep patterns. Idiosyncratic reactions to phenobarbital include allergic dermatitis, Stevens–Johnson syndrome, serum sickness, hepatic failure, agranulocytosis, and aplastic anemia. Folate deficiency in patients treated with antiepileptic drugs is claimed to be associated with behavioral changes. Phenobarbital is known to exacerbate acute intermittent porphyria.

Induction of hepatic oxidative metabolism by phenobarbital is a fundamental mechanism for drug interaction. Vitamin D metabolism is induced by phenobarbital; thus, handicapped and non-ambulatory children receiving this drug or other enzyme-inducing antiepileptic drugs may develop osteopenia or osteoporosis; vitamin D supplementation is important in these children. Phenobarbital alters absorption and reduces metabolism of vitamin K. Neonates of mothers treated with phenobarbital need vitamin K supplementation to prevent neonatal hemorrhagic disease. Prophylactic vitamin K must be given during the last month of gestation, at the beginning of labor, and to the infant at birth.

Long-term phenobarbital treatment may cause connective tissue changes, with coarsened facial features, Dupuytren's contracture, Ledderhose syndrome (plantar fibromas), and frozen shoulder. Sedative effects of phenobarbital may exacerbate absence, atonic, and myoclonic seizures, although other mechanisms may be operating. Sudden withholding of doses of short-acting barbiturates may precipitate drug withdrawal seizures or even status epilepticus. Phenobarbital's slow rate of clearance makes such acute seizures less of a problem, but dose tapering is recommended if discontinuation is planned. Some children may experience mild withdrawal symptoms, including tremor, sweating, restlessness, irritability, weight loss, disruption of sleep, and even psychiatric manifestations. Infants of mothers treated with phenobarbital may manifest irritability, hypotonia, and vomiting for several days after delivery.

Phenytoin

Phenytoin is a weak organic acid, poorly soluble in water, and available as a sodium salt or free acid. It is metabolized by hepatic enzymes that are capacity limited. This system is commonly saturated at serum concentrations of 8–10 μg/mL. The saturation kinetics of phenytoin results in large changes in total serum concentrations with small changes in the maintenance dose. The half-life increases with higher plasma concentrations. Because of the saturation kinetics, those changes must be made with care. Another challenge to phenytoin use is its alteration of steady state by interactions with other drugs.

Dose-related side effects of phenytoin include nystagmus, ataxia, altered coordination, cognitive changes, and dyskinesia. Infrequently, children may become irritable or hyperactive. Children rarely develop nystagmus even when they are overtly ataxic and have elevated serum levels of phenytoin. A constellation of anorexia, weight loss, and vomiting in a child should suggest phenytoin toxicity. Although not strictly a pharmacological problem, phenytoin causes some drug-specific effects that do not appear to be related to dose.

Facial features may coarsen and body hair will change in texture and become dark in color. Acne may develop and worsen, and gingival hypertrophy is common. Use of phenytoin monotherapy and strict dental hygiene will minimize gingival hypertrophy. Other effects of long-term phenytoin use are osteopenia, osteoporosis, and lymphadenopathy. Folate deficiency may be severe enough to cause megaloblastic anemia: a transient encephalopathy is said to occur by a similar mechanism. Prolonged exposure to high plasma levels of phenytoin has been linked to cerebellar atrophy.

Idiosyncratic reactions that may be fatal include allergic dermatitis, hepatotoxicity, serum sickness reaction, and aplastic anemia. Drug-induced lupus erythematosus reactions have been observed.

Pregabalin [21]

Pregabalin binds to the alpha-2/delta site (an auxiliary subunit of the voltage-gated calcium channel) in central nervous system tissues. Dose-related adverse effects in controlled trials as adjunctive therapy for adult patients with partial-onset seizures included digestive system and central nervous system side effects. These consist of increased appetite with weight gain, peripheral edema, dizziness, somnolence, ataxia, tremor, blurred vision, and diplopia. Adverse reactions leading to discontinuation are dizziness, ataxia, and somnolence.

Rare post-marketing reports of angioedema and a hypersensitivity reaction have been noted. Immediate discontinuation of pregabalin in patients with these symptoms is recommended.

Rufinamide [22]

Rufinamide is a triazole derivative structurally unrelated to any currently marketed antiepileptic drug. Rufinamide has been granted orphan drug status for adjunctive treatment of patients with Lennox–Gastaut syndrome. The precise mechanism by which rufinamide exerts its antiepileptic effects is unknown, but it centers around modulation of activity of the sodium channel. Based on the clinical trials, rufinamide appears to be well tolerated. The adverse experiences most commonly associated with discontinuation of rufinamide (>1%) were similar in adults and children: dizziness, fatigue, and headache. In clinical trials, the majority of the adverse events were judged to be mild or moderate, often transient in nature, and largely occurring during the titration phase. The most common adverse events (occurring in more than 5%) pooled from all studies of patients with epilepsy were headache, dizziness, fatigue, somnolence, and nausea. Children appear to report fewer adverse events than adults. In all pediatric trials, with a fixed titration dose of 45 mg/kg/day, only somnolence, vomiting, and headache were associated with rufinamide administration. Importantly, there is no increased incidence of neuropsychiatric side effects. This side-effect profile of rufinamide is similar to other drugs that affect the sodium channel (e.g., primarily non-specific gastrointestinal and central nervous system side effects). An antiepileptic drug hypersensitivity syndrome has occurred in association with rufinamide therapy, and if a serious rash related to rufinamide is suspected, the drug should be discontinued and alternative treatment started. In adolescents and adults, cognitive assessments were performed at baseline and after 3 months, and none of the cognitive tests for psychomotor speed, attention, or working memory demonstrated any significant worsening at any dose of rufinamide studied. In a placebo-controlled study of the QT interval, a higher percentage of subjects taking rufinamide had a QT shortening greater than 20 ms compared with placebo, but none had a reduction below 300 ms. Patients with potassium channelopathy associated with familial short QT syndrome cannot be treated with rufinamide. Caution is advised when administering rufinamide with other drugs or diseases that shorten the QT interval (e.g., digoxin toxicity, hypercalcemia, hyperkalemia, and acidosis). No changes in laboratory data were observed.

Topiramate [23]

Topiramate has a monosaccharide-type structure. The drug has multiple mechanisms of action, including influence of sodium and chloride channels, blocking non-*N*-methyl-D-aspartate (NMDA) glutamate receptors and inhibiting carbonic anhydrase. Treatment-emergent adverse effects with add-on studies revealed ataxia, impaired concentration, confusion, dizziness, fatigue, paresthesias, somnolence, and abnormal thinking. Nephrolithiasis and dose-related weight loss are potential problems that require discussion with patients. Many side effects in studies were caused by forced titration to higher doses. Adverse cognitive effects occur at higher doses; however, slowing the pace of dose increase reduces the impact on cognitive function.

Serious rashes have occurred. Reports of acute secondary angle-closure glaucoma require cautioning of patients to report ocular pain or altered visual acuity immediately. This typically presents as acute onset of near-sightedness early on. As with other drugs that alter carbonic anhydrase, oligohydrosis with hyperthermia has been reported, and this is probably more common in children, especially in hot weather. Children require careful monitoring for this problem, and limitation of outside exposure in hot weather while on this medication. An encephalopathy has been reported in patients who take topiramate combined with valproate.

Tiagabine

The most commonly identified side effects in the pivotal trials conducted with tiagabine included dizziness, asthenia, muscle weakness, nervousness, tremor, impaired concentration, lethargy, and depression. These occur during dose titration. Reasons for withdrawals from the trials included the occurrence of confusion, somnolence, ataxia, and dizziness. Hepatic clearance of this medication indicates the need to reduce the dose in patients with liver disease.

Valproate

Gastrointestinal effects commonly accompany initiation of valproate treatment, and include nausea, diarrhea, abdominal pain, or even vomiting. Administration of the drug at meal times or administration of a delayed-release or slow-release form of the drug cause abatement of the symptoms in most patients. Three dose-related effects occur commonly. Tremor with intention and at rest is age and dose related, but this symptom is found less in children. Bodyweight gain is another side effect, with 20–50% of patients reporting this problem. Patients report appetite stimulation, and weight change may lead to discontinuation of the drug. Hair loss is not uncommon but is often transient. Supplementation with multivitamins containing zinc and biotin may protect the hair.

Thrombocytopenia occurs in a pattern that suggests it is dose related. Platelet counts will vary without dose changes and are commonly asymptomatic. Petechial hemorrhage and ecchymosis do occur, necessitating lowering the dose or even discontinuing the drug. Transient thrombocytopenia may occur in the setting of a viral infection, and may be more commonly associated with chicken pox.

Other less frequently encountered side effects include sedation or encephalopathy. Acute encephalopathy and even coma may develop on initial exposure to valproate. Upon investigation, these patients may be severely acidotic and may have elevated organic acid excretion. Valproate is known to sequester coenzyme A; therefore, such patients are suspected of having a partially compensated defect in the mitochondrial beta-oxidation enzymes. Dermatological abnormalities are unusual, but may be severe.

Acute hemorrhagic pancreatitis may develop in younger patients, and a fatal outcome has been reported. Abdominal pain reported by patients receiving valproate should lead to the measurement of serum amylase and lipase levels.

Hyperammonemia may occur in the absence of hepatic dysfunction, possibly caused by inhibition of either nitrogen elimination or urea synthesis. In rare instances, an insufficiency of urea cycle enzymes, such as ornithine transcarbamylase deficiency, may be present.

Age-related changes in the pharmacokinetics of valproate should be anticipated because of the high percentage of the drug that is protein bound. Valproate's acid is a branch-chain carboxylic acid that may be metabolized via either mitochondrial pathways or cytoplasmic enzymes. Dehydrogenation of valproate results in the accumulation of 2-en, 3-en, and 4-en valproate compounds. Synthesis of the 4-en metabolites is highest in infants and declines with age. The 2-en compound has anticonvulsant potency. Valproic acid binds albumin at high- and low-affinity sites. This binding is saturable causing the free fractions to increase with dose, and more dramatically as serum levels exceed 90 μg/mL.

A review of patients developing hepatotoxicity from treatment with valproate suggests that the highest risk is in children younger than 2 years being treated with several antiepileptic drugs. Additional risk factors are presumed metabolic disorders or severe epilepsy complicating mental retardation and organic brain disease. Most clinicians, however, consider this pattern of incidence too restrictive or insufficiently detailed to allow identification at highest risk. Management strategies are further complicated by the fact that routine laboratory monitoring does not predict the development of fulminant and irreversible hepatic failure. Some patients who develop fatal hepatic toxic reactions have never exhibited abnormalities on specific hepatic function tests. Conversely, abnormalities of serum ammonia, carnitine, fibrinogen, and hepatic function tests have been reported to occur without the presence of clinically significant hepatotoxic reactions. Therefore, reporting of clinical symptoms and identification of high-risk patients are more reliable means of monitoring. Vomiting is an initial symptom in serious cases. Nausea, vomiting, and anorexia with lethargy, drowsiness, and coma are critical symptoms and must be evaluated immediately. Although early drug discontinuation may reverse hepatotoxic reactions in some patients, fatalities may still result. Some patients have required liver transplantation. No biochemical marker has been identified to differentiate those who survive from those with a fatal outcome. Patients with hepatic failure have been rescued by intravenous carnitine supplementation. Measurement of urinary organic acids and a metabolic evaluation are recommended in high-risk patients or in any patient without an established reason for mental retardation and seizures.

Identifying high-risk patients was supported by Dreifuss and colleagues [24]. Most all of the cases of hepatic toxicity occurred in the first 6 months of treatment, but some patients developed hepatic toxicity up to 2 years after initiation. Children under 2 years of age receiving polytherapy with antiepileptic drugs had a 1 in 500–800 chance of a fatal hepatotoxic event. Negative predictors were also documented. Patients at negligible risk are those older than 10 years treated with valproate alone and free of indications of underlying metabolic and neurological disorders. Children at intermediate risk were those between 2 and 10 years of age on monotherapy, and all patients requiring polytherapy.

Patients reported with fatal hepatotoxicity had, in the majority of cases, neurological abnormalities including mental retardation, encephalopathy, and decline of neurological function. In those rare reported cases of patients older than 21 years, one-half had degenerative diseases of the nervous system. In two other reports, one-half of patients who had fatalities were neurologically abnormal, and in another series, all patients in the 11–20-year-old age group were neurologically abnormal. A more recent review identifies only 7 of 26 adults reported with fatal hepatic failure from valproate to be considered neurologically normal.

Specific biochemical disorders associated with valproate hepatotoxicity include urea cycle defects, organic acidurias, multiple carboxylase deficiency, mitochondrial or respiratory chain dysfunction, cytochrome aa3 deficiency in muscle, pyruvate carboxylase deficiency, and hepatic pyruvate dehydrogenase complex deficiency. Clinical disorders associated with valproate toxicity include GM1 gangliosidosis type 2, spinocerebellar degeneration, Friedreich ataxia, Laflora body disease, Alpers disease, and mitochondrial encephalopathy with ragged red fibers (MERRF syndrome). Patients with such disorders must be identified because of their greater risk for valproate hepatotoxicity.

Vigabatrin [25]

Vigabatrin, also known as gamma-vinyl GABA, increases tissue concentrations of GABA by irreversible inhibition of GABA-transaminase, the enzyme that degrades GABA. The effects on a specific enzyme make pharmacokinetics less relevant.

Severe changes in behavior, with agitation, hallucinations, and altered thinking, are thought to be dose related. Depression is a potential problem in all patients. General adverse events are those expected with an antiepileptic; drowsiness, irritability, ataxia, and headaches have been observed.

Loss of peripheral retinal function and vision is of concern. Both children and adults treated with vigabatrin have been reported with a concentrically constricted visual field. If this visual field constriction occurs, it appears not to resolve after the drug is discontinued.

Use of this drug should be restricted to children with infantile spasms and those with severe and intractable complex partial seizures. In these patients with severely refractory seizures the risk of visual loss should be outweighed by the need of treatment for seizures.

Zonisamide

Zonisamide is a sulfonamide drug that may cross-react in patients known to be allergic to sulfa-containing compounds. Adverse effects including drowsiness, altered thinking, anorexia, dizziness, ataxia, fatigue, somnolence, confusion, and poor concentration were seen in clinical trials. Zonisamide has been associated with nephrolithiasis. Children may develop oligohydrosis and hyperthermia. Parents must be taught to be vigilant when the child is exposed to a hot environment, and provide skin moisture to aid in convection cooling. Children with a history of renal stones or a family history of such should be informed of the risk of nephrolithiasis and must be advised to remain adequately hydrated.

11.3 At-risk profiles and monitoring

One strategy to minimize the risk of serious adverse effects is to identify high-risk patients by constructing clinic profiles from reports of idiopathic drug reactions. For example, the risk of hepatotoxicity from valproate is too non-specific to be of much practical help; however, at-risk patients are less than 2 years old, are being treated with other antiepileptic drugs, and have known metabolic disease with developmental delay. Patients fitting this profile need detailed laboratory screening for the presence of metabolic disorders, including measurement of serum lactate, serum pyruvate, serum carnitine, serum uric acid, routine hematological and chemical tests, urinary organic acid levels, and possible genetic screening for mitochondrial defects (*POLG1*, the polymerase gamma A gene) [26]. Prothrombin time, partial thromboplastin time, and determination of arterial blood gases and ammonia levels are also useful tests.

The risk of hypersensitivity, including Stevens–Johnson syndrome and toxic epidermal necrolysis, has been identified to markedly increase in those with the HLA-B∗1502 allele of the human leukocyte antigen [13] This allele occurs predominantly in persons of Han Chinese, Filipino, Malaysian, South Asian Indian, and Thai decent. Physicians have been advised by the FDA to screen Asian patients for this allele prior to prescribing carbamazepine and to consider the risk in using phenytoin or fosphenytoin in these patients. Cross-reactivity and sensitivity between carbamazepine, phenytoin, phenobarbital, lamotrigine, and oxcarbazepine does occur.

After the antiepileptic drug is selected, the physician must review its relative benefits and risks, documenting this discussion in the patient's medical record. This process forms the basis for informal informed consent. Patients should be the told the criteria by which their child will be evaluated for success, and be reminded of the trial and error of drug selection and the methods for changing drugs. The family must know the nature of the medication side effects, what may need to be tolerated, and how side effects influence drug titration. Serious, life-threatening, idiosyncratic effects must be explained clearly but within the context of rarity. Although the family and the patient must be ready to report symptoms, the physician must identify patients who lack advocates or have impaired communication. These patients may require a monitoring strategy (Box 11.1). A screening program may be useful in some high-risk patients.

Box 11.1 Recommendations for monitoring

1. Obtain screening laboratory studies before initiation of antiepileptic drug treatment. Baseline studies provide a benchmark and could identify patients with special risk factors that could influence drug selection.
2. Blood and urine monitoring in otherwise healthy and asymptomatic patients is unnecessary [28,29].
3. Identify high-risk patients before treatment:
   - Presumptive biochemical or genetic disorders.
   - Altered systemic health.
   - Neurodegenerative disease.
   - History of significant adverse drug reactions.
   - Patients without an advocate:
     - those unable to communicate require a different strategy;
     - patients with multiple handicaps.
4. For newly introduced drugs, follow recommended guidelines for monitoring until the numbers of children treated increase and data become available.

As new drugs become available, physicians have an obligation to review source documents for those medications and advise on a strategy of treatment and monitoring. Side-effect data tend to be limited when a new drug is first introduced, so patients should be given as much information as possible and the drug should be initiated cautiously. Baseline data should be obtained, the patient must be prepared to contact the physician if they experience adverse events, and the physician must facilitate that communication. Chemical and hematological monitoring may be recommended in the material developed by the manufacturer in concert with the FDA. It may be wise to follow those guidelines until broader clinical experiences are available. Table 11.3 summarizes screening laboratory tests that may aid in detection of adverse effects of antiepileptic drugs.

Finally, in early 2008, the FDA issued an alert regarding suicidality and the use of antiepileptic drugs [27]. Parents and caregivers for adolescents and older children must be aware of this problem, and patients' behavior monitored. Based upon a meta-analysis of 199 placebo-controlled trials including 11 antiepileptic drugs, the FDA found approximately twice the risk of suicidal thoughts or behavior in those taking antiepileptic drugs as compared to placebo (0.43% vs 0.22%, respectively). The FDA interpreted the findings as likely representing a class effect, generally consistent across medications. Rates differed, however, between the studied antiepileptic drugs, and older antiepileptic drugs were not included in the analysis. Demographic factors (e.g., age) did not clearly influence risk. These findings prompted labeling changes, and now all antiepileptic drugs carry the class warning for suicidality. In children and adolescents, assessments should include age-appropriate questions regarding risk factors. Age-appropriate standardized inventories may also help assess suicidality. The clinician should also consider the patient's access to antiepileptic drugs, and the potential for overdose. Historically, phenobarbital has been noted to carry the highest risk of suicidality, and this medication along with benzodiazepines should be avoided in those with depression. If older children and adolescents are identified with mood

Table 11.3 Screening laboratory tests to detect adverse drug reactions to antiepileptic drugs

Antiepileptic drug	Laboratory tests
Carbamazepine	CBC, liver enzymes
Ethosuximide	CBC, reticulocyte count
Felbamate	CBC, reticulocyte count, liver enzymes, hepatic panel
Lamotrigine	CBC, liver enzymes, hepatic panel
Oxcarbazepine	Serum sodium
Phenobarbital	CBC, liver enzymes
Phenytoin	CBC, liver enzymes
Topiramate	Urine for microscopic hematuria and renal ultrasound (renal stones), intraocular pressure (glaucoma)
Valproate	CBC, liver enzymes, hepatic panel, serum lipase and amylase (pancreatitis), ammonia, plasma carnitine panel, urine organic acids
Vigabatrin	Visual fields (perimetry)
Zonisamide	Urine for microscopic hematuria and renal ultrasound (renal stones)

CBC, complete blood count with platelet count.

disorders or suicidality, the physician needs to document the level of risk, interventions taken, and plans for monitoring. Psychotherapy and antidepressants are helpful, and referral to a psychiatrist is indicated.

References

[1] Cramer JA, Mintzer S, Wheless J, Mattson RH. Adverse effects of antiepileptic drugs: a brief overview of important issues. *Expert Rev Neurother* 2010;**10**:885–891.

[2] Wheless J. Intractable epilepsy: A survey of patients and caregivers. *Epilepsy Behav* 2006;**8**:756–764.

[3] Johann-Liang R, Wyeth J, Chen M, Cope JU. Pediatric drug surveillance and the Food and Drug Administration's adverse reporting system: an overview of reports, 2003–2007. *Pharmacoepidemiol Drug Saf* 2009;**18**:24–27.

[4] Greenwood RS. Adverse effects of antiepileptic drugs. *Epilepsia* 2000;**41**(Suppl. 2):S42–S52.

[5] Kothare SV, Kaleyias J. The adverse effects of antiepileptic drugs in children. *Expert Opin Drug Saf* 2007;**6**:251–265.

[6] Zaccara F, Franciotta D, Perucca E. Idiosyncratic adverse reactions to antiepileptic drugs. *Epilepsia* 2007;**48**:1223–1244.

[7] Roychowdhury S, Svensson CK. Mechanisms of drug-induced delayed type hypersensitivity reactions in the skin. *AAPS J* 2005;**7**:E834–846.

[8] Gerull R, Nelle M, Schaible T. Toxic epidermal necrolysis and Stevens–Johnson syndrome: a rewiew. *Crit Care Med* 2011;**39**:1531–1532.

[9] Arif H, Buchsbaum R, Weintraub D, *et al.* Comparison and predictors of rash associated with 15 antiepileptic drugs. *Neurology* 2007;**68**:1701–1709.

[10] Samaniego EA, Sheth RD. Bone consequences of epilepsy and antiepileptic medications. *Semin Pediatr Neurol* 2004;**14**:196–200.

[11] Physician's Desk Reference. Oradell, NJ: Medical Economics Co., 2011.

[12] Partikian A, Mitchell WG. Major adverse events associated with treatment of infantile spasms. *J Child Neurol* 2007;**22**:1360–1366.

[13] Hung SI, Chung WH, Liu ZS, *et al.* Common risk allele in aromatic anti-epileptic drug induced Stevens–Johnson syndrome and toxic epidermal necrolysis in Han Chinese. *Pharmacogenomics* 2010;**11**:349–356.

[14] Conry JA, Ng, YT, Paolicchi J. Clobazam in the treatment of Lennox–Gastaut syndrome. *Epilepsia* 2009;**50**:1158–1166.

[15] Faught E. Ezogabine: a new angle on potassium gates. *Epilepsy Curr* 2011;**11**:75–78.

[16] French J, Smith M, Faught E, Brown L. Practice advisory: The use of felbamate in the treatment of patients with intractable epilepsy: report of the Quality Standards Subcommittee of the American Academy of Neurology and the American Epilepsy Society. *Neurology* 1999;**52**:1540–1545.

[17] Chung SS. Lacosamide: new adjunctive treatment option for partial-onset seizures. *Expert Opin Pharmacother* 2010;**11**:1595–1602.

[18] Culy CR, Goa KL. Lamotrigine. A review of its use in childhood epilepsy. *Paediatr Drugs* 2000;**2**:299–330.

[19] Verrotti A, D'Adamo E, Parisi P, *et al.* Levetiracetam in childhood epilepsy. *Paedriat Drugs* 2010;**12**:177–186.

[20] Bang L, Goa K. Oxcarbazepine: a review of its use in children with epilepsy. *Paediatr Drugs* 2003;**5**:557–573.

[21] Zaccara G, Gangemi P, Perucca P, Specchio L. The adverse event profile of pregabalin: a systematic review and meta-analysis of randomized controlled trials. *Epilepsia* 2011;**52**:826–836.

[22] Wheless JW, Conry J, Krauss G, *et al.* Safety and tolerability of rufinamide in children with epilepsy: a pooled analysis of 7 clinical studies. *J Child Neurol* 2009;**24**:1520–1525.

[23] Ormrod D, McClellan K. Topiramate: a review of its use in childhood epilepsy. *Paediatr Drugs* 2001;**3**:293–319.

[24] Bryant AE, Dreifuss FE. Valproic acid hepatic fatalities. III. U.S. experience since 1986. *Neurology* 1996;**46**:465–469.

[25] Wheless JW, Ramsay RE, Collins SD. Vigabatrin. *Neurotherapeutics* 2007;**4**:163–172.

[26] Isohanni P, Hakonen AH, Euro L, *et al.* POLG1 manifestations in childhood. *Neurology* 2011;**76**:811–815.

[27] Hesdorffer DC, Kanner AM. The FDA alert on suicidality and antiepileptic drugs: Fire or false alarm? *Epilepsia* 2009;**50**:978–986.

[28] Pellock JM, Willmore LJ. A rational guide to routine blood monitoring in patients receiving antiepileptic drugs. *Neurology* 1991;**41**:961–964.

[29] Camfield P, Camfield C. Monitoring for adverse effects of antiepileptic drugs. *Epilepsia* 2006;**47**(Suppl. 1):31–34.

12 Vagus nerve stimulation therapy and epilepsy surgery

Kate Van Poppel and James W. Wheless

Department of Pediatric Neurology, University of Tennessee Health Science Center; Le Bonheur Comprehensive Epilepsy Program and Neuroscience Institute, Le Bonheur Children's Hospital, Memphis, TN, USA

Epilepsy and seizures affect at least 2.3 million individuals in the United States. Although antiepileptic drugs (AEDs) are the primary form of treatment, recent outcome surveys reveal only mixed success even with the new AEDs that have become available over the past decade. Approximately one-third of patients have seizures that are unresponsive to pharmacological therapy [1,2] (Figure 12.1). In addition, safety and tolerability issues associated with both the acute and chronic side effects and toxicity complications further diminish the effectiveness of AEDs. Non-adherence to AEDs, which is highly prevalent in the epilepsy population, also diminishes treatment effectiveness and further increases mortality as well as significantly increasing healthcare utilization [3]. Children and adolescents with uncontrolled seizures continue to carry a sad burden of higher mortality rates, higher rates of accidents and injuries, greater incidence of cognitive and psychiatric impairment, poor self-esteem, higher levels of anxiety and depression, and greater social stigmatization or isolation compared with the non-epileptic population. The shortcomings of AEDs in improving overall outcome highlight the need for other treatments (Figures 12.2 and 12.3). Other treatment options are available for select subgroups of patients, including the ketogenic

Epilepsy in Children and Adolescents, First Edition. Edited by James W. Wheless.

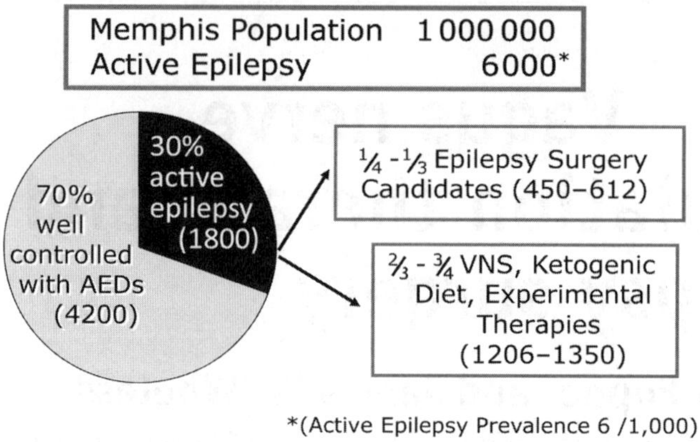

Figure 12.1 Epidemiology of epilepsy treatment. AED, antiepileptic drugs; VNS, vagus nerve stimulation.

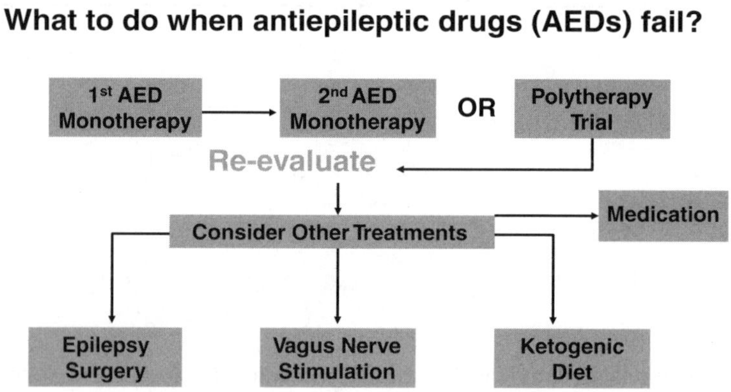

Figure 12.2 Treatment-resistant epilepsy.

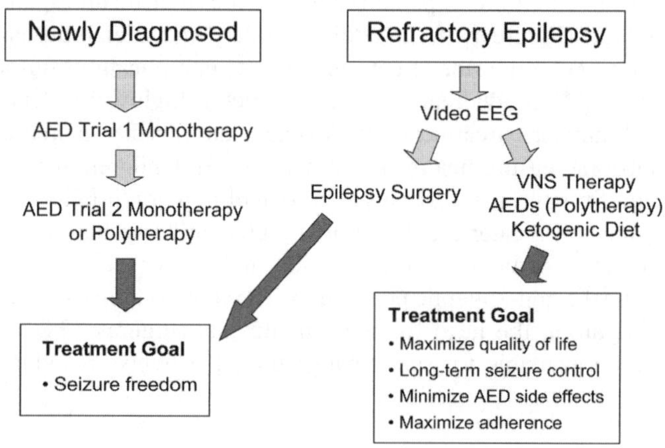

Figure 12.3 Evaluation options and treatment goals for newly diagnosed and refractory epilepsy. AED, antiepileptic drugs; EEG, electroencephalogram; VNS, vagus nerve stimulation.

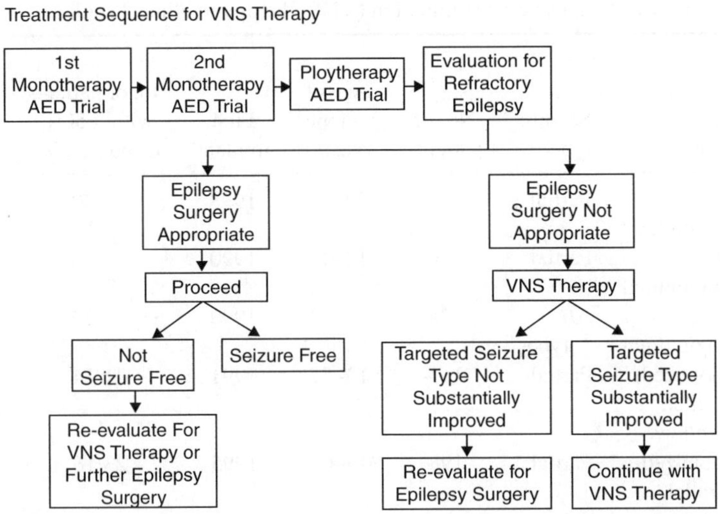

Figure 12.4 Decision algorithm for epilepsy surgery and vagus nerve stimulation (VNS) therapy.

diet (see Chapter 13), epilepsy surgery, and vagus nerve stimulation. In this chapter we will discuss the role of vagus nerve stimulation and epilepsy surgery (Figure 12.4).

12.1 Vagus nerve stimulation

History

The effect of vagus nerve stimulation (VNS) on central nervous system (CNS) activity has been documented, with early attempts in the 1880s linking electrical vagal nerve and cervical sympathetic stimulation and carotid artery compression to the treatment of seizures. In the mid-1980s, Jacob Zabara, a biophysicist at Temple University, again suggested that electrical stimulation of the vagus nerve might prevent seizures. This theory was proved in his first canine studies [4], and a company – Cyberonics, Inc. (Houston, Texas) – was founded in 1987 to develop VNS therapy, which would be delivered by a patented method using a generator device modeled after a cardiac pacemaker.

In 1988, the first patient to have a VNS therapy device implanted became seizure free (Table 12.1) [5]. Five acute-phase clinical studies analyzing the safety and effectiveness of VNS therapy followed (Table 12.2). The first two single-blind trials showed improved

Table 12.1 History of vagus nerve stimulation (VNS) therapy.

1985	First animal studies
1988	First human implant
1992	First randomized active control study (E03) completed
1994	European Community approval
1996	Second randomized active control study (E05) completed
1997	US Food and Drug Administration commercial approval
February 2012	65 000+ implants worldwide for both epilepsy and depression

Table 12.2 Efficacy of vagus nerve stimulation (VNS) therapy in clinical studies.

Study	Design	Seizure type	No. of patients	Age of patients (years)	First implant	No. of patients with >50% response (%)	Mean reduction in seizures/day (%)
E01	Pilot, longitudinal	Partial	11	20–58	1998	30	24*
E02	Pilot, longitudinal	Partial	5	18–42	1990	50	40
E04	Open, longitudinal	All types	124	3–63	1990	29	7*
E03	Randomized, parallel, high/low	Partial	115	13–57	1991	31/14	24*/6
E05	Randomized, parallel, high/low	Partial	198	13–60	1995	23/16	28†/15†

*$P \leq 0.05$ by Student's t test.
†$P < 0.0001$ by analysis of variance.

control in adults with intractable partial seizures who were not candidates for epilepsy surgery [5–7]. The subsequent two randomized, blinded, active-control trials (E03, E05) led to approval of VNS therapy by the US Food and Drug Administration (FDA) in July 1997 for the adjunctive treatment of refractory partial-onset seizures among patients 12 years of age or older [8,9]. VNS therapy also is approved for the treatment of epilepsy without age or seizure-type restrictions (in most countries) and treatment-resistant depression in 68 countries around the world, including member nations of the European Union, Canada, Australia, and China.

The VNS therapy system is made up of a pulse generator, a bipolar VNS lead, a programming wand with accompanying software for an IBM-compatible laptop or hand-held computer, a tunneling tool, and hand-held magnets (Figure 12.5). The generator transmits electrical signals to the vagus nerve through the lead. The software allows placement of the programming wand over the generator for reading and altering stimulation parameters (Table 12.3). Each stimulation period is preceded by 2 s of ramp-up time and followed by 2 s of ramp-down time.

Efficacy

Five clinical studies, including two randomized, controlled, double-blind, pivotal studies, were performed to evaluate the safety and effectiveness of VNS therapy among patients whose partial or generalized seizures were not well controlled by AED therapy. The two controlled pivotal studies (EO3 and EO5) showed statistically significant mean reductions in seizure frequency for patients receiving high stimulation (active treatment group) compared with low stimulation (control group) [8,9]. These findings were seen independent of AEDs, and no factors were identified that predicted response.

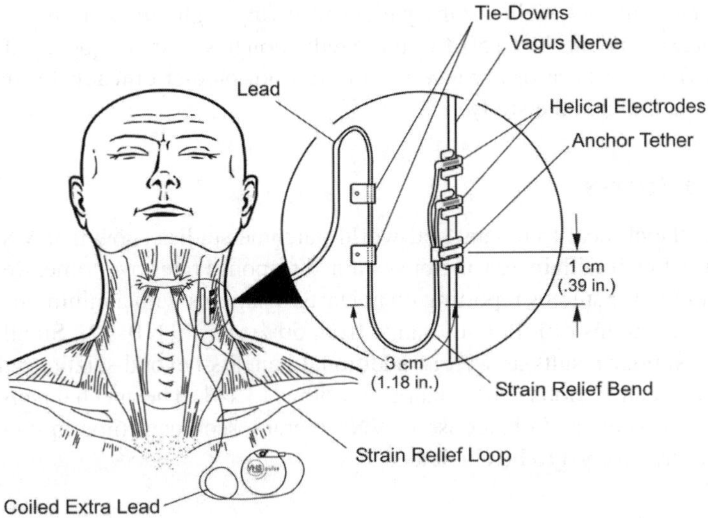

Figure 12.5 Implantable components of the VNS (vagus nerve stimulation) Therapy System.

The two pivotal studies – E03 and E05 – were designed to demonstrate that high (therapeutic) and low (non-therapeutic) stimulation of the vagus nerve had different effects on the frequency of partial seizures. The effects of VNS therapy during the 12-week randomized phases of the studies, which began 2 weeks after implantation, were gauged against 12–16-week baseline periods. E03 acute-study patients [8] ($n = 114$ implanted) had had epilepsy for an average of 22 years. Seizure frequency was reduced by at least half in 31% of patients in the high-stimulation group, compared with 14% in the low-stimulation group. No patients became seizure free during the acute phase, but some reported reduced seizure severity and improved postictal recovery periods. Patients in the high-stimulation group either aborted or decreased 59.8% of seizures with the magnet. No factors were identified that predicted response.

The similarly designed E05 study was the largest prospective controlled trial of a device for epilepsy treatment ever conducted [9]. Patients ($n = 199$) had a median of 0.51 to 0.58

Table 12.3 Vagus nerve stimulation (VNS) variable ranges.

Parameter	Units	Range	Suggested
Output current	Milliamps	0–3.5	>1.50
Signal frequency	Hertz	1–30	20
Pulse width	Microseconds	130–1000	250
ON-time	Seconds	7–60	7*
OFF-time	Minutes	0.2–180	0.3
Magnet Settings			
Output current	Milliamps	0–3.5	>1.75
Pulse width	Microseconds	130–1000	250
ON-time	Seconds	7–60	14

*Other options are 14 sec. on/0.5 min off, or 30 sec. on/3 to 5 min. off.

seizures per day during baseline. One patient receiving high stimulation became seizure free, and 23.4% of patients had a 50% or more reduction in seizure frequency after 3 months of treatment. The presence or absence of aura did not predict efficacy. Of the implanted patients, 99% completed the study.

Real-world outcomes

In addition to the clinical trial data, real-world outcome studies show that VNS therapy is an effective treatment with increasing or sustained response rates over time. Response rates from the literature for studies reporting on at least 50 patients with a minimum of 3 months to more than 12 months of follow-up range from 50% to 59% [10–12]. Small prospective studies report similar results as well as additional benefits beyond seizure reduction such as reduced postictal periods and seizure duration [13,14]. The mechanisms underlying the gradual improvements in response to VNS therapy seen over time in these long-term studies, however, have yet to be elucidated.

Pediatric and special populations

Studies indicate that response to VNS therapy is independent of age, seizure type, or epilepsy syndrome. The largest retrospective pediatric study to date showed the same median reduction in seizure frequency of 51% at 6 months among patients aged 12 to 18 years ($n = 56$) and among those less than 12 years of age ($n = 20$) [15]. Longer-term retrospective studies among pediatric patients treated with VNS therapy showed increasing response rates over time similar to those seen in the real-word outcome data for adults with VNS [16,17]. A retrospective study of 46 children implanted under the age of 18 (median age of 12.1 years) showed median seizure frequency reductions of the order of 60% over 3 years with VNS therapy, with response rates more favorable among patients less than 12 years of age [16]. Particularly favorable results, including reduced seizure frequency and severity and improved quality of life, have been reported among patients in open studies of Lennox–Gastaut syndrome and other refractory childhood epilepsies, such as hypothalamic hamartomas, epileptic encephalopathies, Rett syndrome, and tuberous sclerosis complex [15,18–24]. Verbal performance, alertness, motor and cognitive functions, and general behavior improved, sometimes dramatically [22,25]. A retrospective study [25] showed that improved quality of life (particularly in the area of alertness) was associated with VNS therapy in patients with autism ($n = 59$) or Landau–Kleffner syndrome (LKS; $n = 6$), with more than one-half of the patients in each group also experiencing a 50% or more reduction in seizure frequency at follow-up (12 months of follow-up for autism and 6 months for LKS patients). Studies have also shown both seizure frequency reductions and improved quality of life among both institutionalized and non-institutionalized patients with mental retardation/developmental delay (MRDD) [26]. Another report among three children admitted to the intensive care unit (ICU) after developing status epilepticus showed that VNS therapy allowed early cessation of status and discharge from the ICU [27]. Although the effectiveness of VNS therapy in the treatment of generalized seizures is not well documented, open studies indicate that VNS is a favorable treatment option among this patient population regardless of age.

A study of stimulation parameters among patients of different ages recommended age-related stimulation adjustments based on age-related changes seen in vagus nerve characteristics. Early studies indicated that children might respond more rapidly than adults, with reductions in the interval between stimulations resulting in improved control (see Table 12.3). Additional pediatric studies reported that higher output currents might be required, particularly when lower pulse durations are used [28]. Optimal stimulus parameter settings for patients of various ages or with specific seizure types or syndromes, however, have not yet been defined.

Mechanism of action

The mechanisms by which VNS reduces seizure activity in humans were not known at the time VNS therapy was approved by the FDA. However, considerable progress in mechanistic VNS research has been made. Electrical stimulation of the peripheral vagus nerve requires polysynaptic transmission to mediate the antiseizure effect. The anatomical distribution of vagal projections underlies the therapeutic actions of VNS therapy. Vagal visceral afferents have a diffuse CNS projection, with activation of these pathways broadly affecting neuronal excitability [29].

Experimental studies

The first studies of the antiepileptic effects of VNS were conducted in 1937. Subsequent experiments in cats showed that vagal stimulation produced EEG desynchronization or synchronization, depending on the parameters used. Hypersynchronized cortical and thalamocortical neuronal interactions characterize seizures; therefore, it was postulated that desynchronizing these activities would lead to antiseizure effects of VNS.

Initial work in cats and recent studies of strychnine-induced seizures in the dog, maximal electroshock and pentylenetetrazol-induced seizures in the rat, and the alumina-gel monkey model showed that cervical vagal stimulation decreased interictal epileptiform discharges and shortened or aborted seizures; the antiepileptic effects outlasted the stimulus and depended on its frequency and cumulative duration [30,31]. Most central projections of the vagus nerve terminate in the nucleus of the solitary tract, with extensions to brainstem nuclei, thalamus, amygdala, and hypothalamus. Increased release of gamma-aminobutyric acid (GABA) and glycine by brainstem and subcortical nuclei was proposed as the antiepileptic mechanism of VNS therapy. Brainstem nuclei are known to influence seizure susceptibility; based on animal studies, the nucleus of the tractus solitarius is likely the key brainstem structure involved in transmitting and modulating VNS antiseizure effects.

Animal studies have established three distinct temporal patterns for the antiseizure effects of VNS: (i) acute abortive effects, in which an ongoing seizure is attenuated by VNS; (ii) acute prophylactic effects, in which seizure-inducing agents are less effective in provoking seizures when applied at the end of VNS; and (iii) chronic progressive prophylactic effects, in which total seizure counts are reduced more following chronic VNS stimulation. In addition, animal studies have shown that VNS can antagonize the development of epilepsy in the kindling model of epileptogenesis. Based on these studies, the mechanism of action of VNS therapy appears to be largely distinct from that of medical therapies.

Clinical studies

Initial scalp recording performed in a small number of adults did not demonstrate a significant effect of VNS on EEG total power, median frequency, power in any of the conventional frequency bands, interictal epileptiform activity, or the waking or sleep background rhythms. At seizure onset, however, VNS has terminated both the clinical and the EEG seizure activity [32]. More recent studies have suggested that some patients may have a change in interictal epileptiform discharges (IEDs) with VNS.

Positron emission tomography (PET) $H_2{}^{15}O$ cerebral blood flow (CBF) imaging identifies the neuroanatomical structures recruited by VNS in humans. Acute CBF alterations were correlated with long-term therapeutic response, in an attempt to exclude those regions that show changes in VNS-induced synaptic activity but may not participate in VNS-related antiseizure actions. Decreased seizure frequency was associated with increased CBF only in the right and left thalami. Studies of chronic VNS therapy have shown the same anatomical distribution of CBF [33].

Selection of candidates

In the United States, VNS therapy is indicated as an adjunctive treatment for adults and adolescents 12 years of age or older with refractory partial-onset seizures. In the European Union, VNS therapy is indicated as an adjunctive treatment for patients with partial- or generalized-onset seizures without an age limitation. However, indications for VNS therapy were derived from the clinical trial experience, not from an understanding of its physiological action. Age, sex, and frequency of seizures, secondarily generalized seizures, or interictal EEG spikes do not predict response to VNS therapy. The type or number of coadministered AEDs also do not predict response. Therefore, while children benefit considerably from VNS therapy, randomized controlled studies have not been completed. Patients with other seizure types or epilepsy syndromes also may benefit from VNS therapy.

Although optimal use parameters continue to be defined, candidates should meet the following criteria: (i) medically refractory seizures; (ii) adequate trials of at least two AEDs; (iii) exclusion of non-epileptic events; and (iv) ineligibility for epilepsy surgery (see Figures 12.3 and 12.4). Focal resective surgery (temporal lobectomy or lesional neocortical epilepsy) is preferred for appropriate patients because of its superior seizure-free rate. Recent open studies suggest that VNS therapy may be used among patients considered for corpus callosotomy, producing lower rates of morbidity [34], and among those who have previously undergone epilepsy surgery [15]. Earlier use (within 2 years of seizure onset or after failure of two or three AEDs) of VNS therapy may also produce a higher response rate. Patients with a history of non-adherence to their AED regimens, particularly those on polypharmacy, may also be good candidates for VNS therapy because of the assured compliance and lack of further drug–drug interactions with VNS therapy.

Use of VNS therapy is contraindicated in patients with prior bilateral or left cervical vagotomy, and safety and efficacy have not been established for stimulation of the right vagus nerve. Patients with existing pulmonary or cardiac disease should be evaluated carefully before implantation; chronic obstructive pulmonary disease may increase the risk for dyspnea. Patients with cardiac conduction disorders were not studied in the controlled trials. A cardiologist's evaluation should precede implantation, with post-procedural Holter monitoring performed if clinically indicated. Patients with a history of obstructive sleep apnea should be treated with care, as an increase in apneic events during stimulation is possible. Lowering stimulation frequency (i.e., pulse width and signal frequency to 250 μs and 20 Hz, respectively) may prevent exacerbation of this condition [35].

Initiation and maintenance

Hospitalization for implantation of the device is preceded by evaluations by a neurologist and by a surgeon with experience in the carotid sheath. With the patient typically under general anesthesia, the lead wires are placed on the left cervical vagus nerve and the generator is placed in a subcutaneous pocket in the left upper chest [36,37]. Intraoperative electrical impedance testing ensures integrity of the system. Rare cases of bradycardia, asystole, or both mandate initial lead testing in the operating room. Correct placement of the lead electrodes around the vagus nerve is critical.

Prophylactic antibiotics may be administered both in the operating room and postoperatively. The patient can be discharged after the procedure, which usually lasts less than 1 hour, or can be observed overnight. Discharge education should include care of the incisions and use of the magnet. In clinical studies, the generator's output current was kept at 0 mA for the first 2 weeks; however, programmed stimulation is now being initiated at 0.25 mA in some operating rooms. Dosages of AEDs are generally kept stable for the first 3 months of stimulation unless an early response is noted.

A few weeks after implantation, the patient is examined to confirm wound healing and proper generator operation, either to begin or to continue programming. Output current is increased in 0.25 mA increments until stimulation is comfortable. The subsequent stimulation schedule is determined by patient response. Standard parameter settings range from 20 to 30 Hz at a pulse width of 250 to 500 μs and an output current of 0.25 to 3.5 mA for 30 s "on" time and 5 min "off" time (see Table 12.3 for suggested parameters). At each visit, the generator and the battery are assessed for end of service; the battery's life expectancy of 7 to 10 years depends on the programmed stimulation parameters. If VNS therapy is to be continued, the generator can be replaced at the appropriate time in less than 20 minutes.

VNS may be continued indefinitely and without damage to the vagus nerve as long as the stimulation is less than 50 Hz and the On time remains less than the Off time. The magnet can act as an "off" switch when held or taped over the generator.

Complications and adverse effects

Surgical complications and difficulties are rare. Incisional infections are unusual and generally respond to antibiotic therapy. Fluid accumulation at the generator site with or without infection occurs in 1–2% of implantations and resolves with aspiration and antibiotics; the rare cases of refractory infection require removal of the generator. Unilateral vocal cord paralysis, which accompanies approximately 1% of implants, may be caused by excess manipulation of the vagus nerve, and subsequent damage to the vagal artery and its reinforcing arterioles; in most cases, it remits completely over several weeks.

Common side effects, which occur primarily when the stimulator is actually delivering a pulse (Table 12.4), are dose dependent and usually mild or absent when VNS parameters are appropriately programmed; many patients become accustomed to them with time. Most patients experience hoarseness or a change in vocal quality and tingling over the left cervical region on delivery of the electrical pulse. Subjective dyspnea or a sensation of muscle tightening in the neck may occur, without changes on pulmonary function testing. Cough or throat pain during stimulus delivery sometimes necessitates a reduction in current or pulse width.

Table 12.4 Common side effects of vagus nerve stimulation (VNS).

	Study (see Table 12.2)	
Adverse event	E03 and E05 patients ($n = 314$; 591 device years) >3 months' follow-up, no. of patients (%)*	E03 and E05 patients with high stimulation ($n = 152$) >3 months' follow-up, no. of patients (%)*
Voice alteration	156 (50)	91 (60)
Increased coughing	129 (41)	57 (38)
Paresthesia	87 (28)	32 (21)
Dyspnea	55 (18)	32 (21)
Dyspepsia	36 (12)	22 (15)
Laryngismus	10 (3.2)	9 (5.9)

*Number of patients reporting the adverse event at least once in the E03 and E05 randomized studies.

Despite the widespread visceral efferent projections of the vagus nerve, systemic effects are rare. No substantial effects on cardiac function were reported during clinical studies. The clinical studies demonstrated no clinically relevant effects on the gastrointestinal system, serum chemistries, AED concentrations, vital signs, or weight.

Rare reported side effects associated with VNS therapy include diarrhea, sternocleidomastoid muscle spasm, phrenic nerve stimulation, tonsillar pain, emergent psychiatric disorders, and prominent drooling and vomiting. Children with a history of dysphagia may experience swallowing difficulties during VNS therapy; using a magnet to turn off the stimulator during mealtimes may help. The majority of side effects, including many of the rare incidents reported, are amenable to stimulus modifications, which could include changes in output current and/or pulse width.

Advantages and disadvantages

Many patients maintained on VNS therapy can decrease their total AED burden, which typically results in a more alert patient who, while still receiving polytherapy, is without the cognitive or systemic side effects typically associated with multiple therapies. Therefore, use of AED monotherapy with VNS therapy may produce a better risk-to-benefit ratio than therapy with two AEDs. Even when AEDs cannot be substantially decreased or withdrawn, however, VNS therapy may allow amelioration of seizures with no risk of toxic organ reactions, drug interactions or failures, allergies, rashes, and other systemic adverse effects or cognitive side effects; in some patients, memory, alertness, mood, and communication have been shown to improve. Improvements in quality of life independent of treatment effect on seizure frequency, as well as increased daytime vigilance, have also been reported. In addition, because the beneficial results are maintained without active patient participation, VNS therapy may be an ideal treatment for the partially compliant. Teratogenesis is not expected with VNS therapy. Although no controlled studies of VNS therapy in pregnancy have been conducted, animal studies showed no harm to fertility or to the fetus. Finally, VNS therapy can both prevent and abort seizures. The ability to trigger the device externally (with the magnet) and to interrupt the seizure or improve the postictal phase empowers the patient and provides a sense of control over epilepsy.

Cost-effectiveness studies indicate that VNS therapy provides a substantial cost-saving benefit to hospitals over the long-term course of treatment. These savings are sustained over time and are sufficient to cover or exceed the cost of the device. With VNS therapy over time, further savings can be seen in significant reductions in healthcare utilization and time spent on epilepsy-related matters.

According to the manufacturer of the device, a transmit-and-receive head coil magnetic resonance imaging (MRI; 1.5 or 3 tesla) should be performed rather than a full-body MRI, with the generator programmed to 0 mA for the procedure and returned to the original settings thereafter. Diathermy, which could heat the system above safe levels and thereby cause either temporary or permanent tissue or nerve damage, should be avoided in patients receiving VNS therapy.

12.2 Epilepsy surgery

Introduction

Children with medically intractable epilepsy represent a population for which neurosurgical intervention may allow a patient to gain seizure control and in some cases even a cure. This may offer an opportunity for significant improvement in the patient's quality of life [38]. Surgery for epilepsy was first described in the sixteenth century by Diveticus, but it was Sir Victor Horsley who founded the practice of epilepsy surgery as it is now practiced. Horsley used clinical examination and seizure semiology to localize the epileptogenic focus, and successfully treated cases of intractable seizures. His clinical findings remain important today, but technological advances now provide multiple tools for better localization, not only of the epileptic focus, but also areas of functional importance. Today, the process of evaluating a child for epilepsy surgery is divided into phases (Figure 12.6). In Phase I, patients are evaluated through non-invasive techniques to establish whether a patient is a candidate for epilepsy surgery. Phase II, which may not be necessary in some instances, involves invasive electrode monitoring for more precise localization of the epileptogenic zone in relation to functional cortex. Finally, Phase III involves the actual epilepsy surgery.

Patient selection and referral

Patients who are referred to epilepsy centers for presurgical evaluation carry a diagnosis of intractable epilepsy, which has different connotations to different practitioners. An appropriate diagnosis of intractable epilepsy can be made when a patient has failed two or more antiepileptic drugs that have been used at optimal doses [39]. The decision to refer a patient for possible surgery also depends on how detrimental the epilepsy is to the child. Intractability has also been defined by seizure frequency of at least one seizure per month for the past year. A patient who has failed three medications, but has only one seizure every 6 months may not be a good surgical candidate. Yet, if this same child is suffering decline in neurocognitive skills, the need to go forward with epilepsy surgery evaluation becomes much greater. Some children suffer regression not only from the ongoing epilepsy but also from the burden of excessive medication. Other factors to consider include the burden of the patient's current treatment, such as side effects of medications, and also the impact of the patient's ongoing epilepsy on their psychosocial functioning [40].

A special population specific to pediatric epilepsy surgery, which requires prompt referral, is the group of infants and young children with catastrophic epilepsy. Catastrophic epilepsies, such as infantile spasms, lead to developmental stagnation and even decline. Although these patients may have generalized EEG findings and seizure types, epilepsy

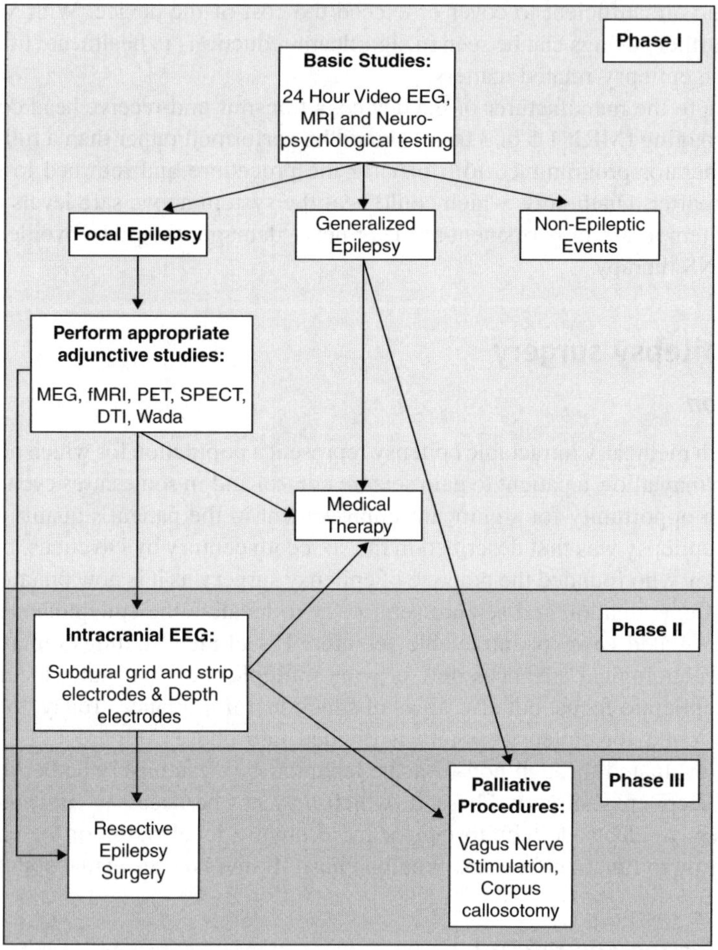

Figure 12.6 All patients begin evaluation for epilepsy surgery in Phase I. Based on the data obtained in Phase I patients may be determined to be poor surgical candidates and will be treated with medical therapy. Patients with unclear localization, discordant non-invasive studies, or lesions near eloquent cortical areas may go to Phase II for intracranial monitoring to gather further information prior to the decision to proceed with a Phase III procedure. Patients with clearly localized lesions and adjunctive studies confirming the epileptogenic zone may be able to go directly from Phase I to Phase III for resective surgery. DTI, diffusion tensor imaging; EEG, electroencephalography; fMRI, functional magnetic resonance imaging; MRI, magnetic resonance imaging; MEG, magnetoencephalography; PET, positron emission tomography; SPECT, single photon emission computed tomography; Wada, intra-carotid amobarbital test.

may be caused by an early focal brain lesion, such as encephalomalacia from infarction or infection, Sturge–Weber syndrome, or tuberous sclerosis complex [41]. These cases are amenable to surgical resection of a focal lesion or hemispherectomy, either of which might not only offer seizure improvement but also allow for progression of development [42]. In children, early surgery may be critical to the patient's long-term neurocognitive outcome, so early referral for evaluation is imperative.

Patients with intractable seizures should be referred to a comprehensive epilepsy center for further evaluation. A comprehensive pediatric epilepsy center should have the personnel and services required to perform complex neurodiagnostic testing and invasive diagnostic testing, and be able to offer all surgical options with a neurosurgeon experienced in epilepsy surgery. This team includes a neurologist who is trained specifically in clinical neurophysiology and video-EEG monitoring, as well as, a neuropsychologist with specialization in clinical neuropsychology [43].

Phase I evaluation: non-invasive evaluation

The goals of the non-invasive evaluation are multiple. In this stage, the child should undergo testing including at a minimum video-EEG monitoring, MRI of the brain (with a specific epilepsy protocol), and neuropsychological testing. Other non-invasive studies, including high-density EEG, magnetoencephalography (MEG), functional MRI (fMRI), positron emission tomography (PET), and single photon emission computed tomography (SPECT), may also be performed in this stage, but this should be tailored to the needs of each individual patient.

Defining the seizure events

The first goal is to determine if the patient is truly having epileptic events. In childhood there are many paroxysmal events that are mistaken for seizure including night terrors, tics, cardiac events, stereotypies, breath-holding spells, and staring spells due to inattention. Also children with known epilepsy may be found to have better control than their parents realize, as cautious parents may begin noting normal childhood behavior such as inattentive staring as seizure events.

Once it has been determined that a patient is truly having seizures, the type of seizure and also the epilepsy syndrome may be better defined. This knowledge will allow the practitioner to decide if the patient is a candidate for surgical intervention. Generalized seizures generally do not lend themselves to surgical resection, although there may be other surgical options for this group of patients. There are also focal epilepsy syndromes, such as benign rolandic epilepsy, which will be outgrown, therefore surgical procedures would not be indicated.

Defining the epileptogenic focus

In patients with focal onset seizures, the next step is to define as precisely as possible the localization of the epileptogenic zone. This is the region that, if resected, would lead to seizure freedom. Video-EEG and MRI are critical for defining this region. With EEG the epileptologist can use interictal EEG abnormalities and the region of seizure onset during seizures to localize the epileptogenic zone.

High-quality MRI with an appropriate epilepsy protocol is also extremely important. Locating a lesion is helpful in determining the likely epileptogenic zone. Having a lesion that can be visualized with MRI also improves the likelihood of successful seizure control two- or three-fold compared to non-lesional cases where the focus has been defined by neurophysiological and functional studies [44]. However, in pediatric patients the frequency of pathology such as cortical dysplasia, which is frequently more diffuse and ill-defined, makes even lesional cases more difficult. MRI should be performed with a 1.5 tesla or higher strength magnet and include an epilepsy protocol with thin slices through the mesial temporal structures. A neuroradiologist trained in evaluation of MRI for epilepsy patients may also improve the yield of identifying a lesion on imaging.

Although MRI and video-EEG (VEEG) are the primary modalities for locating the epileptogenic zone, other radiological and neurophysiological studies may also be used when needed, including PET, SPECT, and MEG.

Nuclear medicine studies may be helpful in defining the epileptogenic focus also. Fluorodeoxyglucose-PET (FDG-PET) evaluates the glucose metabolism of the brain. In epilepsy, the hallmark of an epileptogenic focus is interictal reduction in glucose metabolism, which can be visualized as an area of decreased FDG uptake on PET. SPECT studies use cerebral blood flow to create images. Epileptic foci will have decreased cerebral blood flow on interictal studies, and with injection of isotope during an ictal event will have increased cerebral blood flow. Interictal and ictal SPECT scans are subtracted from each other and then co-registered to MRI to produce the most reliable localization of the epileptogenic zone. It is critical that the ictal-SPECT be evaluated with ongoing VEEG monitoring as postictal studies may not be reliable in actually predicting the epileptogenic region. Although these studies are helpful, it is important that they be used cautiously and in conjunction with EEG and MRI findings.

MEG is a newer technology that measures the magnetic flux produced by electrical potentials in activated neurons. This activity is similar to the EEG recording of electrical potentials; however, it is not affected by intervening tissue such as scalp and bone, allowing for a better evaluation of epileptic foci [45]. MEG data can also be used to evaluate areas of functional cortex in a similar manner. Once the MEG data are obtained they can be co-registered to the patient's MRI to produce magnetic source imaging (MSI). This allows for an accurate spatial localization within 1–4 mm from the anatomical brain source when compared with intracranial EEG. These data can be used in conjunction with EEG to define the neurophysiological epileptic focus. Studies have also shown that resection of MEG dipoles may predict better seizure outcomes in patients with non-lesional epilepsy [46].

These adjunctive studies are most useful in non-lesional and multifocal cases where MRI has not been as helpful with delineating an area of anatomical abnormality. These adjunctive studies are also useful when an MRI lesion is present but EEG findings do not correlate with the lesion. These studies are also helpful for extra-temporal resections where outcomes are not generally as good due to restriction of the areas that can be resected.

Neuropsychological testing should be performed. Testing has two goals: (i) identifying areas of cognitive dysfunction with localization to a specific region of functional cortex; and (ii) establishing a baseline level of developmental or cognitive function prior to intervention. For example, an adolescent with isolated impairment of verbal memory would have localized dysfunction in the dominant temporal lobe. This type of information helps with localization of the epileptogenic zone, as areas responsible for epilepsy may lead to material specific dysfunction.

Defining functional or eloquent cortex

If a patient has a localizable area of seizure focus then the decision to go forward with resective surgery depends on whether the procedure can be performed without causing significant injury. Localizing areas of functional cortex such as the motor strip, Broca's and Wernicke's areas, and visual cortex may be critical in a given patient. These have variability in their individual locations, which must be established, as they may be near the area to be resected. This knowledge aids in multiple areas of resective epilepsy surgery: (i) making the decision to go forward with surgery (discussing risks, benefits with the family); (ii) determining whether the patient needs a Phase II procedure; and (iii) creating a safe surgical plan and approach.

Non-invasive studies that can assist in localizing function include fMRI and MEG. Both of these modalities can be used to define motor, sensory, language, and visual cortex. fMRI uses changes in oxyhemoglobin (blood oxygen-level-dependent (BOLD) signal) during tasks to define regions that are active [47]. Since fMRI is dependent on blood flow, highly vascular lesions and brain tumors can affect the reliability of the study. Also fMRI can be confounded by patients with frequent daily seizures due to poor reliability in the postictal period. MEG/MSI data can also be used for localization of functional cortex providing very accurate localization to within 4–10 mm of the actual area of activation when compared to direct cortical stimulation. In patients, with metal implants such as VNS or braces, MEG potentials may not be picked up due to artifact. MEG functional studies can be limited by patients with very active interictal epileptiform discharges, which obscure the functional potentials one is trying to detect. Diffusion tensor imaging (DTI) can be used as an adjunct to fMRI or MEG by defining the tracts of white matter making critical connections such as the visual tracts and radiations or the corticospinal tract [22]. This information can be invaluable in surgical planning and reduce potential functional complications.

Phase II evaluation: invasive evaluation

For some patients, Phase I testing may answer all of the questions to establish that a person is a good surgical candidate. This group of patients may be able to forgo invasive monitoring and "skip" phase II. For example, in studies of patients with tumor-related epilepsy, completeness of the resection has been found to be more important than results from mapping [47]. There are multiple situations where intra-cranial monitoring may be necessary:

1. Patients with studies providing potentially discordant localization.
2. Patients without a discrete MRI lesion.
3. Patients with an epileptogenic zone in close proximity to areas of functional cortex such as language or vision.

Intra-carotid amobarbital testing (IAT)

The intra-carotid amobarbital test (IAT), or Wada test, is the gold standard for localization of the dominant hemisphere for language and also may be used to evaluate memory function. It is well known that hand dominance can predict the hemisphere of language dominance; however, there are some patients in whom language is not located in the same hemisphere as hand dominance. This is particularly true in patients who are left-handed or who have suffered early injury to one hemisphere, which is a fairly common etiology for children with epilepsy [48]. Patients with epilepsy generally have a higher rate of atypical language lateralization. Use of non-invasive methods for functional mapping is making the need for IAT less common. MEG and fMRI have been studied in comparison to WADA with good results, and MEG data have also been shown to be concordant with cortical stimulation

[49]. Both MEG and fMRI are not only able to lateralize language but also to localize language to a particular region of the hemisphere.

Not only does IAT carry serious risk, although uncommon, of complications such as stroke and hemorrhage, it is an invasive procedure that requires significant cooperation. IAT is possible in young children and patients with neurocognitive disabilities; however, in some cases it may not be an option and results should always be interpreted with caution. Although IAT is not a perfect test and there are other studies that can localize memory and language, IAT is the only test available that can indicate whether a person can function without a particular hemisphere. IAT is still used in cases of bilateral dominance or equivocal findings on functional imaging studies or in patients with a high likelihood of atypical language lateralization.

Intracranial monitoring

Placement of intracranial electrodes is truly the definition of Phase II evaluation of epilepsy surgery, as well as the gold standard for localization of the epileptogenic zone. As mentioned previously, not all patients will require this step in their evaluation based on results from Phase I. It is important to remember that this step is another diagnostic evaluation, and in some cases is a critical step in determining if the patient is a resective surgical candidate. Patients and their families need to recognize that although surgery is being performed, there is a possibility that the data obtained may indicate that resective surgery is not an option, or that only part of the epileptogenic zone can be resected, because of its close relationship to eloquent cortex. In these cases, the electrodes are removed and the patient continues seizure management with antiepileptic drugs or pursues palliative surgical options such as vagus nerve stimulation.

Intracranial EEG (ICEEG) monitoring is an important tool for localization of the epileptogenic zone, allowing for more precise localization. On scalp EEG, approximately 6 cm^2 of cortex discharging simultaneously is required to generate a scalp potential, which may be too inexact for precise localization, especially when near critical functional areas. Also scalp EEG cannot adequately record from some structures, such as inferior orbital frontal and mesial temporal cortex, and may show only epileptiform activity in a wide field due to rapid spread. ICEEG produces a larger signal and may show more focal interictal discharges and seizure onset compared to scalp EEG [50].

While ICEEG can have many advantages over scalp EEG, the precise placement of the electrodes is critical to actually recording the epileptiform potentials of interest, and capturing the true area of seizure onset. This can be challenging since many patients require intracranial monitoring because the location of the epileptogenic zone is unclear. It is important to have a working hypothesis for the most likely location of the epileptogenic zone and cover the areas of interest based on seizure semiology, scalp EEG findings, and studies such as MEG, SPECT, and PET. Possible functional cortical areas should also be taken into account for coverage in order to allow bedside cortical stimulation for further localization of eloquent cortex.

Intracranial electrodes also allow for cortical stimulation, which can be used to define motor regions or language cortex and actually create a map on the electrodes depicting functional locations (Figure 12.7).

ICEEG electrodes can be placed in strip or grid arrays on the surface of the cortex, and depth electrodes can be placed to target deeper structures. Depth electrodes and subdural strip electrodes may be placed through a burr hole; however, grid arrays require craniotomy

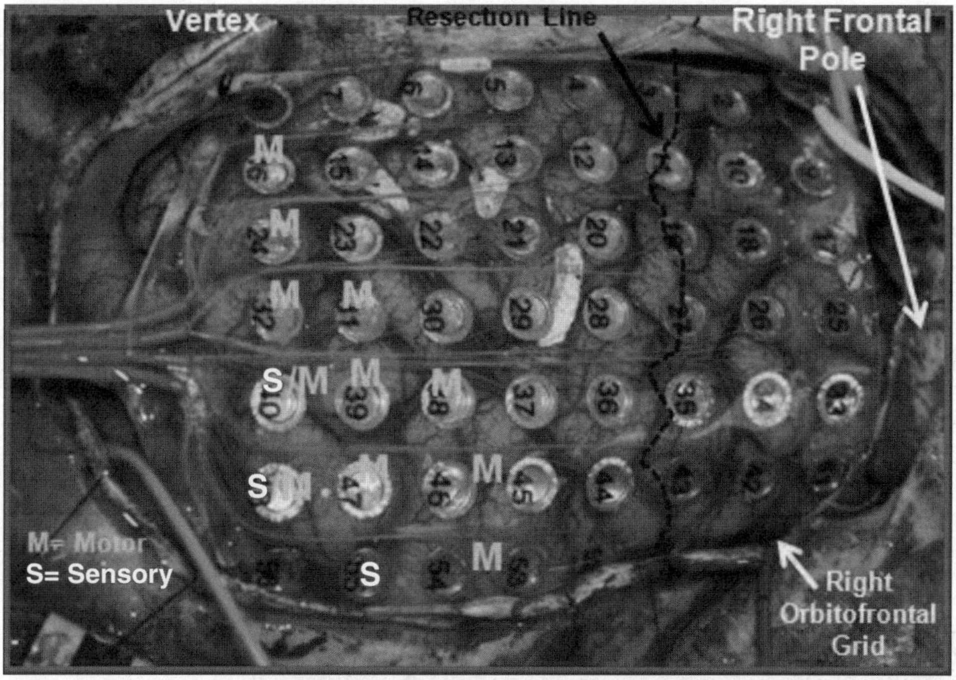

Figure 12.7 Subdural grids placed over the right frontal and anterior parietal lobes allow for motor and sensory cortex mapping using electrocorticography. The grids are also used for intracranial EEG monitoring, which will help determine areas of cortex most likely to be responsible for seizure generation. This creates a "map" on the grid for planning the extent of resection allowing for more successful and safer outcomes. M, motor; S, sensory.

over the area that is likely to require resection. Intraoperative placement of electrodes requires the surgeon to place grids according to the plan created with the epileptologist for optimal coverage and balance this with the safety and feasibility of the operative procedure. Some plans may need to be adjusted based on the anatomical differences among patients such as large veins or venous lakes, which increase the risk of complications. The use of stereotactic technology can aid the surgeon in appropriate placement of electrodes. Intracranial monitoring can carry significant risk. Commonly patients suffer minor issues such as nausea, headache, and fever. More serious complications include infection, epidural hematoma, increased intracranial pressure and stroke, as well as death. Relatively minor complications including cerebrospinal fluid (CSF) leaks and transient neurological deficits can also occur. Permanent deficits are rare. These risks may decline as the surgeon's experience increases, but are higher in patients with prolonged grid placement, greater number of grids, performance of burr holes in addition to craniotomy, older age, and left-sided insertion of grids. Overall, pediatric patients tolerate intracranial monitoring well.

Phase III: resection

Planning the actual resection requires close cooperation with an epileptologist to determine the area of resection. All of the data obtained from the previous phases are used to accurately predict the epileptogenic zone. Outcome studies show that completeness of resection of the epileptogenic zone is the best prognostic feature for good outcome [51], so planning the extent of the resection is very important. However, this must be balanced by the limitations created by surrounding eloquent functional cortex defined during Phase I and II studies.

The use of neuronavigational technology can be very helpful in obtaining an optimal surgical outcome. Data from phase II studies such as MEG, fMRI, and DTI can be co-registered to the navigational system imaging allowing the surgeon to have real-time intraoperative localization of functional cortex. Also MEG epileptiform dipoles can be co-registered to the neuronavigational system to allow better localization intraoperatively of the actual epileptogenic focus (Figure 12.8).

During the resective procedure, intraoperative electrocorticography (ECoG) can be performed to evaluate the epileptiform and non-epileptiform activity and better localize the area to be resected. ECoG is performed by laying electrode strips over areas of cortex for EEG recording. This technique is frequently used in patients who did not require intracranial monitoring to confirm the area of resection. There are also significant data showing that post-resection ECoG may be predictive of seizure outcome [52]. In cases of cortical dysplasia, which is a common pathological finding in pediatric epilepsy, this is especially true. Cortical dysplasia is poorly defined by imaging, and use of ECoG can help define the borders of the lesion leading to better outcomes. Electrode strips can also be used for

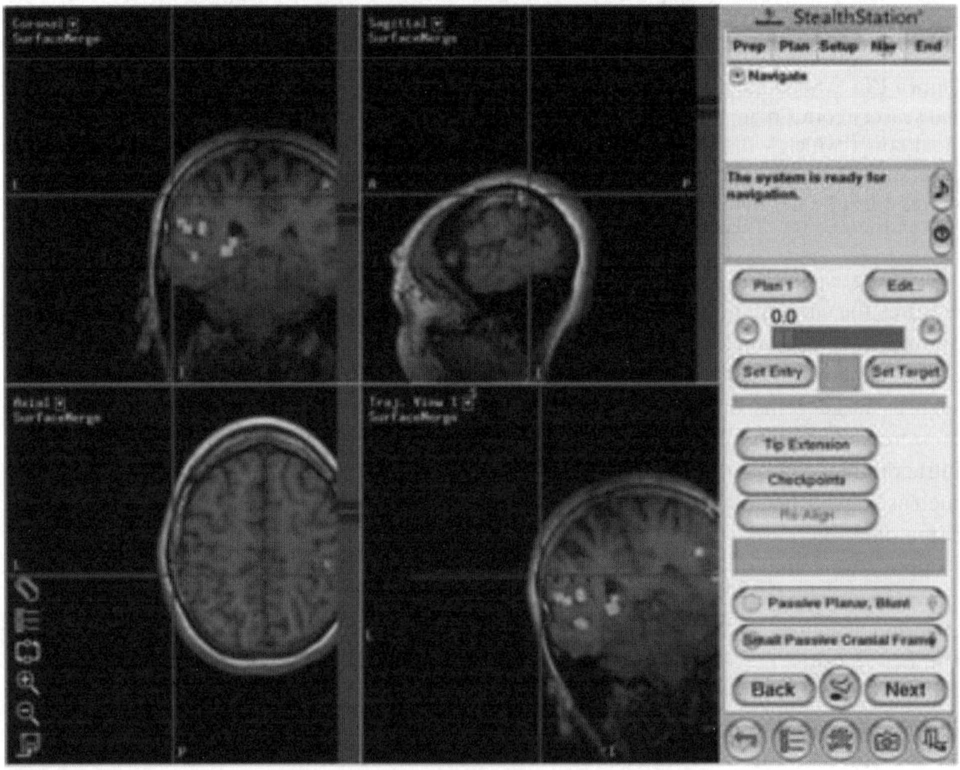

Figure 12.8 Magnetoencephalography (MEG)/magnetic source imaging (MSI) data can be co-registered to intraoperative neuronavigational systems to provide guidance intraoperatively. Epileptiform activity detected by MEG is noted in the left hemisphere.

cortical stimulation to localize functional cortex while in the operating room. In pediatric patients this technique is useful for motor cortex localization because it does not require awake craniotomy.

Temporal lobectomy

While temporal lobectomy (Figure 12.9) is the best known and most commonly performed resective epilepsy surgery, its use in pediatrics is less than in adults, and represents management of a different disease process compared to the common adult procedure. In adults, mesial temporal sclerosis (MTS) is the most common reason for temporal lobe resection. In children, however, neocortical temporal lobe epilepsy is more frequent and MTS is relatively rare. Cortical dysplasia of the neocortical temporal lobe is the most common etiology in children, and when MTS is present it is frequently associated with another pathological abnormality such as cortical dysplasia or low-grade neoplasm, so-called dual pathology. Other pathological findings include vascular malformations, gliosis from perinatal injury, and tuberous sclerosis lesions.

Several surgical approaches may apply in cases of temporal lobe epilepsy, including traditional anterior temporal lobectomy (ATL), amygdalohippocampectomy (AH), lesionectomy with hippocampectomy, or lateral temporal lesionectomy. The decision to perform a lateral temporal lobe resection versus a procedure for resection of the mesial temporal structures will be dictated by the patient's seizure semiology and MRI findings. In children, however, it appears that ATL produces significantly better outcomes compared to more limited resections, and neuropsychological performance was not significantly affected with ATL [53]. These findings may be due to the fact that childhood temporal lobe epilepsy does not generally have the same etiology as that in adults.

Risks of temporal lobe resection include impairment of memory or language when resecting the dominant temporal lobe or dysfunction of visuospatial memory function with non-dominant temporal resection. Memory and language should be evaluated and lateralized to avoid alterations in memory or speech function after temporal lobectomy; however, in children the risk of long-term cognitive affects appears to be less, and many children

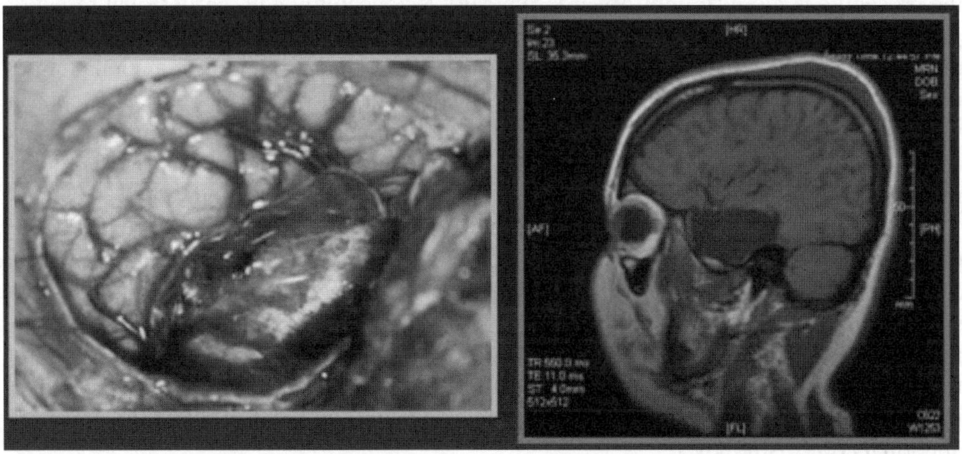

Figure 12.9 Right temporal lobectomy.

may actually improve with better seizure control and fewer antiepileptic medications. In predicting the risk of postoperative memory impairment, studies have shown that alteration in memory is more likely to occur, with testing showing good memory ipsilateral to the resection or poor memory contralateral to the resection. Neuropsychological testing is the most helpful study in making this determination, along with data from IAT. Patients may also have visual field deficits following ATL due to interruption of the optic radiations. Use of DTI preoperatively to define the optic radiations may be helpful in surgical planning to reduce this risk. In clear-cut cases, using non-invasive studies, temporal lobectomy is a resection that may be performed without a phase II procedure.

Extra-temporal resection

In pediatric populations extra-temporal resections represent a much higher proportion of the cases requiring surgical intervention compared to adults. Extra-temporal lobe epilepsy (ETLE) is seen in only 30–40% of the resections for adults but in children may represent as much as 50% of the cases in childhood and 90% of the cases in infants. ETLE is also one of the most challenging forms of epilepsy surgery in regards to both localization and resection. The challenges of extra-temporal resection arise from the pathology, which often is more diffuse in nature and frequently abuts eloquent cortex without clear margins. In contrast to temporal lobe resection, where the anatomical regions involved in seizure generation are well established (e.g., hippocampus, amygdala), the offending cortex in ETLE is specific to each individual patient. This makes each resection extremely variable based on the needs of the patient.

Frontal lobe epilepsy is the most common extra-temporal site, with parietal and occipital epileptogenic zones being more rare. At times multilobar procedures are also required. Hypothalamic hamartoma may also arise as a source for seizures, and is specific to childhood. These patients have gelastic epilepsy as well as severe encephalopathy, both of which may be reversible with resection of the hamartoma.

Extra-temporal resections are most frequently lesionectomies. MRI may reveal abnormalities such as cortical dysplasia, low-grade tumor, vascular malformation, or gliosis from previous injury [54]. When the lesion on MRI correlates well with neurophysiological data the procedure is more straightforward. Typically lesionectomy with perilesional resection provides good outcomes. ECoG can be used to guide the extent of resection surrounding the lesion. However, even with a clearly defined lesion, the surrounding functional cortex may represent a significant barrier to safely obtaining a full resection. Cortical dysplasia, which may be seen on MRI, also represents a surgical challenge. Although there may be a lesion, the borders of these developmental malformations are not generally well defined, making it difficult to determine the extent needed for adequate resection.

In non-lesional cases, focal topectomy is performed. These procedures are guided purely on the basis of neurophysiological data, such as EEG, MEG, PET, and SPECT. These studies will define the area of the epileptogenic zone and guide resection. Intraoperative stereotactic guidance can be very helpful in these cases when MEG and SPECT data are co-registered to the neuronavigational system. Topectomies are also limited by surrounding functional cortex and underlying white matter tracts, which must be avoided to reduce the risk of neurological sequelae. Overall, outcomes will be better if all of the presumed abnormal cortex is removed.

Risks specific to extra-temporal lobe resections are based on the area to be resected. Frontal lobe lesions must be evaluated to avoid functional cortex such as the primary motor strip and Broca's area. The supplementary motor area may be resected but can produce a signifcant transient neurological deficit with contralateral hemiparesis, hemineglect, and mutism, which resolves typically over 2–3 weeks. Parietal lobe resection can produce sensory impairment or Gerstmann's syndrome, which may be transient, but if primary sensory cortex is injured the deficit may be permanent. Occipital lobe resections can frequently produce visual field defects. Limited resections in conjunction with multiple subpial transections may minimize the size of the deficit.

Hemispherectomy

Hemispherectomy is a procedure that is seldom performed in adult populations, but in pediatric epilepsy has been able to provide some of the clearest successes for pediatric patients, not only in regards to seizure control but also for cognitive outcomes. This procedure has achieved dramatic success for infants with catastrophic epilepsy. Candidates for hemispherectomy have very specific criteria including unilateral seizures, extensive lesion involving only one hemisphere, generally with maximal motor deficits, and in optimal cases, visual deficits. Exceptions to these rules are made at times but outcomes may be affected. When there are bilateral seizures or MRI abnormalities the likelihood of seizure control is diminished. If hemispherectomy is performed in a patient without a complete functional injury preoperatively, they will have a contralateral hemiparesis and hemianopsia following resection. This scenario most commonly arises in patients with Rasmussen's encephalitis who have not yet reached maximal deficit. Many patients who require hemispherectomy have had early injury to one hemisphere, such as perinatal infarction. Other etiologies include diffuse hemispheric developmental malformation, Sturge–Weber syndrome, hemimegaloencephaly, and Rasmussen's encephalitis. Patients generally do well with little to no new motor impairment and no change in their ability to ambulate. Infants who undergo the procedure may still go on to ambulate [55]. After hemispherectomy many patients have improvement in cognitive development or halting of developmental decline. It is believed this occurs by stopping the ongoing epileptiform activity of the injured hemisphere, which interferes with the function of the undamaged hemisphere.

Functional hemispherectomy typically involves a full temporal lobectomy, but more limited resections with hemispherotomy are also performed. Outcome is technically dependent on acquiring complete disconnection [56]. Complications include chemical meningitis, hydrocephalus requiring shunting and transfusion, which occur more frequently in small children. Some patients may have new permanent neurological deficits but these are generally expected in those cases. Mortality is a greater risk with this procedure compared to other resective epilepsy surgery, with some studies showing mortality rates as high as 7%.

Corpus callosotomy

Corpus callosotomy is a palliative surgical disconnection procedure that is effective in the treatment of medically intractable epilepsy in select patient populations [57]. Corpus callosotomy disrupts the hemispheric synchrony that is critical in the expression of some generalized seizures such as atonic, tonic, and generalized tonic-clonic seizures. This procedure effectively treats epileptic seizures that cannot be helped by cortical resection. In general, the purpose of corpus callosotomy is to palliate the patient's intractable seizure condition by decreasing or abolishing the most incapacitating of the generalized seizures and improving the patient's quality of life [58]. The best response has been observed in patients with drop attacks presenting as tonic and atonic seizures (many of which have Lennox–Gastaut syndrome). Corpus callosotomy has also yielded a significant reduction of generalized tonic-clonic seizures. Patients with secondarily generalized tonic-clonic seizures in the presence of electroencephalographic evidence of secondary bilateral synchrony and clinical or neuroradiological evidence of focality derive greater benefits than those with generalized tonic-clonic seizures without these characteristics. Children with complex partial seizures are less likely to respond to this procedure. Corpus callosotomy may be performed as a partial resection involving the anterior 75%, or a complete section. In patients with secondary generalized tonic-clonic seizures, a complete callosotomy is superior to partial callosotomy. A complete corpus callosotomy should be considered as the initial procedure in lower-functioning children affected by atonic, tonic, or myoclonic seizures [59–61]. Additionally, children with significant unilateral hemispheric disease may have a complete callosotomy performed as the initial procedure with little risk of producing a disconnection syndrome. Higher functioning children with atonic seizures only could be approached initially with the anterior 75% corpus callosotomy, which could be completed later if indicated. The primary use of the corpus callosotomy is the treatment of patients with Lennox–Gastaut syndrome. Although vagus nerve stimulation therapy has increased in use in the treatment of the various seizure types associated with Lennox–Gastaut syndrome, no head to head studies have compared this treatment to corpus callosotomy, and some children may benefit from both procedures being performed, in a step-wise manner.

Complications of corpus callosotomy are varying degrees of the acute disconnection syndrome, which is often resolved by hospital discharge. This may be characterized by bladder incontinence, apathy, lethargy, and mutism in the first few days after surgery, and this is always transient. Rarely epidural hematoma, infection (e.g., osteomyelitis), or hydrocephalus may occur.

Surgical outcomes

Outcomes have classically been evaluated based on the frequency of seizures post-resection; however, in children it is important to recognize that improvement in cognitive skills and velocity of development or cessation of decline is probably even more important. A meta-analysis by Tonini *et al.* showed that the strongest predictors of good seizure outcome were MTS, tumors, MRI abnormality, EEG and MRI correlation, and extensive resection [62]. Studies have also shown that pathological findings also affect outcome, with tumor resections producing 82% seizure freedom and resections of cortical dysplasias only 52% [63].

Overall, pediatric patients can have significant improvement in their cognitive skills; however, there may not always be improvement in developmental and cognitive outcomes in every individual and some patients may even show decline following surgery. Children with epilepsy frequently have behavioral problems, and studies have shown significant improvement in behavior in some children after surgery. Quality of life can be greatly improved for both the patients and their families. The most significant factor in improving quality of life is generally the extent of seizure control [64].

12.3 Conclusions

Epilepsy surgery in children offers patients with refractory seizure disorders the possibility of seizure freedom with subsequent improvement in many aspects of their lives including cognitive skills and overall quality of life. Early referral for surgery in infants and children with catastrophic epilepsy or declining development is extremely important, since early intervention may change the overall developmental outcome for that child. Successful surgery requires close cooperation between a neurosurgeon and a neurologist trained specifically in epilepsy and neurophysiology. Technology now provides many modalities for evaluating not only the source of epileptogenesis but also the functional cortex, creating new opportunities for non-invasive evaluation of children. Children can have good seizure outcomes similar to those of adults, but children may have less risk of permanent neurological sequelae due to the functional plasticity of the developing brain. With continued advancement of non-invasive technology and imaging modalities, these challenging surgeries are becoming safer and more effective.

References

[1] Kwan P, Brodie MJ. Early identification of refractory epilepsy. *N Engl J Med* 2000;**342**:314–319.

[2] Mohanraj R, Brodie MJ. Diagnosing refractory epilepsy: response to sequential treatment schedules. *Eur J Neurol* 2006;**13**:277–282.

[3] Faught E, Duh MS, Weiner JR, Guerin A, Cunnington MC. Nonadherence to antiepileptic drugs and increased mortality: findings from the RANSOM Study. *Neurology* 2008;**71**:1572–1578.

[4] Zabara J. Inhibition of experimental seizures in canines by repetitive vagal stimulation. *Epilepsia* 1992;**33**:1005–1012.

[5] Penry JK, Dean JC. Prevention of intractable partial seizures by intermittent vagal stimulation in humans: preliminary results. *Epilepsia* 1990;**31**(Suppl. 2):S40–S43.

[6] Uthman BM, Wilder BJ, Penry JK, *et al.* Treatment of epilepsy by stimulation of the vagus nerve. *Neurology* 1993;**43**:1338–1345.

[7] *VNS Therapy Physician's Manual*. Cyberonics, Inc., 2006. http://www.vnstherapy.com/epilepsy/hcp/manuals/default.aspx.

[8] Handforth A, DeGiorgio CM, Schachter SC, *et al.* Vagus nerve stimulation therapy for partial-onset seizures: a randomized active-control trial. *Neurology* 1998;**51**:48–55.

[9] [No authors listed] A randomized controlled trial of chronic vagus nerve stimulation for treatment of medically intractable seizures. The Vagus Nerve Stimulation Study Group. *Neurology* 1995;**45**:224–230.

[10] Renfroe JB, Wheless JW. Earlier use of adjunctive vagus nerve stimulation therapy for refractory epilepsy. *Neurology* 2002;**59**:S26–S30.

[11] Labar D. Vagus nerve stimulation for 1 year in 269 patients on unchanged antiepileptic drugs. *Seizure* 2004;**13**:392–398.

[12] De Herdt V, Boon P, Ceulemans B, *et al.* Vagus nerve stimulation for refractory epilepsy: a Belgian multicenter study. *Eur J Paediatr Neurol* 2007;**11**:261–269.

[13] Ardesch JJ, Buschman HP, Wagener-Schimmel LJ, van der Aa HE, Hageman G. Vagus nerve stimulation for medically refractory epilepsy: a long-term follow-up study. *Seizure* 2007;**16**:579–585.

[14] Abubakr A, Wambacq I. Long-term outcome of vagus nerve stimulation therapy in patients with refractory epilepsy. *J Clin Neurosci* 2008;**15**:127–129.

[15] Helmers SL, Wheless JW, Frost M, *et al.* Vagus nerve stimulation therapy in pediatric patients with refractory epilepsy: retrospective study. *J Child Neurol* 2001;**16**:843–848.
[16] Alexopoulos AV, Kotagal P, Loddenkemper T, Hammel J, Bingaman WE. Long-term results with vagus nerve stimulation in children with pharmacoresistant epilepsy. *Seizure* 2006;**15**:491–503.
[17] Benifla M, Rutka JT, Logan W, Donner EJ. Vagal nerve stimulation for refractory epilepsy in children: indications and experience at The Hospital for Sick Children. *Childs Nerv Syst* 2006;**22**:1018–1026.
[18] Frost M, Gates J, Helmers SL, *et al.* Vagus nerve stimulation in children with refractory seizures associated with Lennox–Gastaut syndrome. *Epilepsia* 2001;**42**:1148–1152.
[19] Parain D, Penniello MJ, Berquen P, Delangre T, Billard C, Murphy JV. Vagal nerve stimulation in tuberous sclerosis complex patients. *Pediatr Neurol* 2001;**25**:213–216.
[20] Murphy JV, Wheless JW, Schmoll CM. Left vagal nerve stimulation in six patients with hypothalamic hamartomas. *Pediatr Neurol* 2000;**23**:167–168.
[21] Aldenkamp AP, Majoie HJM, Berfelo MW, *et al.* Long-term effects of 24-month treatment with vagus nerve stimulation on behaviour in children with Lennox–Gastaut syndrome. *Epilepsy Behav* 2002;**3**:475–479.
[22] Wilfong AA, Schultz RJ. Vagus nerve stimulation for treatment of epilepsy in Rett syndrome. *Dev Med Child Neurol* 2006;**48**:683–686.
[23] Major P, Thiele EA. Vagus nerve stimulation for intractable epilepsy in tuberous sclerosis complex. *Epilepsy Behav* 2008;**13**:357–60.
[24] You SJ, Kang HC, Ko TS, *et al.* Comparison of corpus callosotomy and vagus nerve stimulation in children with Lennox–Gastaut syndrome. *Brain Dev* 2008;**30**:195–199.
[25] Park YD. The effects of vagus nerve stimulation therapy on patients with intractable seizures and either Landau–Kleffner syndrome or autism. *Epilepsy Behav* 2003;**4**:286–290.
[26] Andriola MR, Vitale SA. Vagus nerve stimulation in the developmentally disabled. *Epilepsy Behav* 2001;**2**:129–134.
[27] Zamponi N, Rychlicki F, Corpaci L, Cesaroni E, Trignani R. Vagus nerve stimulation (VNS) is effective in treating catastrophic epilepsy in very young children. *Neurosurg Rev* 2008;**31**:291–297
[28] Heck C, Helmers SL, DeGiorgio CM. Vagus nerve stimulation therapy, epilepsy, and device parameters: scientific basis and recommendations for use. *Neurology* 2002;**59**:S31–S37.
[29] Henry TR. Therapeutic mechanisms of vagus nerve stimulation. *Neurology* 2002;**59**:S3–S14.
[30] Lockard JS, Congdon WC, DuCharme LL. Feasibility and safety of vagal stimulation in monkey model. *Epilepsia* 1990;**31**(Suppl. 2):S20–S26.
[31] McLachlan RS. Suppression of interictal spikes and seizures by stimulation of the vagus nerve. *Epilepsia* 1993;**34**:918–923.
[32] Hammond EJ, Uthman BM, Reid SA, Wilder BJ, Ramsay RE. Vagus nerve stimulation in humans: neurophysiological studies and electrophysiological monitoring. *Epilepsia* 1990;**31**(Suppl. 2):S51–S59.
[33] Henry TR, Votaw JR, Bakay RAE, *et al.* Vagus nerve stimulation-induced cerebral blood flow changes differ in acute and chronic therapy of complex partial seizures. *Epilepsia* 1998;**39**:92.
[34] Baumgartner JE, Clifton GL, Wheless JW, *et al.* Corpus callosotomy. *Techniques Neurosurg* 1995;**1**:45–51.
[35] Malow BA, Edwards J, Marzec M, Sagher O, Fromes G. Effects of vagus nerve stimulation on respiration during sleep: a pilot study. *Neurology* 2000;**55**:1450–1454.
[36] Reid SA. Surgical technique for implantation of the neurocybernetic prosthesis. *Epilepsia* 1990;**31**(Suppl. 2):S38–S39.
[37] Amar AP, Heck CN, Levy ML, *et al.* An institutional experience with cervical vagus nerve trunk stimulation for medically refractory epilepsy: rationale, technique, and outcome. *Neurosurgery* 1998;**43**:1265–1276; discussion 1276–1280.

[38] Sabaz M, Lawson JA, Carins DR, *et al.* The impact of epilepsy surgery on quality of life in children. *Neurology* 2006;**66**:547–556.
[39] Brodie MJ, Kwan P. Staged approach to epilepsy management. *Neurology* 2002;**58**(Suppl. 5):S2–S8.
[40] Cross JH, Jayakar P, Nordli D, *et al.* Proposed criteria for referral and evaluation of children for epilepsy surgery: Recommendations of the subcommission for pediatric epilepsy surgery. *Epilepsia* 2006;**47**:952–959.
[41] Wyllie E, Lachhwani DK, Gupta A, *et al.* Successful surgery for epilepsy due to early brain lesions despite generalized EEG findings. *Neurology* 2007;**69**:389–397.
[42] Asarnow RF, LoPresti C, Guthrie D, *et al.* Developmental outcomes in children receiving resection surgery for medically intractable infantile spasms. *Dev Med Child Neurol* 1997;**39**:430–440.
[43] Gumnit RJ, Walczak TS, National Association of Epilepsy Centers. Guidelines for essential services, personnel, and facilities in specialized epilepsy centers in the United States. *Epilepsia* 2001;**42**:804–814.
[44] Tellez-Zenteno JF, Hernandez RL, Moien-Afshari F, Wiebe S. Surgical outcomes in lesional and non-lesional epilepsy: a systematic review and meta-analysis. *Epilepsy Res* 2010;**89**:310–318.
[45] Wheless J, Castillo E, Maggio V, *et al.* Magnetoencephalography (MEG) and magnetic source imaging (MSI). *The Neurologist* 2004;**10**:138–153.
[46] Ramachandran-Nair R, Otsubo H, Shroff MM, *et al.* MEG predicts outcome following surgery for intractable epilepsy in children with normal or nonfocal MRI findings. *Epilepsia* 2007;**48**:149–157.
[47] Khajavi, K, Comair, YG, Wyllie E, *et al.* Surgical management of pediatric tumor-associated epilepsy. *J Child Neurol* 1999;**14**:15–25.
[48] Szabo CA, Wyllie E. Intracarotid amobarbital testing for language and memory dominance in children. *Epilepsy Res* 1993;**15**:239–246.
[49] Panagiotis GS, Papanicolaou AC, Breier JI, *et al.* Localization of language-specific cortex by using magnetic source imaging and electrical stimulation mapping. *J Neurosurg* 1999;**91**:787–796.
[50] Nair DR, Burgess R, McIntyre CC, Luders H. Chronic subdural electrodes in the management of epilepsy. *Clin Neurophys* 2008;**119**:11–28.
[51] Paolicchi JM, Jayakar P, Dean P, *et al.* Predictors of outcome in pediatric epilepsy surgery. *Neurology* 2000;**54**:642.
[52] Gallentine WB, Mikati MA. Intraoperative electrocorticography and cortical stimulation in children. *J Clin Neurophys* 2009;**26**:95–108.
[53] Clusmann H, Kral T, Gleissner U, *et al.* Analysis of different types of resection for pediatric patients with temporal lobe epilepsy. *Neurosurgery* 2004;**54**:847–860.
[54] Sinclair DB, Aronyk K, Snyder T, *et al.* Extratemporal resection for children. *Pediatr Neurol* 2004;**30**:177–185.
[55] Delalande O, Bulteau C, Dellatolas G, *et al.* Vertical parasagittal hemispherotomy: surgical procedures and clinical long-term outcomes in a population of 83 children. *Neurosurgery* 2007;**60**(2; Suppl. 1):19–32.
[56] Gonzalez-Martinez JA, Gupta A, Kotagal P, *et al.* Hemispherectomy for catastrophic epilepsy in infants. *Epilepsia* 2005;**46**:1518–1525.
[57] Asadi-Poova AA, Sharan A, Nei M, Sperling MR. Corpus callosotomy. *Epilepsy Behav* 2008;**13**:271–278.
[58] Wheless JW. Managing severe epilepsy syndromes of early childhood. *J Child Neurol* 2009;**24**:24S–32S.
[59] Sorenson JM, Wheless JW, Baumgartner JE, *et al.* Corpus callosotomy for medically intractable seizures. *Pediatr Neurosurg* 1997;**27**:260–267.
[60] Jalilian L, Limbrick DD, Steger-May K, *et al.* Complete versus anterior two-thirds corpus callosotomy in children: analysis of outcome. *J Neurosurg Pediatr* 2010;**6**:257–266.

[61] Rahimi SY, Park YD, Witcher MR, *et al*. Corpus callosotomy for treatment of pediatric epilepsy in the modern era. *Pediatr Neurosurg* 2007;**43**:202–208.

[62] Tonini C, Beghi E, Berg AT, *et al*. Predictors of epilepsy surgery outcome: a meta-analysis. *Epilepsy Res* 2004;**62**:75–87.

[63] Wyllie E, Comair YG, Kotagal P, *et al*. Seizure outcome after epilepsy surgery in children and adolescents. *Ann Neurol* 1998;**44**:740–748.

[64] Sabaz M, Lawson JA, Cairns DR, *et al*. The impact of epilepsy surgery on quality of life in children. *Neurology* 2006;**66**:557–561.

13 Dietary therapies to treat epilepsy

James W. Wheless

Department of Pediatric Neurology, University of Tennessee Health Science Center; Le Bonheur Comprehensive Epilepsy Program and Neuroscience Institute, Le Bonheur Children's Hospital, Memphis, TN, USA

Seizure disorders in childhood represent a frequently occurring neurological problem. The incidence of epilepsy in children and adolescents ranges from 50 to 100 per 100 000. Antiepileptic drugs are the primary treatment modality and provide good seizure control in most children. However, more than 25% of children with seizure disorders have uncontrolled seizures (i.e., treatment-resistant epilepsy) or suffer significant adverse effects secondary to medication. Some children benefit from neurostimulation devices or surgical therapy (see Box 13.1 for a listing of all treatment options). The ketogenic diet has proven to be an effective alternative treatment for many children with epilepsy [1]. An independent review of the role of the efficacy of the ketogenic diet by the Blue Cross and Blue Shield Technology Assessment Center [2] concluded that "the ketogenic diet appears efficacious in reducing the frequency of seizures in children with refractory epilepsy . . . this improvement is in the range of, or greater than, that reported with the addition of newer AEDs (antiepileptic drugs)." This evaluation verifies the efficacy and the utility of the ketogenic diet even in the modern era with many more medication treatment options available. In this chapter the history of the development of the diet, current understanding of the biochemistry of ketone body formation and its relation to the anticonvulsant effect of the diet, considerations

Epilepsy in Children and Adolescents, First Edition. Edited by James W. Wheless.

Box 13.1 Treatment options for children with epilepsy*

- Medical therapy
- Neurostimulation devices
  - Vagus nerve stimulation (VNS therapy)
- Epilepsy surgery
- Dietary therapy:
  - ketogenic diet
  - modified Atkins diet
  - low glycemic index diet

*Listed in order of relative use, may be used in combination or alone.

related to patient selection, and diet efficacy, complications, advantages, and disadvantages are reviewed.

13.1 History

Since biblical times, fasting has been used to treat many diseases, including seizures. Contemporary accounts of fasting were also reported earlier in the twentieth century, the first being the patient of an osteopathic physician, Hugh Conklin. This child did not respond to the conventional treatment of the day, which was a combination of bromides and phenobarbital. Conklin managed this child's seizures with prayer and fasting, producing dramatic improvement in seizure control during the period of starvation. However, when the period of starvation was terminated, the seizures returned. The child's uncle, a pediatrician, enlisted the aid of John Howland at Johns Hopkins Hospital to understand how starvation and fasting controlled seizures and how one could maintain the beneficial effects of fasting. Concurrently, Wilder at the Mayo Clinic suggested that a diet high in fat and low in carbohydrates could maintain ketosis and its accompanying acidosis longer than fasting. Wilder was also the first to coin the term *ketogenic diet* [3]. The beneficial effects of this diet were initially recorded by investigators from Johns Hopkins University, the Mayo Clinic, and Harvard University.

Until 1938, the ketogenic diet was one of the few available therapies for epilepsy. The ketogenic diet fell into disfavor when researchers turned their attention to new antiepileptic drug development. Use of the ketogenic diet decreased greatly until it received national media attention in October 1994 when NBC Dateline aired a program on the ketogenic diet (Charlie Foundation to Help Cure Pediatric Epilepsy). This renewed public and scientific interest has led to a better understanding of the use of the ketogenic diet, inclusion in the American Academy of Pediatrics textbook on pediatric nutrition [4], publication of a textbook devoted to the ketogenic diet [5], an international consensus statement on clinical implementation [6], and worldwide use [7].

13.2 Efficacy

Initial reports began to appear in the 1920s and 1930s that documented the efficacy of the ketogenic diet. These were all retrospective reports; some entailed a small number of patients and many provided few clinical details or specification of epilepsy syndrome type. The studies clearly demonstrated that some patients had improved seizure control on the diet. Meta-analysis of the published data is not possible given the differences in study design, sparse clinical details, and the lack of any standardized definitions of what is meant by a "good" or "partial" response to the diet [8] (see Table 13.1 for outcome data from recent studies). Despite these limitations from some of the older studies, the literature supports the view that the diet improved seizure control in selected children. About one-third to one-half of children appeared to have had an excellent response to the diet, defined by cessation or marked reduction in seizure activity. About 10% of children become seizure free after initiation of the ketogenic diet, and typically stop the diet after 2 years. Of those children who become seizure free, a minority have recurrence after the diet is stopped. Risk factors that increase the likelihood of recurrence are: EEG epileptiform abnormalities (obtained within 12 months of diet discontinuation), a focal abnormality on MRI, lower initial seizure frequency, and tuberous sclerosis complex. When the diet is discontinued, it is usually due to lack of efficacy. It appeared that younger children were more likely to have a more favorable response than older children because these children were able to produce more elevated serum ketones and adhered to the diet's regimen.

Recent studies attest to the efficacy and safety of the ketogenic diet in infants. Nordli *et al.* retrospectively reviewed their experience with 32 infants who had been treated with the ketogenic diet, 17 of whom had infantile spasms [9]. Most infants (71%) were able to maintain strong ketosis. The overall effectiveness of the diet in infants was similar to that reported for older children; 19.4% became seizure-free, and an additional 35.5% had >50% reduction in seizure frequency. The diet was particularly effective for children with infantile spasms. In 2010, the Johns Hopkins Hospital reported their 14-year experience with 104 consecutive infants prospectively started on the ketogenic diet [10]. Thirty-seven percent became spasm free for at least a 6-month period, within a median 2.4 months of starting the ketogenic diet. A normal EEG was eventually obtained in 18%, and 17% showed resolution of hypsarrhythmia.

A few early studies evaluated use of the ketogenic diet in adults (Table 13.2). Some revealed improved seizure control, but subsequent reports concluded that the diet is not particularly beneficial in adolescents and adults with epilepsy. Reasons cited for this were poor dietary compliance, types of seizures seen in these age groups, and the developmental differences in the ability of the brain to use ketone bodies. As a result, past studies suggested that the optimum age of response to the diet may be in young children before the onset of adolescence. Recent studies have challenged the belief that older patients could not maintain therapeutic ketosis, could not comply with the rigors of the diet, and that the ketogenic diet was less efficacious in this age group. Mady *et al.* reviewed their experience with 45 adolescents who had been on the ketogenic diet for an average duration of 1.2 years [11]. They found no evidence to support the beliefs that the diet was not efficacious and too restrictive in this age group. Adolescents with multiple seizure types did best, and simple and complex partial seizures had the poorest response. The retention rate for motivated adolescents on the diet was not significantly different than reports in younger children.

Table 13.1 Efficacy of the ketogenic diet in the modern era.

Author	No. of patients	Age (years) of patients	Seizure type*	Diet*	Success rate (%)	Comments
Vining EPG, 1996	51	1–8	230 szs/month average (IS, SP, GTC, AB, CP, A, M)	KD	At 1 year 53% off diet ($^1/_2$ poor seizure control, $^1/_2$ poor tolerance), 40% of original group had a ≥50% decrease in seizure frequency and 10% were seizure free	Prospective, multicentered Failed average of seven drugs previously
Freeman JM, 1998	150	1–16	410 szs/month average (AB, M, A, IS, GTC)	KD	At 1 year, 55% remained on diet, of original group 43% had ≥50% decrease in seizure frequency, 7% were seizure-free	Prospective, 70% had IQ or DQ <69, prior trials of 6.2 AEDs (average)
Hemingway C, 2001	150	1–16 (mean 5.3)	Multiple seizure types	KD	83 on at 1 year, 58 on at >24 moths, 30 on >3 years. Of original 150, 13% seizure-free, 14% had 90–99% seizure decrease, many off or on fewer AEDs	Prospective, 3–6-year follow-up of Freeman JM, 1998
Maydell BV, 2001	143	0.34–29 (mean 7.5)	Multiple types, 34 focal onset, 100 generalized, Average 23.8 seizures/day	KD	68% on at 1 year, 16% seizure-free, 10% had 90–99% seizure decrease, 47% on fewer AEDs	Retrospective, 83 patients had mental retardation
Coppola G, 2002	56	1–23 (mean 10.4)	CP, GTC, LGS, M, GT, SMEI, AA	KD	Mean duration 5 months. At 12 months only 5 patients (8.9%) on diet and all of them had a >50% to <90% seizure reduction. None seizure free at 1 year	Prospective, multi-center. 96.4% had MR, 67% had CP, and 16% had microcephaly

Kang, HC, 2005	199	0.5–17.5	IS, LGS, PE, GE, SMEI, LKS, EIEE	KD	At 1 year 54% off diet (~$^1/_2$ intolerance or side effects, $^1/_2$ poor seizure control); 41% of the original group had a ≥50% decrease in seizure frequency and 25% were seizure free	Retrospective, Korean Partial onset and symptomatic etiology had frequent relapse after discontinuation
Freeman, 2009	20	1–7	LGS – A	KD	At 1 year, 60% remained on diet, 65% of those had ≥50% seizure reduction, 30% were seizure free	Prospective
Neal EG, 2009	73	2–16	LGS, IS, PE, A, M, GE	KD, MCT	3-month trial, at that time 54/73 on KD; 38% of total had >50% seizure reduction and 7% had >90% improvement. One child seizure free	UK, prospective, randomized trial of KD vs current treatment. Mean 11.6 seizures/day at baseline
Hong AM, 2010	104	1.2 (mean)	IS	KD	37% spasm-free for 6 months within 2.4 months (median) of starting diet. 18% had EEG normalize and 17% had resolution of hypsarrhythmia	Prospective

*A, atonic; AA, atypical absence; AB, absence; AEDs, antiepileptic drugs; CP, cerebral palsy; CP, complex partial; DQ, development quotient; EIEE, early infantile epileptic encephalopathy; GE, generalized epilepsy; GT, generalized tonic; GTC, generalized tonic-clonic; IQ, intelligence quotient; IS, infantile spasms; KD, classic ketogenic diet; LGS, Lennox–Gastaut syndrome; LKS, Landau–Kleffner syndrome; M, myoclonic; MCT, medium-chain triglyceride diet; MR, mental retardation; PE, partial epilepsy; SMEI, severe myoclonic epilepsy of infancy (Dravet syndrome); SP, simple partial.

Table 13.2 Efficacy of the ketogenic diet in adolescents and adults.

Author	Number of patients	Age (years)	Seizure type	Diet	Success rate (%)	Comments
Barborka CJ, 1928	49	17–42	GM, PM	KD	16% seizure free; 22% improved; 27% not benefitted; 35% did not cooperate and stay on diet	No patients with symptomatic epilepsy. Only 5 on an AED (PB)*. 3–36 month follow-up
Barborka CJ, 1930	100	16–51	GM, PM	KD	12% seizure free; 44% improved; 44% not benefited	No patients with symptomatic epilepsy. 3–60 month follow-up
Bastible C, 1931	45	19–57	GM, PM	KD	Of those staying on diet 7% seizure free; 72% improved; 21% seizures increased. 16/45 unable to maintain diet	All institutionalized females, diagnosed with "epileptic insanity," without known etiology. 6-month follow-up Best response seen in those with least "mental disorder"
Notkin J, 1934	20	22–47	GM	KD	No improvement in any, 90% had an increase in seizure number	All institutionalized patients and off AEDs, no known etiology. Average time on the diet 11 months
Sirven J, 1999	11	19–45	PE, GE	KD	9% seizure-free, 46% had >50% decrease in seizure number, 9% slight seizure decrease, 36% discontinued diet	All symptomatic epilepsy. 8-month follow-up
Mady MA, 2003	45	12–19	MT, LGS, CP, GTC, AB, M, A, SP	KD	20 remained on diet at 1 year, of these 6 had >90% efficacy, 7 had 50–90% efficacy	Average duration 1.2 years
Mosek A, 2009	9	23–36	PE	KD	None seizure free. 2/8 had >50% seizure reduction at 12 weeks	Only 2 maintained for 12 weeks (and they were dependent on family members for their food supply)

A, atonic; AB, absence; AED, antiepileptic drug; CP, complex partial; GE, generalized epilepsy; GM, grand mal; GTC, generalized tonic-clonic; KD, classic ketogenic diet; LGS, Lennox–Gastaut syndrome; MT, multiple seizure types; PB, phenobarbital; PE, partial epilepsy; PM, petit mal; SGTC, secondary GTC; SP, simple partial.

The first multicenter prospective study of the efficacy of the ketogenic diet was based on data collected at seven comprehensive epilepsy centers [12]. All children had intractable epilepsy, averaging 230 seizures per month. It was found that 10% of treated patients were seizure free at 1 year. A greater than 50% decrease in seizure frequency was observed at 3 months in 54% of patients. This improvement was maintained at 6 (53% controlled) and 12 months (49% controlled) after initiation of the diet. Patient age, seizure type, and EEG abnormalities were not related to outcome. Approximately 47% remained on the diet for at least 1 year. Reasons for discontinuation included insufficient seizure control, inability to medically tolerate the diet, concurrent medical illnesses, or inability to tolerate the restrictive nature of the dietary regimen. Although the number of patients was small, the study demonstrated that the diet could be effectively used in different epilepsy centers with different support staff, and that children and their families were able to comply with the diet when it was effective. The study also confirmed results similar to those reported over the past five decades.

The first large prospective evaluation of the ketogenic diet was conducted in 150 consecutive children ages 1 to 16 years (mean age 5.3 years) [13]. The children were followed for a minimum of 1 year, had previously been on an average of 6.24 medications, and were on a mean of 1.97 medications at the diet's initiation. Seventy percent of children had an intelligence or a developmental quotient of <69. The children averaged 410 seizures per month before the ketogenic diet. At 6 months, 71% remained on the diet and 32% had a >90% decrease in seizures. At 1 year, 55% remained on the diet, 7% were seizure-free, and 27% had a >90% decrease in seizure frequency. There was no statistically significant difference in seizure control based on age, sex, or seizure type, although none had purely partial seizures. Most of those discontinuing the diet did so because it was either insufficiently effective or too restrictive.

All of the prior reports of efficacy for the ketogenic diet were open-label trials (retrospective or prospective). Only one randomized, blinded crossover study has been performed. This study evaluated the efficacy for atonic-myoclonic or drop seizures associated with Lennox–Gastaut syndrome [14]. This documented it was feasible to perform a larger, blinded, placebo-controlled, crossover trial in this population with frequent seizures. Twenty children, experiencing at least 15 atonic seizures per day, were fasted for 36 hours, then received the ketogenic diet for 1 week in conjunction with a solution of glucose or saccharin. They were then crossed over to the other arm for an additional week. Physicians and parents were blinded to the solution composition and level of ketosis. Fasting and the ketogenic diet had a significant effect on decreasing the numbers of atonic seizures, which was only partially reversed with the addition of the glucose solution (urine ketones present at trace to moderate amounts: 15–60 mg/dL). The improvement in seizure control seen in the glucose arm may explain the effectiveness of the less restrictive diets (Atkins-like and low glycemic).

A single randomized controlled trial of the ketogenic diet has been performed in children ages 2 to 16 years old [15]. Children with various seizure types or epilepsy syndromes experiencing daily seizures were recruited. They were randomly assigned to receive the ketogenic diet immediately ($n = 73$), or after a 3-month delay, with no other changes in their treatment ($n = 72$, control group). Children were also randomly assigned to the classic or the medium-chain triglyceride (MCT) ketogenic diet. After 3 months, the mean percentage of baseline seizures was significantly lower ($P < 0.0001$) in the diet group (62%) than in the controls (136.9%). The children in the diet group had a mean of 13.3 seizures per day at baseline, and after 3 months of treatment, one was seizure-free, 28 (38%) had a >50% reduction in seizures, and 5 (7%) had a >90% reduction. Efficacy was the same for symptomatic generalized or symptomatic focal epilepsies. The most common adverse events were constipation, vomiting, lack of energy, and hunger.

The same authors report on the 1-year follow-up of those children randomized to the classic or MCT versions of the ketogenic diet [16]. Of the 125 children who started the diets, data from 64 were available at 6 months, and from 47 at 12 months. At 12 months there was no significant difference between groups in number achieving >50% (17.8% vs 22.2%) or >90% (9.6% vs 9.7%) seizure reduction. There was no significant difference in tolerability except increased reports of lack of energy after 3 months, and vomiting after 12 months, both in the classical group.

In recent years, two alternative diet regimens that are less restrictive and may be more palatable in nature have emerged: the modified Atkins diet and a low glycemic index treatment (Figure 13.1). No prospective, comparative trials have been performed between the three treatments to evaluate relative efficacy and side-effect profiles. The Atkins diet is less restrictive than the ketogenic diet, and induces a metabolic ketosis. A modified Atkins diet was created at Johns Hopkins Hospital for patients reluctant to start on a traditional ketogenic diet. The modified Atkins diet is similar in fat composition to a 1:1 ketogenic ratio diet, with approximately 65% of the calories from fat sources. This treatment can be started as an outpatient, with guidance from a nutritionist. Studies in children, adolescents, and adults reveal that 45% have a 50–90% seizure reduction, and slightly over 25% have a >90% seizure reduction (Table 13.3).

The low glycemic index treatment was designed at the Massachusetts General Hospital as a regimen that would be less restrictive than the ketogenic diet, but keep the principle of minimizing the blood glucose [17]. Approximately 20–30% of calories are from protein, and 60–70% from fat. Total carbohydrates are gradually decreased to 40–60 g/day (about 10% of calories), using foods with a low glycemic index. In a retrospective review, of 76 children on the low glycemic index diet, the percentage who achieved a >50% seizure reduction from baseline seizure frequency was 42%, 50%, 54%, 64%, and 66% of the population with follow-up at 1, 3, 6, 9, and 12 months, respectively. Efficacy did not differ with regard to partial-onset or generalized seizure types. Increased efficacy was correlated with lower serum glucose levels at the 1- and 12-month follow-up visits. Side effects were minimal, with only three patients reporting transient lethargy. Children were placed on

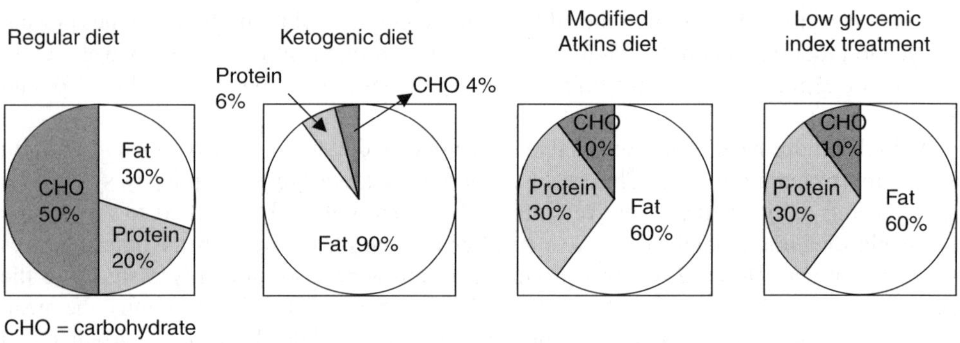

Figure 13.1 Composition of diets.

Table 13.3 Efficacy of the modified Atkins diet.

Author	Number of patients	Age (years)	Seizure type	Success rate (%)	Comments
Kossoff EH, 2006	20	3–18 (mean 8.1)	Not given	At 6 months, 65% had >50% improvement; 35% had >90% improvement (4/7 seizure free)	Prospective. 16/20 (80%) completed 6 months. 11/20 remained on diet at 10 months
Kang HC, 2007	14	2–14	CP, LGS, Doose syndrome	At 6 months, only 7 on diet, but 5/7 (36%) had >50% seizure reduction and 3/7 seizure free	Prospective
Kossoff EH, 2007	20	4–15 (mean 7.5)	CP, generalized or multifocal epilepsy	12 completed 6-month trial. 10 (50%) had >50% improvement and 7 (35%) >90% (2 seizure free)	Prospective, randomized, crossover study (10 vs 20 g of carbohydrate/day). 10 g/day more likely to have >50% seizure reduction at 3 months
Carrette E, 2008	8	31–55 (mean 41.8)	CP, LGS	3 completed 6-month trial, 1/3 (12.5%) showed >50% seizure reduction	Prospective
Kossoff EH, 2008	30	18–53 (median 31)	CP, AB, multiple types	14 completed the 6-month study; 8 (30%) had >50% improvement, 1 seizure free	Prospective, open label
Weber S, 2009	15	2/17 (median 10)	CP, LGS, AB, JME, Doose syndrome	12 completed the 6-month study, 6 (40%) had >50% improvement, 2 (13%) had >90%	Prospective, open label
Porta, 2009	10	0.5–15	CP, IS, LGS, GTC	5 completed, median duration 3 months; 2 (20%) had >50% improvement at 6 months	Retrospective

AB, absence; CP, complex partial or partial onset +/– secondary generalization; GTC, generalized tonic-clonic; IS, infantile spasms; JME, juvenile myoclonic epilepsy; LGS, Lennox–Gastaut syndrome.

the low glycemic treatment for several reasons: (i) families thought their child could not comply with the ketogenic diet; (ii) there was a greater than 2-week wait for admission to initiate the ketogenic diet; or (iii) they were unable to tolerate the restrictive nature of the ketogenic diet, so they were transitioned to the low glycemic treatment. These reports raise important questions about the level of restrictions on protein and calories imposed by the ketogenic diet, and there may be a subgroup of patients who benefit from less restrictive diets. Dietary therapies may become even more valuable in the therapy of epilepsy when the mechanisms underlying their success are understood.

13.3 Mechanism of action

While clinical reports detailed the efficacy of the ketogenic diet, several theories emerged to explain the diet's mechanism of action [18]. Animal models and human evidence suggest a prominent role of ketonemia [19]. However, despite its prolonged use and proven value, the exact mechanism of action of the diet remains unknown [20].

Oxidation of fatty acids: ketogenesis

Ketonemia is essential for the ketogenic diet to work. Ketonemia occurs as a result of fatty acid oxidation during fasting or while on the ketogenic diet. Fatty acids are both oxidized to and synthesized from acetyl-CoA. However, these are not reverse processes. Fatty acid biosynthesis (lipogenesis) takes place in the cytosol, whereas fatty acid oxidation occurs in mitochondria and generates ATP. The oxidizable substrate may come from dietary sources (ketogenic diet) or from mobilization of peripheral adipose stores (starvation) (Figure 13.2). The brain does not directly use fatty acids but readily oxidizes ketone bodies. Increased fatty acid oxidation leading to ketone body (acetoacetate and beta-hydroxybutyrate) formation by the liver is characteristic of starvation or the ketogenic diet (Figure 13.3). Glucose, present in small concentrations, is necessary to facilitate ketone body metabolism. This is referred to as the permissive effect of glucose, and is explained metabolically by the conversion of glucose-derived pyruvate to oxaloacetate. Oxaloacetate is the key rate-limiting metabolite of the tricarboxylic acid (TCA) cycle, and is necessary for the condensation reaction with acetyl-coenzyme A to form citrate. Acetoacetate continually undergoes spontaneous decarboxylation to yield acetone, which is volatilized in the lungs and gives the breath its characteristic odor. The ratio of beta-hydroxybutyrate to acetoacetate in blood varies

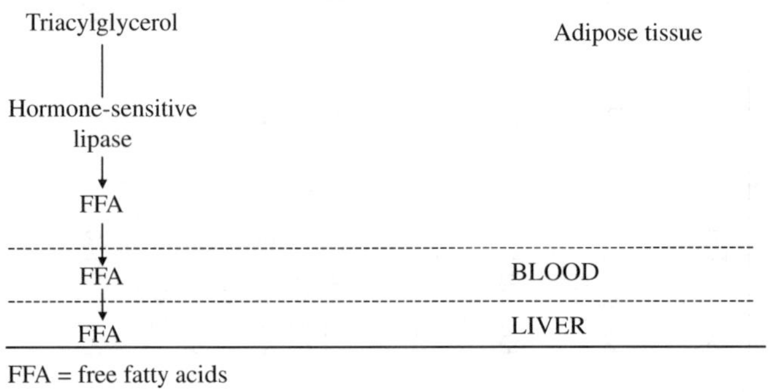

Figure 13.2 Initial steps in ketogenesis: lipolysis.

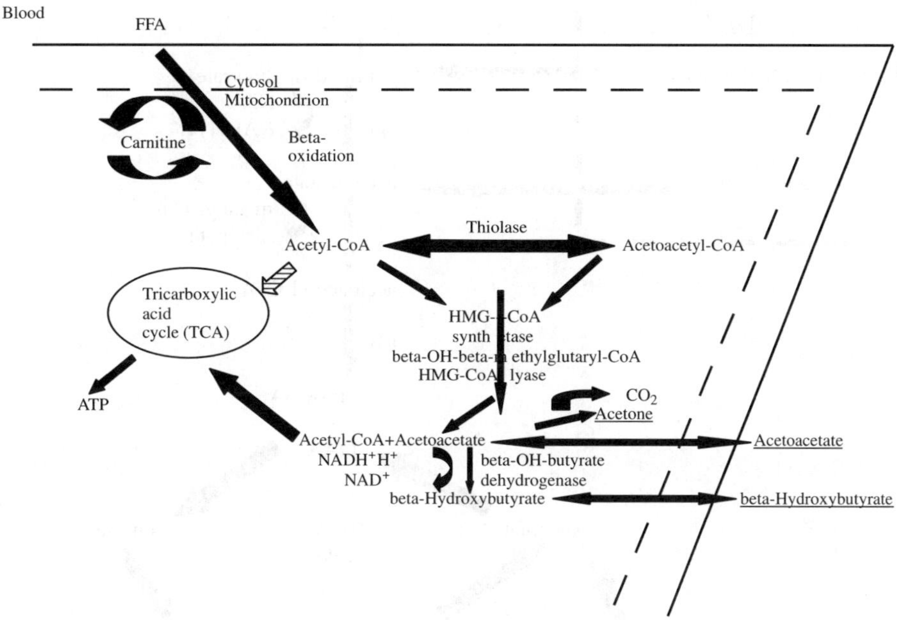

Figure 13.3 Ketogenesis in the liver. FFA (free fatty acids) from the circulation enter the hepatocyte, then cross the mitochondrial membrane by carnitine transport (long-chain fatty acids) or diffusion (short- and medium-chain fatty acids). CoA, eoenzyme A; HMG, hydroxymethylglutaryl-.

between 1:1 and 10:1; the concentration of total ketone bodies in the blood does not normally exceed 0.2 mmol/L.

The liver is the only organ capable of synthesizing significant quantities of ketone bodies that are released into the blood (Figure 13.3). The liver is equipped with an active enzymatic mechanism for the production of acetoacetate. Once formed, acetoacetate cannot be significantly metabolized back to fatty acids in the liver because the latter lacks the enzyme 3-oxoacid-CoA transferase. This accounts for the net production of ketone bodies by the liver. Ketone bodies are then transported to and oxidized in extrahepatic tissues proportionately to their concentration in the blood. Oxidation and brain influx rates of ketone bodies are proportional to their blood concentration to approximately 12 mmol/L. At this level, the oxidative machinery and uptake mechanisms of the cell are saturated.

Glucose is the principal source for brain metabolism. Under certain conditions (e.g., fasting, ketogenic diet), the human brain uses ketone bodies for fuel, with the movement of ketone bodies into the brain dependent on a monocarboxylic transport system. Acetoacetate and beta-hydroxybutyrate are metabolized primarily in the mitochondrial compartment. In the brain the main pathway for the conversion of acetoacetate to acetoacetyl-CoA involves succinyl-CoA (Figure 13.4). Acetoacetyl-CoA is split to acetyl-CoA and oxidized in the tricarboxylic acid cycle. The enzymes that break down beta-hydroxybutyrate and acetoacetate into acetyl-CoA are regulated developmentally, with maximal expression early in life. Ketone bodies serve not only as a source of energy (from their oxidation) but also contribute to certain cerebral metabolic pathways normally dependent on glucose metabolism (i.e., glutamate, gamma-aminobutyrate (GABA)). Tricarboxylic acid cycle activity is governed by the availability of oxaloacetate and the rate-limiting enzyme, alpha-ketoglutarate dehydrogenase. Alpha-ketoglutarate dehydrogenase is regulated by the concentration of

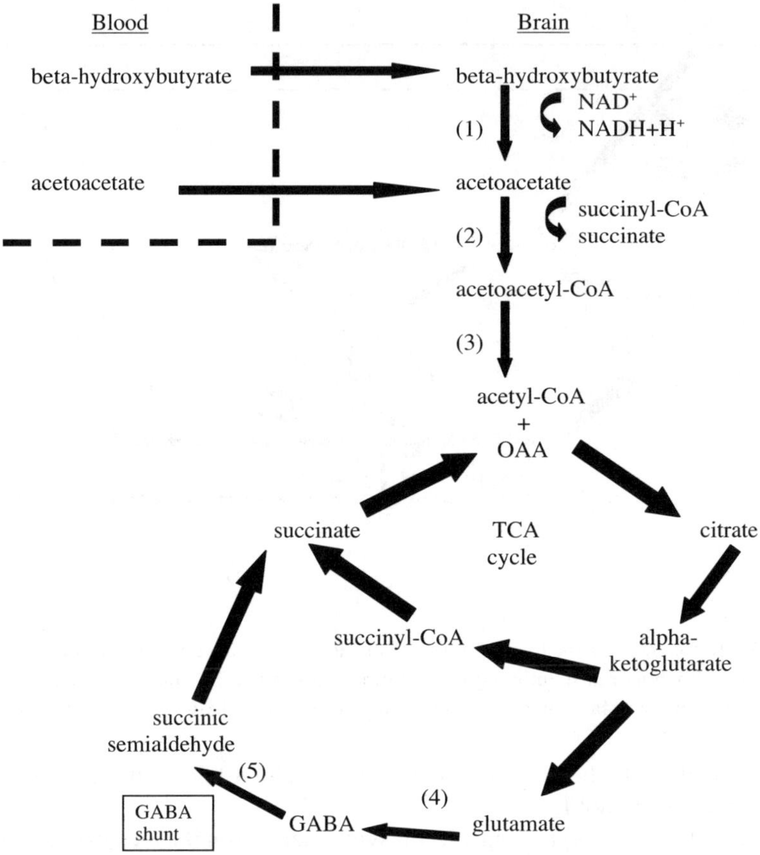

GABA, gamma-aminobutyrate; OAA, oxaloacetate; TCA, tricarboxlyic acid cycle; 1, beta-hydroxybutyrate dehydrogenase; 2, 3-oxoacid-coenzyme A (CoA) transferase; 3, acetoacetyl-CoA thiolase; 4, glutamic acid decarboxylase (GAD); 5, GABA-transaminase.

Figure 13.4 Ketone body utilization and oxidation in the brain.

succinyl-CoA. Increased alpha-ketoglutarate and decreased succinyl-CoA imply maximal tricarboxylic acid cycle activity. Fatty acid oxidation increases brain ATP concentration. Elevation of brain ATP concentration has been verified in an animal model of the ketogenic diet and suggests that the ketogenic diet improves cerebral energetics. Increased cerebral energy reserves have been hypothesized to be important for the anticonvulsant effect. Another mechanism may be alteration of the synthesis or function of GABA. Increases in alpha-ketoglutarate when on the diet may increase input into the $GABA_A$ shunt. The addition of beta-hydroxybutyrate to cultured rat astrocytes suppresses GABA-transaminase in time- and dose-dependent manners [21]. Recent human studies correlate GABA receptor stimulation with increased energy demand, probably at the synaptic or glial cell level. Activation of GABA pathways, although inhibitory, requires increased energetic demand. The ketogenic diet increases cerebral energetics, potentially helping to meet this demand and will increase the overall GABA inhibitory effects by activating certain GABA receptor subtypes. Many epilepsies may involve disruptions of brain energy homeostasis, leading to potential management through dietary elevations of ketone bodies and reduction of glucose.

Clinical studies

Although the exact mechanism of action of the ketogenic diet is unknown, it is generally accepted that for the diet to be successful, the child must remain in ketosis and generate ketone bodies. Ketonemia is necessary but not sufficient for ketogenic diet-induced seizure control. Urine ketones are the only readily available inexpensive approach to ketone assessment, and typically the desired range is 80–160 mmol/L. Seizure control correlates significantly with serum beta-hydroxybutyrate levels greater than 4 mmol/L, although urine ketones of 160 mmol/L can be found when blood beta-hydroxybutyrate levels exceed 2 mmol/L. It is also accepted that the classic ketogenic diet produces the greatest amount of ketone bodies. Despite the fact that ketone bodies partially replace glucose for cerebral metabolism, cerebral glucose levels are unaltered. Ketones from the circulation are transported across the blood–brain barrier by facilitated diffusion, using a monocarboxylate transport system. The efficacy of the diet in childhood and the apparent slightly lower efficacy in older children and adults may be due to maturational changes in this transport system. A child's ability to extract ketones from the blood into the brain is four to five times greater than that seen in adults. This developmentally based ability to extract ketones from the blood may, in part, explain why the diet is more successful in children. However, even adult animals placed on the ketogenic diet can upregulate brain monocarboxylate transporter levels. Magnetic resonance spectroscopy (MRS) has also been used to study changes in cerebral energetics induced by the ketogenic diet. Alteration of the TCA cycle activity by ketosis, resulting in an increased ATP:ADP ratio or greater cerebral energy, has been hypothesized to have an anticonvulsant effect. This hypothesis is supported by recent experiments in patients with Lennox–Gastaut syndrome that used magnetic resonance spectroscopy (MRS; ^{31}P) to document improvement in cerebral energy metabolism on the ketogenic diet.

Additionally, during chronic ketosis, adaptive mechanisms occur that increase the cerebral extraction of ketone bodies. These mechanisms may explain why ketosis develops promptly within several days after initiation of the diet but the anticonvulsant effect may be delayed for 1 to 2 weeks. This observation suggests that ketosis per se is insufficient to explain the anticonvulsant effect. Once ketone bodies are extracted, it is postulated that there is a secondary biochemical change or a cascade of biochemical effects that have some form of anticonvulsant effect.

Experimental studies

In the last 15 years there has been an explosion of basic research, which has led to an increased understanding of the ketogenic diet and its effect on brain chemistry. At the present time, there are several animal models used to study the effects of the ketogenic diet [19]. In general, these animal models demonstrate that the ketogenic diet provides protection for partial-onset seizures with secondary generalization and generalized myoclonic, tonic, and tonic-clonic seizures, providing laboratory evidence that the diet is effective against a variety of seizure types. However, some studies have failed to show a protective effect of the ketogenic diet in models where animals were acutely challenged with a convulsant stimulus (kainic acid, strychnine, maximal electroconvulsive shock, flurothyl or pentylenetetrazol mouse models). The discrepancy is probably explained by the fact that the latter studies did not test the diet in animals with spontaneous seizures. The relative efficacy of the ketogenic diet in differing animal models suggests that different areas of the brain might be affected more than others, and this could relate to localized differences in the function of GABA, other neurotransmitters (e.g., norepinephrine), or protein phosphorylation.

Despite differences in ketogenic diet protocols and laboratory models, collectively they show improvement in control of multiple seizure types by increasing seizure threshold. Additionally, the response of most seizure types to the ketogenic diet implies that the diet exerts a general suppressant effect on neuronal excitability.

13.4 Selection of candidates for the diet

Indications for the use of the ketogenic diet have unfortunately grown out of experience, not from understanding of its physiologialc action. Despite the fact that several thousand patients have been treated, there currently are no consensus criteria as to which patients are candidates for the diet (see Tables 13.1–13.3). Many seizure types appear to respond to the ketogenic diet. In general, several groups of children are potential candidates for treatment. These include children with the following:

1. Medically intractable seizures.
2. Poor tolerance or significant side effects from antiepileptic drugs.
3. Intractable seizures who are being considered for epilepsy surgery (i.e., callosotomy; non-lesional, extra-temporal resections).
4. Specific neurometabolic disorders or neurological syndromes (Box 13.2).

One must also consider the age of the patient in children with medically intractable epilepsy or in those who have serious side effects from medication. As previously discussed, successful outcomes have been experienced in children ages 1 to 12 years. In

Box 13.2 Specific conditions treated with the ketogenic diet

- Glucose transporter deficiency syndrome* (GLUT1-DS, *SLC2A1* gene, McKusick 138140)
- Pyruvate dehydrogenase complex deficiency* (McKusick 312170)
  - Associated with Leigh syndrome
  - Associated with lactic acidosis and cerebral dysgenesis
- Succinic semialdehyde dehydrogenase (SSADH) deficiency
- Phosphofructokinase deficiency
- Mitochondrial respiratory chain complex defects
- Ketotic hypoglycemia
- Glycogenosis type V (McArdle disease)
- Acquired epileptiform opercular syndrome
- Acquired epileptic aphasia (Landau–Kleffner syndrome)
- Rett syndrome
- Tuberous sclerosis complex

*The ketogenic diet is specifically indicated for these two metabolic disorders.

older children, it is often more difficult to maintain ketosis. Seizure type appears to be less important. Almost all seizure types respond to the ketogenic diet. The success of the diet in children is determined far more by circumstances within the home than by the epilepsy itself. The ketogenic diet is a strictly regulated medical diet. Its success depends on the detailed accuracy and consistency with which the regimen is carried out within the home. Continued support, monitoring, and education by a team of professionals (including physicians, dietitians, nurses, and social workers) are necessary.

The diet could be used preferentially in selected candidates who are being considered for corpus callosotomy, non-lesional resections, or extra-temporal resections. In those patients in whom a malignancy or vascular malformation is detected, surgery is preferable. Additional research is needed in this area.

The ketogenic diet may be the preferred initial therapy in children with seizures and specific metabolic defects or seizures associated with specific neurological syndromes (see Box 13.2 and Figure 13.5).

For some patients, the ketogenic diet is contraindicated (Box 13.3). When indicated, obtaining a metabolic screen, including urine amino and organic acids, serum amino acids, lactate, pyruvate, and carnitine profile should be performed before starting the ketogenic

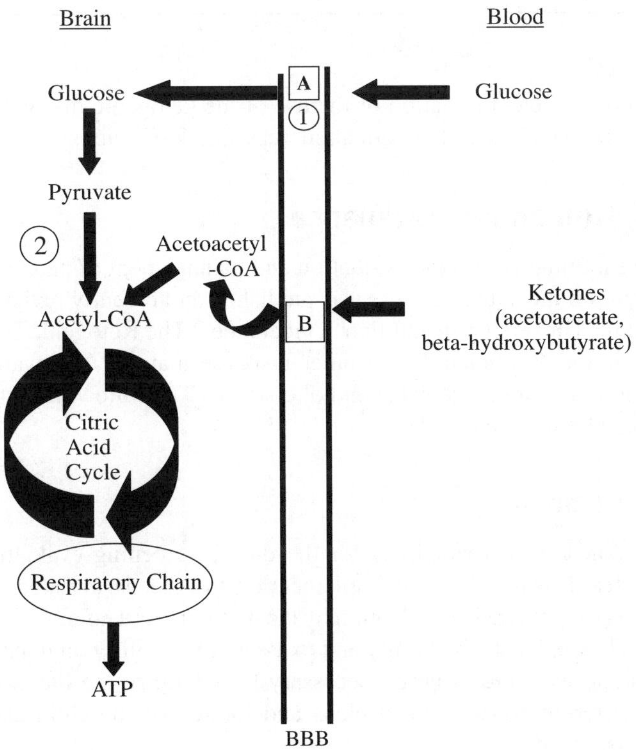

Figure 13.5 Metabolic defects and the ketogenic diet. Glucose enters the brain via (A) the glucose transporter, GLUT1; ketones penetrate the blood–brain barrier (BBB) via (B) the medium-chain triglyceride transporter, MCT-1-transporter. 1: GLUT1 deficiency syndrome is caused by a defect in glucose transport into the brain. 2: Pyruvate dehydrogenase deficiency impairs acetyl-CoA production. The ketogenic diet bypasses these two defects and provides acetyl-CoA for brain energy production.

Box 13.3 Specific contraindications to the ketogenic diet

- Pyruvate carboxylase deficiency
- Organic acidurias
- Selected mitochondrial disease
- Porphyria
- Defects in fatty acid oxidation:
  - Short-chain acyl dehydrogenase deficiency (SCAD)
  - Medium-chain acyl dehydrogenase deficiency (MCAD)
  - Long-chain acyl dehydrogenase deficiency (LCAD)
  - Medium-chain 3-hydroxyacyl-CoA deficiency
  - Long-chain 3-hydroxyacyl-CoA deficiency
- Carnitine deficiency (primary)
- Carnitine palmitoyltransferase (CPT) I or II deficiency
- Carnitine translocase deficiency
- Glutaric aciduria, type II
- Pyruvate dehydrogenase phosphate deficiency

diet [22]. In addition, the combination of the use of the ketogenic diet with topiramate or zonisamide appears to be associated with an increased risk of acidosis.

13.5 Initiation and maintenance

A comprehensive monograph on the evaluation and management of patients being considered for placement on the ketogenic diet was published and recently revised by Kossoff *et al.* at Johns Hopkins University. In addition, a videotape, "The Ketogenic Diet for Families, Dietitians, Nurses and Physicians," and other resource material are available from The Charlie Foundation (see Resource list at end of chapter). The following is a brief overview of how the diet can be implemented.

Pre-hospital evaluation

Once a child is considered a candidate for the diet, a screening evaluation by selected members of the team responsible for implementing the diet is initiated. This screening usually includes a comprehensive evaluation by the dietitians and nursing staff. The purpose of this evaluation is to educate the family and to assess their ability on many levels to carry out the rigorous and exacting program necessary to maximize the diet's success. At the same time, the different types of meal plans and foods that the child can eat and their preparation are discussed.

Hospitalization

The child is typically scheduled for elective admission to the hospital for initiation of the ketogenic diet (Box 13.4), although, in recent years, both retrospective and prospective

Box 13.4 Initiation of the ketogenic diet

Hospitalization for 3 days

Day 1

Maintenance fluids
Check urine ketones each void
Check finger-stick blood glucose every 6 hours
Initial EEG, labs
Simplify AED regimen, change to low- or carbohydrate-free medicine formulation
Nutrition consult
Education

Day 2

4:1 ratio (3:1 in infants), 1/3 of total calories using eggnog for 2–3 meals, then 2/3 of total calories for 2–3 meals.
Stop finger-stick blood glucose checks.

Day 3

First regular meal on 4:1 ratio.
Discharge – AED regimen
B vitamins, sugar-free multivitamins
Calcium supplements

AED, antiepileptic drug.
May start the ketogenic diet on the first day, after a brief or no initial fast.

studies have documented the feasibility of initiating the diet as an outpatient. However, the intense educational process afforded by inpatient initiation may be preferable for some families and ketogenic diet centers. Additionally, inpatient initiation allows observation of the child's initial response to the diet and possible immediate adverse effects. Parents are told to view this treatment as a 6–8-week trial. When effective, the ketogenic diet works quickly, typically within the first 1–2 weeks. The time to improvement was significantly quicker (mean 5 vs 14 days, $P < 0.01$) in those children who are fasted at onset, but there is no difference (vs non-fasting) in long-term outcome. If there is no seizure reduction after 6–8 weeks, the ketogenic diet can be discontinued. During this time the patient must adhere strictly to the diet, with proof of persistent ketosis. The frequency of seizures usually decreases gradually, but reversal of the effect can occur rapidly. Weeks of hard work can be undone if a child eats a cookie or a piece of candy. If the seizures are improved, this usually is sufficient motivation for the parents to continue. If there are any questions that the child may have an underlying metabolic disease that could be exacerbated by the initial fast, an appropriate evaluation should be performed before initiating the diet. The day before hospital admission, the parents are asked to eliminate carbohydrates from the child's diet. The child eats foods that contain only protein or fat. After dinner, the child begins fasting with only non-caloric, non-caffeinated beverages given. On the first hospital day, a wake-and-sleep EEG may be performed. Laboratory studies (complete blood count (CBC), platelet count, chemistry panel, and antiepileptic drug levels) are obtained either before or at the time of admission. During this time the child receives maintenance fluids and may have one caffeine-free diet drink per day. Blood glucose levels are checked every 6 hours. The dietitian uses this time to further review meal plans and the child's food preferences and eating habits with the parents. On Day 1 the child is started on the ketogenic diet using a 3:1 or 4:1 ratio (fat to protein plus carbohydrate), depending on the child's age. A ketogenic eggnog is used for the initial feedings. The child receives three meals at one-third the total calories, is advanced as tolerated to two-thirds of the total calories for three meals (Day 2), and then eats his or her first full meal. Before discharge the parents prepare their first ketogenic meal for their child under the supervision of the dietitian. At discharge the parents have several meal plans for their child and are instructed to monitor the urine ketones on a daily basis and record all seizures. Individual decisions are made during the hospital stay if the antiepileptic drug regimen will be simplified. The child is given a prescription for sugar-free multivitamin, mineral, and calcium supplements and instructed to begin these at home. Supplementation with vitamin D and calcium prevents osteomalacia and decreased bone mass while on the ketogenic diet. Inadvertent administration of carbohydrates may occur when intercurrent illnesses are treated. Parents and pediatricians must appreciate that decongestants, antipyretics, and antibiotics are often contained in carbohydrate-containing vehicles. The child is then seen regularly for follow-up (Box 13.5). Special attention should be paid to the serum albumin and total protein concentration to make sure that the diet is providing enough protein. Cholesterol and triglyceride levels typically rise when the diet is started, but the diet may be continued unless the cholesterol level rises above 1000 mg/dL and consistently stays there. It is not unusual to see minor elevations in the direct bilirubin. Decisions regarding withdrawal of antiepileptic drugs depend on the child's response to the diet and the family's perception of lack of efficacy and side effects. Early reduction (during diet initiation or the first month thereafter) of antiepileptic drugs appears to be safe and well tolerated; however, it offers no definite advantage compared with a late taper. At follow-up, the dietitian also reviews the parental concerns with implementing the diet and makes adjustments in the meal plan as necessary to maintain the child in maximum ketosis. In children who can be successfully withdrawn from antiepileptic drug therapy and are seizure free for 2 years on the ketogenic diet (about 10% of treated children), an EEG is repeated and the ketogenic diet is slowly withdrawn over 1 year. Many of these families elect to continue a low-carbohydrate diet, concerned that seizures may recur.

13.6 Complications

It needs to be stressed to parents that the diet is a form of medical therapy, and as such, although relatively safe, it is not without side effects [22]. However, only 6–17% of patients discontinued the diet for medical reasons. Like antiepileptic drugs, the ketogenic diet has an adverse event profile, consisting of possible complications seen during initiation

Box 13.5 Ketogenic diet maintenance visits

One month

Neurologist, dietitian, nurse, social worker
Adjust diet as needed
Labs: CBC, platelets; CMP; AED level(s); serum lipid and carnitine profiles
Urine calcium, creatinine and urine analysis

Three, six, and twelve months

Neurologist, dietitian, nurse
Labs: CBC, platelets, CMP; serum lipid and carnitine profiles
AED level(s) if needed, urine analysis with calcium, creatinine
New meals

Maintain for 2 years (seizure free) (shorter time interval for infantile spasms)

Wean over 1 year

$3^1/_2$:1 for 3 months → 3:1 for 3 months →
$2^1/_2$:1 for 3 months → 2:1 for 3 months →
Off

Check labs mentioned above at 3, 6, and 12 months, then every 4–6 months after that, and at other times as clinically indicated.
AED, antiepileptic drug; CBC, complete blood count; CMP, comprehensive metabolic profile.

(Table 13.4) or maintenance (Table 13.5) [22]. If the child has an unrecognized metabolic defect, a catastrophic event could occur during the fasting phase (see Box 13.3). Other adverse events can occur during the initial hospital stay, and, if recognized, are usually easily treated (see Table 13.4). A number of adverse events can occur during the maintenance phase. Many can be prevented with close monitoring, vitamin supplementation, and anticipatory treatment. Fatigue occurs in many children during initiation of the diet but is prolonged in only a small number. Children with gastroesophageal reflux, especially if they have cerebral palsy, may have increased gastroesophageal reflux while on the diet. The high fat content decreases gastric emptying, which promotes gastroesophageal reflux. This problem usually can be managed medically. Close attention to growth measurements, laboratory data, and medical supervision is indicated in infants on the ketogenic diet. A prospective cohort study of 237 children, with an average length of follow-up of 308 days, analyzed height and weight measurements (age- and sex-appropriate) over time on the ketogenic diet. A small decrease in height scores was observed in the first 6 months, with larger changes by 2 years. There was a drop in weight in the first 3 months, and after this, the

Table 13.4 Possible adverse events during initiation of the ketogenic diet.*

Adverse event	Monitoring/treatment strategy
Dehydration	Encourage fluids (do not limit fluids to less than 75% of maintenance); intravenous fluids if necessary (without dextrose)
Hypoglycemia	Check blood sugars every 6 hours until the diet is initiated; if symptomatic or blood sugar <30 mg/dL, give orange juice. Screen for metabolic errors in advance
Vomiting	Intravenous fluids; give orange juice

*The adverse event on the left side is linked to the monitoring and/or treatment strategy on the right side of the table.

weight remained constant in children who started the diet below the 50% for their weight, while it continued to decrease in children starting above the 50%. Very young children (0–2 years) grew poorly on the diet, while older children (7–10 years) grew almost normally.

Several laboratory abnormalities have been reported in children on the ketogenic diet, although none has been found to have clinical significance. Patients on the ketogenic diet are in a chronic acidotic state, putting them at risk for osteopenia. Supplementation of vitamin D and calcium were not sufficient to prevent bone mineral content loss. Increased supplementation and periodic surveillance with dual energy X-ray absorptiometry may be needed to prevent or treat the loss of bone mineral content in children treated with

Table 13.5 Possible adverse events during maintenance of the ketogenic diet.*

Adverse event	Monitoring/treatment strategy
Constipation	Polyethylene glycol, mineral oil, suppositories
Exacerbation of gastroesophageal reflux disease	Medical management
Poor growth	Check albumin, total protein Adequate protein Monitor height, weight
Kidney stones	Urine dipstick for blood, renal ultrasonography Analyze stone (specific treatment) Increase fluids, alkalinize urine
Dyslipidemia, hyperlipidemia	Check liver function tests, lipid profile; if sustained elevations of cholesterol/triglycerides, adjust diet and/or treat
Prolonged QT interval, cardiomyopathy	Electrocardiography, echocardiography, check serum selenium level
Excessive bruising	Complete blood count, platelet count
Optic neuropathy	B vitamins
Elevated very-long-chain fatty acids	Check prior to ketogenic diet if clinically suspected
Vitamin D deficiency, osteomalacia	Vitamin D, calcium supplement; bone mineral density/densitrometry
Trace mineral deficiencies	Copper, selenium, zinc

*The adverse event on the left side is linked to the suggested treatment and/or monitoring strategy on the right side of the table.

the ketogenic diet. Serum cholesterol and triglycerides may increase, especially during the first 6 months, tend to plateau by 6 months, then decline and require routine monitoring. Adjustments to the diet (e.g., increased protein and polyunsaturated fat) can be made in children with significantly high cholesterol and triglyceride concentrations. Supplementation with magnesium, zinc, calcium, vitamin D, and B vitamins is recommended to avoid deficiency-related disease states. The ketogenic diet is deficient in several trace minerals, and if children are maintained on the diet for more than 2 years, these need to be supplemented.

Serious complications of the ketogenic diet are rare, and typically consist of single reports: Fanconi renal tubular acidosis (co-treatment with valproate), severe hypoproteinemia, marked increase in liver function tests (co-treatment with valproate), cardiomyopathy, prolonged QTc, acute hemorrhagic pancreatitis, basal ganglia injury, scurvy, lipoid pneumonia, and fatal propofol infusion syndrome.

A single, retrospective chart review reports maintenance of efficacy and tolerability with long-term use of the ketogenic diet (duration of 6–12 years, $n = 28$) [23]. However, side effects of decreased growth (23/28), kidney stones (7/28), and fractures (6/28) occurred, and careful monitoring with strategies to minimize these complications are suggested. Lipid profiles were not significantly affected.

13.7 The ketogenic diet in the twenty-first century

More than 80 years have passed since the ketogenic diet was initially used, and many more therapies are now available for children with epilepsy. The ketogenic diet compares favorably with other new treatments that have been introduced to treat epilepsy. The question that remains unanswered is, "When in the course of therapy for a child with intractable epilepsy should the ketogenic diet be used?" Currently, it is not used until children have failed multiple medications and are not considered surgical candidates. However, in some epilepsy syndromes the diet should be offered as a treatment strategy after failure of one or two drugs. If the child has an epilepsy syndrome that is often resistant to current therapy, at the time of the initial therapeutic discussions, the ketogenic diet should be mentioned as an alternative therapy if the seizures are not controlled on medication. This is especially true in children who are not good candidates for epilepsy surgery or whose parents do not wish to have epilepsy surgery. It is critical that those taking care of children with seizures be aware of all the treatment options and refer children whose seizures are not controlled to centers specializing in the care of such children [24]. For many such children the ketogenic diet continues to represent a therapeutic alternative.

References

[1] Wheless JW. The ketogenic diet: fa(c)t or fiction. *J Child Neurol* 1995;**10**:419–423.

[2] Lefevre F, Aronson N. Ketogenic diet for the treatment of refractory epilepsy in children: a systematic review of efficacy. *Pediatrics* 2000;**105**:e46. Available at: http://www.pediatrics.org/cgi/content/full/105/4/e46.

[3] Wheless JW. History and origin of the ketogenic diet. In: Stafstrom CE, Rho JM (eds), *Epilepsy and the Ketogenic Diet*. Totawa, NJ: Humana Press, Inc., 2004; pp. 31–50.

[4] Kleinman RE (ed.). *The Ketogenic Diet. Pediatric Nutrition Handbook*, 6th edn. Chicago, IL: American Academy of Pediatrics, 2009; pp. 1021–1040.

[5] Stafstrom CE, Rho JM (eds). *Epilepsy and the Ketogenic Diet*. Totawa, NJ: Humana Press, Inc., 2004.

[6] Kossoff EH, Zupec-Kania BA, Amark PE, *et al*. Optimal clinical management of children receiving the ketogenic diet: recommendations of the International Ketogenic Diet Study Group. *Epilepsia* 2009;**50**:304–317.

[7] Kossoff EH, McGrogan. Worldwide use of the ketogenic diet. *Epilepsia* 2005;**46**:280–289.

[8] Prasad AN, Stafstrom CF, Holmes GL. Alternative epilepsy therapies: the ketogenic diet, immunoglobulins, and steroids. *Epilepsia* 1996;**37**:S81–S95.

[9] Nordli DR, Kuroda MM, Carroll J, *et al*. Experience with the ketogenic diet in infants. *Pediatrics* 2001;**108**:129–133.

[10] Hong AM, Turner Z, Hamdy RF, Kossoff EH. Infantile spasms treated with the ketogenic diet: prospective single center experience in 104 consecutive infants. *Epilepsia* 2010;**51**:1403–1407.

[11] Mady MA, Kossoff EH, McGregor AL, *et al*. The ketogenic diet: adolescents can do it, too. *Epilepsia* 2003;**44**:847–851.

[12] Vining EPG, Freeman JM, Ballaban-Gil K, *et al*. A multi-center study of the efficacy of the ketogenic diet. *Arch Neurol* 1998;**55**:1433–1437.

[13] Freeman JM, Vining EPG, Pillas DJ, *et al*. The efficacy of the ketogenic diet – 1998: A prospective evaluation of intervention in 150 children. *Pediatrics* 1998;**102**:1358–1363.

[14] Freeman JM. The ketogenic diet: additional information from a crossover study. *J Child Neurol* 2009;**24**:509–512.

[15] Neal EG, Chaffe HM, Schwartz RH, *et al*. The ketogenic diet for the treatment of childhood epilepsy: a randomized controlled trial. *Lancet Neurol* 2008;**7**:500–506.

[16] Neal EG, Chaffe HM, Schwartz RH, *et al*. A randomized trial of classical and medium chain triglyceride ketogenic diets in the treatment of childhood epilepsy. *Epilepsia* 2009;**50**:1109–1117.

[17] Pfeifer HH, Lyczkowski DA, Thiele EA. Low glycemic index treatment implementation and new insights into efficacy. *Epilepsia* 2008;**49**:42–45.

[18] Schwartzkroin PA. Mechanisms underlying the anti-epileptic efficacy of the ketogenic diet. *Epilepsy Res* 1999;**37**:171–180.

[19] Stafstrom CE. Animal models of the ketogenic diet: what have we learned, what can we learn? *Epilepsy Res* 1999;**37**:241–259.

[20] Nordli DR Jr, DeVivo DC. The ketogenic diet revisited: back to the future. *Epilepsia* 1997;**38**:743–749.

[21] Suzuki Y, Takahashi H, Fukuda M, *et al*. β-hydroxybutyrate alters GABA- transaminase activity in cultured astrocytes. *Brain Res* 2009;**1268**:17–23.

[22] Wheless JW. The ketogenic diet: an effective medical therapy with side-effects. *J Child Neurol* 2001;**16**:633–635.

[23] Groesbeck DK, Bluml RM, Kossoff EH. Long-term use of the ketogenic diet in the treatment of epilepsy. *Dev Med Child Neurol* 2006;**48**:978–981.

[24] The National Association of Epilepsy Centers. The National Association of Epilepsy Centers Guidelines for diagnosis and treatment in specialized epilepsy centers. *Epilepsia* 1990;**31**:S1–S12.

Resources

Videotapes on the ketogenic diet for families, dietitians, nurses, and physicians. The Charlie Foundation to Help Cure Pediatric Epilepsy, 501 10th Street, Santa Monica, CA 90402; Fax (310) 393-2347. (www.charliefoundation.org).

Kossoff EH, Freeman J, Turner Z, Rubenstein J. *Ketogenic Diets: Treatments for Epilepsy and Other Disorders*, 5th edn. New York: Demos, 2011. Demos, 386 Park Avenue South, Suite 301, New York City, NY 10016; Tel: (800) 532-8663.

Snyder D. *Keto Kid*. New York: Demos, 2007.
Zupec-Kania BA. *Ketogenic Diet: Parent's Guide*. Santa Monica, CA: The Charlie Foundation, 2009 (www.charliefoundation.org).
The ketogenic diet. In: Kleinman RE (ed.), *Pediatric Nutrition Handbook*, 6th edn [Policy of the American Academy of Pediatrics]. Elk Grove Village, IL: American Academy of Pediatrics, 2009; pp. 1021–1040.

Websites

The Charlie Foundation (www.charliefoundation.org).
Matthew's Friends (www.matthewsfriends.org).
KetoCaluculator (www.ketocalculator.com).
Epilepsy Therapy Project (www.epilepsy.com/ketonews).
Atkins Diet (www.atkins.com/recipes.aspx).

Section 4

Generalized seizures and generalized epilepsy syndromes

Amy L. McGregor

14 Idiopathic generalized epilepsies

Amy L. McGregor

Department of Pediatrics, Division of Child Neurology, Le Bonheur Comprehensive Epilepsy Program, University of Tennessee Health Science Center, Memphis, TN, USA

The term idiopathic generalized epilepsy, also historically referred to as primary generalized epilepsy, is being re-evaluated, as is the classification of these syndromes. However, the syndromes classically referred to as idiopathic generalized epilepsies share several characteristics that differentiate them from other epilepsy syndromes.

Idiopathic epilepsies were defined by the International League Against Epilepsy (ILAE) in 1989 as epilepsies with a presumed genetic etiology, an age-related onset, and specific clinical and electrographic features [1]. According to the 1989 ILAE definition of idiopathic generalized epilepsy (IGE), individuals with IGE have a normal neurological exam and neuroimaging; their background EEG rhythm is normal, but there may be generalized epileptiform discharges that increase in slow-wave sleep; and their seizures are generalized clinically and electrographically (Box 14.1). Specifically, the EEG shows generalized discharges that are bilaterally synchronous and symmetric, including spikes, polyspikes, spike-waves, and polyspike-waves $\geq$3 Hz. The first clinical changes suggest initial involvement of both hemispheres. Also, there is no etiology except a genetic one, similar to other idiopathic epilepsies. Using this definition, idiopathic generalized epilepsies represent approximately 15–20% of all epilepsies [2].

Epilepsy in Children and Adolescents, First Edition. Edited by James W. Wheless.

Box 14.1 International League Against Epilepsy (ILAE) definition of idiopathic generalized epilepsies (1989) [1]

- Generalized seizures (semiology and EEG)
- Typical EEG:
  - normal background
  - generalized features of epileptiform discharges
  - increase in slow-wave sleep
- Normal examination
- Neuroimaging normal
- No etiology (except genetic)

In 2010, an ILAE statement proposed elimination of the term "idiopathic" and use of the term "genetic" instead [3]. This statement recommended that the term genetic be used if the epilepsy is thought to have a genetic cause and seizures are a major feature of the condition. In the past, the term idiopathic carried the connotation of being pharmacoresponsive and benign. The 2010 ILAE statement refuted this. Furthermore, severe myoclonic epilepsy of infancy/Dravet syndrome, which is associated with pharmacoresistant seizures and was not previously classified as an idiopathic epilepsy, is considered a genetic epilepsy in the 2010 ILAE classification.

The 2010 ILAE report also recommended changing the definition of generalized seizures. It stated that generalized seizures may be asymmetric and do not have to involve the whole cortex. Instead, they are thought to begin and rapidly spread within bilateral networks, which may include cortical and subcortical structures. The 2010 ILAE classification of seizures lists the types of generalized seizures as tonic-clonic, absence, myoclonic, clonic, tonic, and atonic. Absence seizures are further divided into typical, atypical, and absence seizures with special features, such as myoclonic absence and eyelid myoclonia. Myoclonic seizures are subdivided into myoclonic, myoclonic-atonic, and myoclonic-tonic seizures. (The term myoclonic-atonic replaced the term myoclonic-astatic.)

Since the implications of the 2010 ILAE statement are not fully clear and earlier terminology was used to study these conditions, this chapter will primarily use definitions from prior to this statement. Furthermore, severe myoclonic epilepsy of infancy/Dravet syndrome and epilepsy with myoclonic-atonic seizures (Doose syndrome) are described in Chapter 15 with symptomatic generalized epilepsy/epilepsies with encephalopathy.

14.1 Clinical features

In IGE, the main seizure types are: typical absence, myoclonic, and generalized tonic-clonic seizures. Patients may have one, a combination of two, or all three of these seizure types [4]. The predominant seizure type can help to determine the diagnosis [5]. Seizures often occur upon awakening, and sleep deprivation is a trigger for seizures [4].

Historically, children with IGE have been thought to be neurologically normal. However, more recently, studies with neuropsychological testing have revealed abnormalities [6,7].

Description of seizures

Absence seizures

Typical absence seizures begin and end quickly, lasting 3 to 30 seconds. They are characterized by impairment of consciousness and a characteristic EEG, specifically generalized >2.5 Hz, typically 3–4.5 Hz, spike/polyspike-slow-wave discharges. They can be triggered by hyperventilation [8] (Figure 14.1).

Absence seizures arise from thalamocortical networks, which also generate sleep spindles [9,10].

Myoclonic seizures

Myoclonic seizures are quick jerks due to involuntary muscle contraction as a result of abnormal neuronal activity in the brain. Typically, generalized epileptiform discharges are seen [4].

Generalized tonic-clonic seizures

Generalized tonic-clonic seizures (GTC) begin with bilateral tonic contraction of skeletal muscles and then evolve into clonic contractions. They are usually associated with

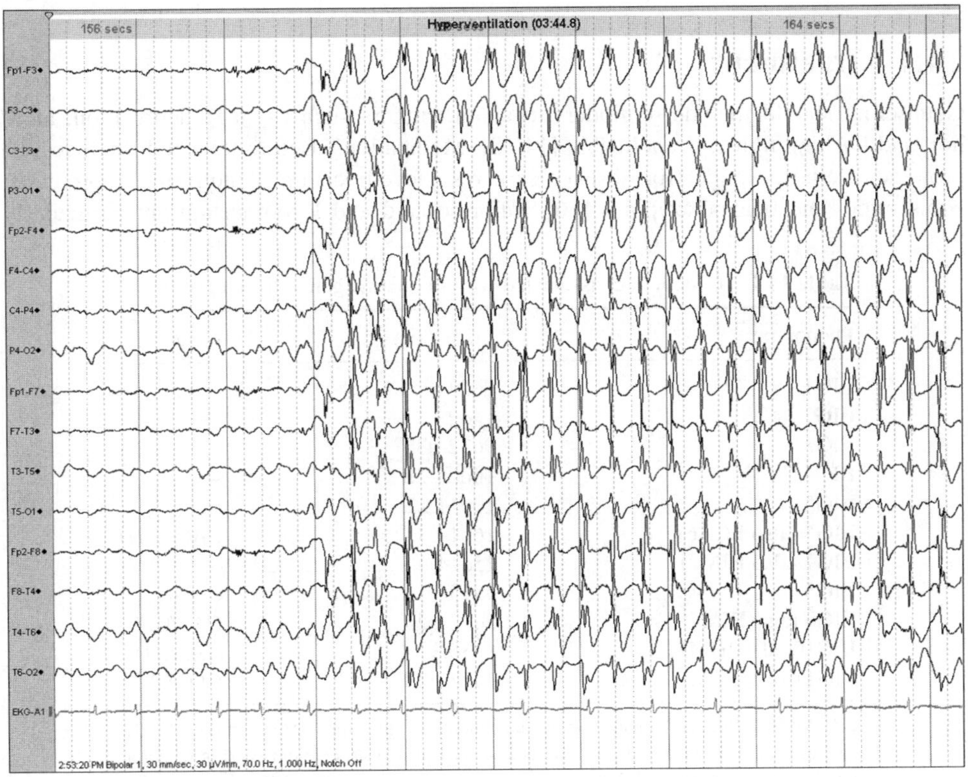

Figure 14.1 An absence seizure triggered by hyperventilation (characteristic generalized 3 Hz spike-and-slow-wave complexes).

autonomic signs and are followed by a postictal period. Patients are amnestic for the event. EEG changes are generalized and essentially synchronous and symmetric [4].

14.2 Natural history

Idiopathic generalized epilepsies tend to present in children and adolescents [4]. Many of the IGEs are life-long, but some, such as childhood absence epilepsy (CAE) may be limited [8]. Typically, seizure control occurs in 80–90% of patients with IGE [11].

14.3 Genetics

Multiple genetic loci are associated with idiopathic generalized epilepsies (Table 14.1). Mutations in genes encoding voltage-gated calcium channels (*CACNA1H* and *CACNB4*), calcium-sensing receptor (*CASR*), GABA-A receptor delta peptide (*GABRD*), and a chloride receptor (*CLCN2*) have all been associated with IGE [12].

Mutations in the chloride channel 2 (*CLCN2*) gene on chromosome 3q27-28 result in multiple IGE phenotypes such as juvenile absence epilepsy, juvenile myoclonic epilepsy, and epilepsy with grand mal seizures upon awakening. It is thought that abnormal function of the CLCN2 ion channel could impact transmembrane chloride movements associated with GABA-ergic synaptic transmission, resulting in excitability [13].

14.4 Treatment

Counseling should include reminders to avoid triggers such as sleep deprivation, alcohol, and flashing lights, if applicable [14,15]. Medications used to treat IGE include valproic acid, ethosuximide (for absence seizures), levetiracetam, lamotrigine, topiramate, zonisamide, and benzodiazepines [16]. Valproic acid and levetiracetam are particularly

Table 14.1 Genetic loci associated with idiopathic generalized epilepsy.

Phenotype	Locus/loci	Gene
EIG1	8q24	–
EIG2	14q23	–
EIG3	9q32-q33	–
EIG4	10q25-26	–
EIG5	10p11.22	–
EIG6 (also ECA6)	16p13.3	*CACNA1H*
EIG7 (also EJM2)	15q14	–
EIG8	3q13	*CASR*
EIG9 (also EJM6)	2q22-q23	*CACNB4*
EIG10 (also EJM7)	1p36.3	*GABRD*
EIG11 (also EJM8)	3q27-q28	*CLCN2*

CACNA1H, calcium channel, voltage-dependent, T type, alpha-1H subunit; *CACNB4*, calcium channel, voltage-dependent, beta-4 subunit; *CASR*, calcium-sensing receptor; *CLCN2*, chloride channel 2; ECA, epilepsy, childhood absence; EIG, epilepsy, idiopathic generalized; EJM, epilepsy, juvenile myoclonic; *GABRD*, $GABA_A$ receptor, delta polypeptide; IGE, idiopathic generalized epilepsy.

useful in patients with photosensitivity [15]. Carbamazepine, oxcarbazepine, phenytoin, gabapentin, pregabalin, and tiagabine should be avoided as they are either ineffective or exacerbate absence and/or myoclonic seizures [11]. (Treatment is discussed further below.)

Drug withdrawal, after a prolonged seizure-free period (e.g., 2 years) and following a normal EEG, is much more likely to be successful in CAE than other IGEs [17]. As many as 30% of patients with IGE may not respond to valproic acid or other antiepileptic medications. Factors associated with medication failure include non-adherence, psychiatric conditions, early onset of epilepsy, and generalized tonic-clonic seizures [18]. Secondary bilateral synchrony needs to be considered if seizures are refractory; frontal lobe epilepsy can be mistaken for IGE [11].

14.5 Classification

There are many types of IGE. The classification has evolved over time and there is a proposal for additional changes. At times, there has been debate whether IGE is in fact one disease rather than a group of multiple syndromes [4]. The classification schemes proposed by the ILAE in 1989 and 2010 are listed in Table 14.2. The age of onset helps to differentiate the syndromes [1].

14.6 Myoclonic epilepsy in infancy

Previously, myoclonic epilepsy of infancy was known as benign myoclonic epilepsy of infancy (BMEI). This is thought to be the earliest age-dependent IGE syndrome [4].

Epidemiology

The age of onset is 6 months to 3 years, and the ratio of males to females is 2:1 [4].

Table 14.2 Idiopathic generalized epilepsy syndromes according to International League Against Epilepsy (ILAE) classification year and age group.

Age of onset	1989 Classification [1]	2010 Classification [3]
Neonatal	Benign neonatal familial convulsions	Benign familial neonatal epilepsy
	Benign neonatal convulsions	–
Infancy	Benign myoclonic epilepsy in infancy	Myoclonic epilepsy in infancy
Childhood	Childhood absence epilepsy	Childhood absence epilepsy
	–	Febrile seizures plus (FS+)
	–	Epilepsy with myoclonic absences
	–	Epilepsy with myoclonic-atonic seizures (Doose syndrome)
Adolescence–adult	Juvenile absence epilepsy	Juvenile absence epilepsy
	Juvenile myoclonic epilepsy	Juvenile myoclonic epilepsy
	Epilepsy with grand mal seizures upon awakening	Epilepsy with generalized tonic-clonic seizures alone

Genetics

Thirty percent of cases have a positive family history for epilepsy or febrile seizures [4].

Clinical manifestations

The main seizure type is myoclonic seizures, which affect the head, limbs (upper extremities more so than lower), shoulders, torso, and eyelids. These may be isolated or repeated; however, they are not in long clusters [19]. In addition, reflex seizures may occur; seizures may be triggered by certain auditory and tactile stimuli. Twenty percent of patients have occasional simple febrile seizures, typically prior to onset of myoclonic seizures. A similar number have rare GTC seizures, which tend to present in the early teens [4].

EEG

The EEG background is normal. During jerks, brief generalized spike/polyspike-and-wave discharges are seen. Discharges and jerks can be seen in response to photic stimulation and during reflex seizures [4].

Natural history

Often seizures remit within a few years; however, photosensitivity may persist and predicts a worse prognosis. Patients with reflex seizures have a better prognosis [4]. Generalized tonic-clonic seizures may occur years later, when patients are in their early teens. Cases of JME following MEI have been reported [20].

Except for 10–20% of patients, development is normal. Lack of treatment is a predictor of worse prognosis [4].

Treatment

Eighty percent of patients become seizure-free on valproic acid [4]. Benzodiazepines have been used in combination with valproic acid in refractory cases [20]. Medications that exacerbate myoclonic jerks should be avoided [19].

14.7 Childhood absence epilepsy (CAE)

Childhood absence epilepsy (CAE), which was referred to as pyknolepsy in the past, is the most common epilepsy syndrome in childhood [21].

Epidemiology

The age of onset of CAE is between 4 and 10 years of age [22]. The peak age is between and 6 and 7 years. More females than males have CAE [1].

Genetics

Childhood absence epilepsy has been associated with mutations in the $GABA_A$ receptor and calcium and chloride channel genes. Specifically, mutations in genes encoding the gamma-aminobutyric acid receptor $\gamma 2$ (GABRG2), gamma-aminobutyric acid receptor α

Table 14.3 Gene loci associated with childhood absence epilepsy.

Phenotype	Locus/loci	Gene
ECA1	8q24	–
ECA2	5q31.1-q33.1	*GABRG2*
ECA3*	–	–
ECA4 (also EJM5)	5q34-q35	*GABRA1*
ECA5	15q11.2-q12	*GABRB3*
ECA6 (also EIG6)	16p13.3	*CACNA1H*

*ECA3 no longer exists because the paper was retracted.
CACNA1H, calcium channel, voltage-dependent, T type, alpha-1H subunit; CAE, childhood absence epilepsy; ECA, epilepsy, childhood absence; EIG, epilepsy, idiopathic generalized; EJM, epilepsy, juvenile myoclonic; *GABRA1*, $GABA_A$ receptor, alpha-1 polypeptide; *GABRB3*, $GABA_A$ receptor, beta-3 polypeptide; *GABRG2*, $GABA_A$ receptor, gamma-2 polypeptide.

(GABRA1), and gamma-aminobutyric acid receptor β3 (GABR3); the calcium channel, voltage-dependent, T-type α 1H subunit (*CACNA1H*) gene; and the chloride channel 2 (*CLCN2*) gene have been found in patients with CAE [13]. Interestingly, the locus for ECA1 (and EIG1) is 8q24, which is also associated with benign neonatal epilepsy 2, an epilepsy syndrome due to mutations in the *KCNQ3* gene that encodes a potassium channel [12] (Table 14.3).

Clinical manifestations

Children with CAE have typical absence seizures, which are described above. Seizures are frequent, occurring multiple times per day, and last 5–15 seconds [22].

EEG

Children with CAE have a normal EEG background. Ictal and interictal activity consists of 3 Hz spike-and-wave discharges [22].

Natural history

Historically, children with CAE have been considered neurologically normal. More recently, studies have shown that these children can have abnormal neuropsychological testing. Inattention is particularly a problem [23]. In addition, children with CAE have more problems with behavioral inhibition, problem-solving, letter fluency, complex motor control, and psychosocial functioning than other children [7].

Absence seizures usually resolve by age 10.5 years, but seizures may continue past puberty [24]. About 15% of patients evolve into juvenile myoclonic epilepsy (JME) [22]. A predictor of lack of remission and progression to JME is development of generalized tonic-clonic seizures or myoclonic seizures while taking antiepileptic medication [25]. Polyspikes also indicate a worse prognosis [11].

Treatment

Children with uncontrolled CAE should avoid activities such as bicycling, roller-blading, skate-boarding, swimming, and climbing. They may resume these activities when their seizures are controlled using the appropriate precautions. For instance, a helmet should be used when riding a bicycle, and children should not swim alone [14].

Efficacy data support the use of ethosuximide, valproic acid, or lamotrigine for CAE [26]. Results of a recent, large, double-blind, randomized controlled trial from the Childhood Absence Epilepsy Study Group indicate that ethosuximide and valproic acid are the more effective treatments, and ethosuximide has less impact on attention; therefore, it is preferred for initial treatment. Unfortunately, in this study, 47% of patients on ethosuximide failed treatment due to persistent seizures (clinical or EEG) or side effects [21]. Previous studies have also shown that if patients have generalized tonic-clonic seizures in addition to absence seizures, ethosuximide alone is usually not sufficient [27].

If a patient with CAE has intractable seizures, consider testing for familial glucose transporter type 1 (GLUT1) deficiency [28,29]. This condition is due to mutations in *SLC2A1*, which has been linked to paroxysmal exertional dyskinesia [30]. Mutations in *SLC2A1* are associated with early-onset absence epilepsy, but early-onset absence epilepsy is not necessarily due to these mutations [31]. Patients with these mutations typically respond to the ketogenic diet [28].

14.8 Juvenile absence epilepsy (JAE)

Juvenile absence epilepsy (JAE) has features of childhood absence epilepsy and juvenile myoclonic epilepsy [11] (Box 14.2).

Epidemiology

The age of onset of JAE is 10 to 16 years, with an average age of onset at 13 years. Males and females are affected equally [5].

Genetics

Mutations in EF-hand domain (C-terminal)-containing 1 (*EFHC1*) and *CLCN2* genes have been associated with juvenile absence epilepsy (EJA1 and EJA2 respectively; Table 14.4). *EFHC1* mutations are also associated with JME, and *CLCN2* mutations are associated with multiple types of idiopathic generalized epilepsy, as mentioned above [13].

Box 14.2 Comparison of juvenile absence epilepsy with childhood absence epilepsy (CAE)

- Age of onset is older (10–16 years versus 4–10 years of age in CAE).
- Equal incidence males = females (rather than females > males).
- Seizures are less frequent, longer, associated with less impairment of consciousness, and less likely to be accompanied by retropulsion.
- Ictal and interictal EEG has faster spike-and-slow-wave complexes, and there are more polyspikes.
- Myoclonic and generalized tonic-clonic seizures are more likely.
- More likely to continue into adulthood.

Table 14.4 Genetic loci associated with juvenile absence epilepsy.

Phenotype	Locus	Gene
EJA1	6p12.3	*EFHC1*
EJA2	3q27-q28	*CLCN2*

CLCN2, chloride channel 2; *EFHC1*, EF-hand domain (C-terminal)-containing 1; EJA, epilepsy, juvenile absence.

Clinical manifestations

The absence seizures in patients with JAE tend to be less frequent, longer-lasting, and less often associated with impairment of consciousness than the absence seizures in patients with CAE. Also, there is less retropulsion with absence seizures in JAE [8].

In addition to absence seizures, most patients also have GTCs [11]. These occur prior to absence seizures in about 25% of patients [5]. GTCs are more common than in CAE, are triggered by sleep deprivation, and tend to occur upon awakening [32]. About 15% of patients with JAE have myoclonic jerks [11].

EEG

The EEG background in JAE is normal. The interictal and ictal patterns are generalized, regular 3.5–4 Hz spike-and-wave discharges that are maximal frontally. These are triggered by hyperventilation, sleep deprivation, and occasionally photic stimulation [32]. Compared with the EEG for CAE, the discharges aren't quite as regular or rhythmic and are often faster (>3 Hz) [8,11] (Figure 14.2). In addition, polyspikes are more prominent in JAE [8].

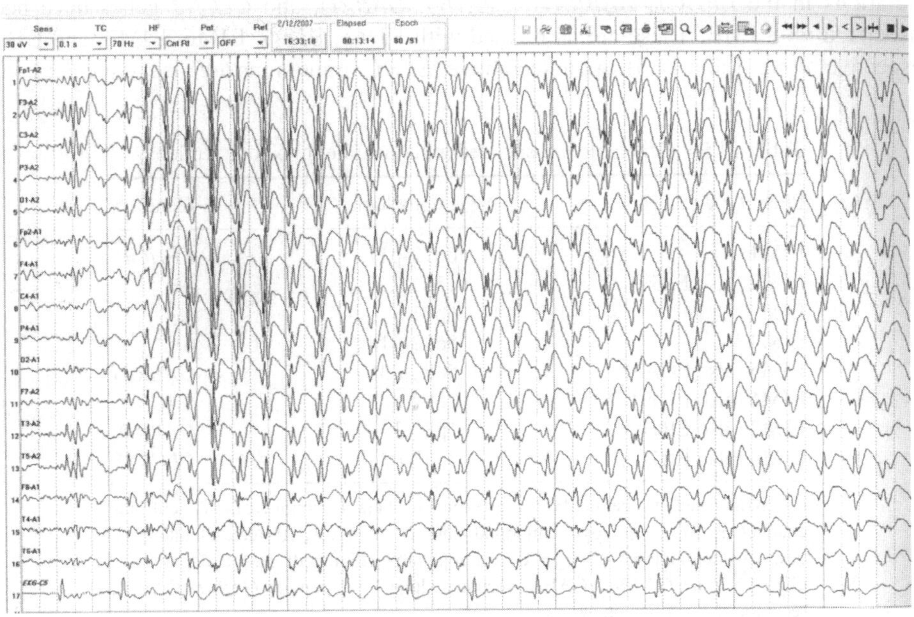

Figure 14.2 EEG of a patient with juvenile absence epilepsy (JAE), depicting absence seizure.

Natural history

Patients with JAE have a good prognosis. They tend to respond to AEDs, but they may require lifelong treatment [5,33].

Treatment

Since it treats absence seizures and GTCs, valproic acid classically has been the drug of choice. Lamotrigine is an alternative if valproic acid is contraindicated. Patients with refractory seizures may respond to the combination of valproic acid and lamotrigine or the addition of ethosuximide [4]. Levetiracetam has also been used. Medications such as carbamazepine, oxcarbazepine, vigabatrin, gabapentin, and pregabalin should be avoided as these can precipitate atypical absence status epilepticus [33].

14.9 Juvenile myoclonic epilepsy (JME)

Juvenile myoclonic epilepsy (JME) is the most common IGE in adolescents and adults [34]. It represents 5–10% of all epilepsies [5].

Epidemiology

The age of onset of JME is 12 to 18 years with an average age of 15 years [5]. Males and females are equally affected [8].

Genetics

Mutations in the *EFHC1*, *GABRA1*, *CACNB4*, *GABRD*, and *CLCN2* genes have been associated with JME. These are associated with EJM1, EJM5, EJM6, EJM7, and EJM8 respectively (see Table 14.5). As noted above, *EFHC1* mutations are also associated with

Table 14.5 Genetic loci associated with juvenile myoclonic epilepsy.

Phenotype	Locus/loci	Gene
EJM1	6p12-p11	*EFHC1*
EJM2 (also EIG7)	15q24	–
EJM3	6p21	–
EJM4	5q12-q14	–
EJM5 (also ECA4)	5q34-q35	*GABRA1*
EJM6 (also EIG9)	2q22-q23	*CACNB4*
EJM7 (also EIG10)	1p36.3	*GABRD*
EJM8 (also EIG11)	3q27-q28	*CLCN2*

CACNB4, calcium channel, voltage-dependent, beta-4 subunit; *CLCN2*, chloride channel 2; ECA, epilepsy, childhood absence; *EFHC1*, EF-hand domain (C-terminal)-containing 1; EIG, epilepsy, idiopathic generalized; EJM, epilepsy, juvenile myoclonic; *GABRA1*, $GABA_A$ receptor, alpha-1 polypeptide; *GABRD*, $GABA_A$ receptor, delta polypeptide.

Box 14.3 Comparison of juvenile myoclonic epilepsy (JME) with juvenile absence epilepsy (JAE)

- Absence seizures are less prominent in JME.
- Myoclonic jerks are more prominent in JME and more likely to occur in the morning.
- The interictal and ictal EEG discharges are typically faster (4–6 Hz versus 3–4 Hz generalized polyspike wave discharges).
- Bursts of interictal discharges are briefer and less likely to be associated with altered consciousness.
- More likely to have photosensitivity.

JAE. Linkage analysis also identified EJM2, EJM3, and EJM4. EJM3 is on 6p21, which is also where *PPR1*, a gene that confers risk for a photoparoxysmal response/photosensitivity, is found [12].

Clinical manifestations

The hallmark of JME is myoclonic jerks, during which consciousness is maintained [34]. These are triggered by sleep deprivation, fatigue, and alcohol and are prominent in the morning. GTC and absence seizures are also seen. GTC seizures occur in over 90% of patients. Frequently these are preceded by myoclonic jerks [32]. Absence seizures occur in about one-third of patients [5]. They are less prominent than in JAE [34] (Box 14.3).

EEG

The EEG background is normal. The interictal pattern is usually 4–6 Hz generalized polyspike-and-wave complexes; however, 3–4 Hz generalized spike-and-slow-wave complexes can be seen [32] (Figure 14.3). JME has the highest rate of photosensitivity among all epilepsies (30–50%) [5,11].

Natural history

Patients respond well to medication, but there is a high risk for relapse if AEDs are discontinued. In general, it is thought that JME requires life-long treatment [14]. Multiple seizure types and EEG asymmetries are indicators of difficult to control JME [18].

Neuropsychological testing has found that JME patients have problems with semantic and verbal fluency [35].

Treatment

Counseling about avoidance of triggers such as sleep deprivation and alcohol is important when treating patients with JME. Historically, the drug of choice has been valproic

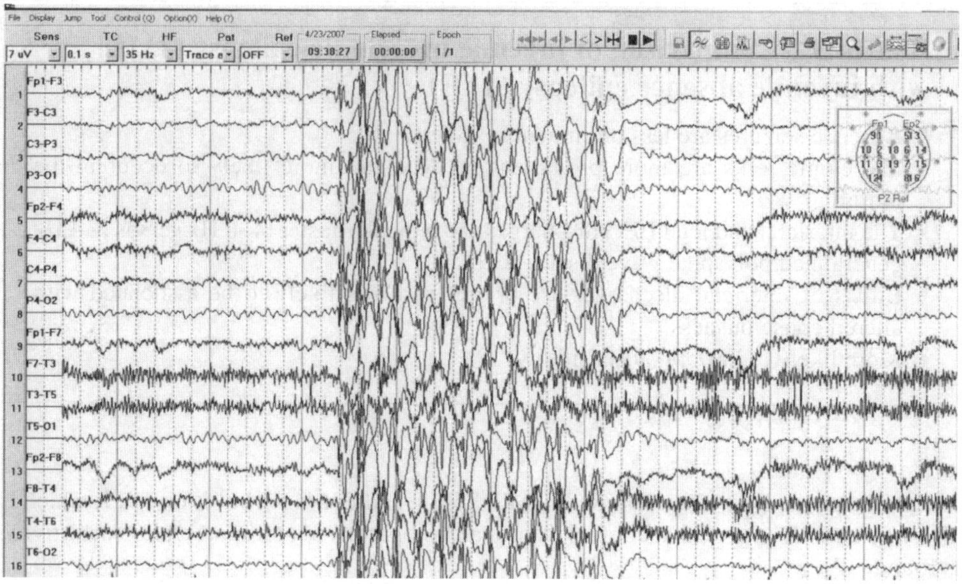

Figure 14.3 Interictal awake EEG in a patient with juvenile myoclonic epilepsy (JME) (middle of figure shows generalized polyspike-and-slow-wave complex lasting 3 seconds).

acid, to which up to 80% of patients respond. Levetiracetam, topiramate, and lamotrigine are alternatives, particularly in woman of child-bearing age due to the risk of congenital defects with valproic acid. However, lamotrigine has been known to worsen myoclonus [36]. Levetiracetam and valproic acid are useful in treating patients with photosensitivity [15].

Carbamazepine, phenytoin, and oxcarbazepine can worsen absence and myoclonic seizures, so they should be avoided. Similarly, gabapentin, pregabalin, tiagabine, and vigabatrin can exacerbate seizures. In fact, tiagabine and vigabatrin can induce absence status epilepticus [36].

14.10 Epilepsy with generalized tonic-clonic seizures alone (IGE-GTCs)

Epilepsy with generalized tonic-clonic seizures alone was recognized as an epilepsy syndrome by the ILAE in 2001 [37]. This includes patients who previously had been classified as epilepsy with grand mal on awakening (EGMA) based upon the 1989 ILAE classification, patients who have GTCs only during sleep (EGMS), and patients who have GTCs at random times of the day (EGMR) [1]. (These abbreviations reflect the previous tendency to refer to GTCs as grand mal seizures.) Further studies about IGE-GTCs as a single entity are needed.

Epidemiology

The age of onset of IGE-GTCs is the oldest among the IGEs. The average age of onset is between 16.6 and 19.5 years. IGE-GTCs are more prevalent in males than females, with some 60% of patients being male [38].

Genetics

Almost 40% of patients with IGE-GTCs have a positive family history [39]. Mutations in the *CLCN2* gene have been found in patients with EGMA [13].

Clinical manifestations

In EGMA, GTCs typically occur within 1 to 2 hours after awakening. Also, they may occur during the evening. More than 80% of patients also have myoclonic jerks and/or absence seizures as well [5]. Sleep deprivation and alcohol are triggers, and patients may have photosensitivity. Photosensitivity is less common in EGMR [38].

EEG

The interictal EEG shows generalized spike-and-wave discharges at greater than 3 Hz, which are maximal frontally. The frequency may become faster with age. As noted above, a photoparoxysmal response is seen more commonly in EGMA [38].

Natural history

A long-term study of patients with IGE-GTC in Nova Scotia found a 75% remission rate (seizure-free, off medication). However, learning and social problems were common [40].

Treatment

As in JME, avoidance of risk factors is important, particularly for EGMA [38]. An expert opinion study regarding treatment of adults with epilepsy found that valproic acid was rated as the treatment of choice; however, lamotrigine and topiramate were also listed as options for initial monotherapy [41]. Levetiracetam was found to be an effective adjunctive medication in a more recent study [42].

14.11 Epilepsy with myoclonic absence

Myoclonic-absence seizures can occur both in this idiopathic syndrome and in symptomatic epilepsies. Symptomatic epilepsies that have myoclonic-absence seizures as a seizure type are not included in this section. Brain magnetic resonance imaging (MRI) and genetic testing, which should be normal in this syndrome, help to exclude symptomatic cases.

Epidemiology

The age of onset for epilepsy with myoclonic absences ranges from 1 to 12 years, with a peak of 7 years [8]. Almost 70% of patients are boys [19].

Genetics

Twenty-five percent of patients have a positive family history [19].

Clinical manifestations

Myoclonic absence seizures are the defining seizure type. These are characterized by myoclonic jerks, typically of the shoulders and extremities, with altered awareness. There often is a tonic component involving the shoulders and deltoid muscles resulting in lifting of the arms. These seizures may last up to 1 minute and occur multiple times per day. During the seizures, 3 Hz generalized polyspike wave discharges (GPSWD) are seen [4].

Other seizure types, such as generalized tonic-clonic or atonic seizures, may occur. If present, these may indicate a worse prognosis and/or a symptomatic epilepsy [4].

EEG

Initially, the EEG background is typically normal. However, it may worsen. The ictal EEG consists of rhythmic 3 Hz GPSWD. The myoclonic jerk occurs at the time of the spike [43].

Natural history

Fifty percent of children with normal cognition at the onset develop cognitive and behavioral problems [43].

Treatment

Valproic acid is a mainstay of treatment. Ethosuximide or lamotrigine may be added. Clonazepam is another option. Acetazolamide has been used in combination in the past [4]. Phenytoin, carbamazepine, oxcarbazepine, vigabatrin, gabapentin, and tiagabine should be avoided [43].

14.12 Epilepsy with myoclonic-atonic seizures/Doose syndrome

Epilepsy with myoclonic-atonic seizures/Doose syndrome, which has also formerly been called epilepsy with myoclonic-astatic seizures, was classified as cryptogenic/symptomatic according to the 1989 ILAE classification [1]. According to the more recent ILAE classifications, including the 2010 classification [3], it is an idiopathic generalized epilepsy; however, here it is discussed in Chapter 15 with the symptomatic generalized epilepsy/epilepsies with encephalopathy for easier comparison and contrast to epilepsies such as Lennox–Gastaut syndrome, from which it must be differentiated.

14.13 Febrile seizures plus (FS+)

The term "febrile seizures plus" evolved from the term "generalized epilepsy with febrile seizures plus" (GEFS+), which was described in 1997. A study of multiple family members with seizures from a large family revealed heterogeneous phenotypes. Within the same family there were individuals with febrile seizures, early febrile seizures, and afebrile seizures, including an individual with myoclonic-astatic epilepsy (now myoclonic-atonic epilepsy). Febrile seizures plus (FS+) was the term used for individuals with early onset of febrile seizures, febrile seizures over age 6 years, or afebrile seizures [44].

Epidemiology

The age of onset is variable. By definition, febrile seizures occur earlier than usual; the median age is 1 year [4]. Prevalence is equal in males and females [45].

Genetics

FS+ was historically considered autosomal dominant with incomplete penetrance, but the inheritance is now thought to be more complex [4]. FS+ has been associated with mutations in voltage-gated sodium channel genes and $GABA_A$ receptor subunit genes. Specifically, it has been linked to mutations in *SCN1A* on 2q24, *SCN1B* on 19q13.1, *SCN9A* on 2q24, *GABRG2* on 5q31.1-q33.1, and *GABRD* on 1p36.3. (Table 14.6). The most severe form of FS+ , Dravet syndrome, has been associated with mutations in *SCN1A* and *GABRG2* genes [12,13].

Clinical manifestations

Clinical manifestations vary from febrile seizures alone to severe epilepsies. The most common phenotype is typical febrile seizures, defined as convulsive activity in children between 3 months and 6 years associated with a temperature greater than 38°C. As would

Table 14.6 Genetic loci associated with febrile seizures plus (FS+).

Phenotype	Locus/loci	Gene
GEFSP1	2q24,19q13.1	*SCN1A, SCN1B*
GEFSP2 (also FEB3A)	2q24	*SCN1A*
GEFSP3 (also FEB8)	5q31.1-q33.1	*GABRG2*
GEFSP4	2p24	–
GEFSP5 (also EIG10)	1p36.3	*GABRD*
GEFSP6	8p23-p21	–
GEFSP7 (also FEB3B)	2q24	*SCN9A*
GEFSP8	6q16.3-q22.31	–

EIG, epilepsy, idiopathic generalized; FEB, febrile seizures, familial; FS+, febrile seizures plus; GEFSP, generalized epilepsy with febrile seizures plus; *GABRD*, $GABA_A$ receptor, delta polypeptide; *GABRG2*, $GABA_A$ receptor, gamma-2 polypeptide; *SCN1A*, sodium channel, neuronal type 1, alpha subunit; *SCN1B*, sodium channel, voltage-gate type I, beta subunit; *SCN9*, sodium channel, voltage-gated, type IX, alpha-subunit.

be expected, the brain MRI is normal in these children. The next most common phenotype is FS+ as defined above. However, patients may have FS+ with absence, myoclonic, or atonic seizures. Furthermore, patients with frontal lobe epilepsy, temporal lobe epilepsy, infantile spasms, myoclonic-atonic epilepsy, and Dravet syndrome have been found in these families [45].

EEG

The EEG findings depend upon the phenotype. Most children have a normal EEG, as would be expected given the most common phenotype (typical febrile seizures). However, the more severe phenotypes, such as myoclonic-atonic epilepsy and Dravet syndrome, have the EEG findings associated with these diagnoses [45].

Natural history

The prognosis depends upon the phenotype. Most children do well; however, children with more severe phenotypes have a worse prognosis, corresponding to their diagnosis [45].

Treatment

Phenotype also impacts treatment. Patients with typical febrile seizures may not require treatment apart from rectal diazepam for rescue therapy. If prophylactic medication is needed, broad-spectrum agents are typically used [45].

14.14 Eyelid myoclonia with absences (EMA)/Jeavons syndrome

Eyelid myoclonia with absences (EMA)/Jeavons syndrome consists of a triad of a specific seizure type, that is, eyelid myoclonia (with or without absence), photosensitivity, and the tendency for eye closure to cause epileptiform discharges and/or seizures. This is considered a reflex epilepsy since specific sensory stimuli cause seizures [4].

Epidemiology

The age of onset ranges from 2 to 14 years, the peak is 6 to 8 years. This occurs twice as often in girls as boys [4].

Genetics

Almost 30% of patients have a family history of epilepsy [46].

Clinical manifestations

Eyelid myoclonia is the characteristic seizure type. Seizures involve fast eyelid jerks (myoclonia) with or without impairment of consciousness (with or without absence). They

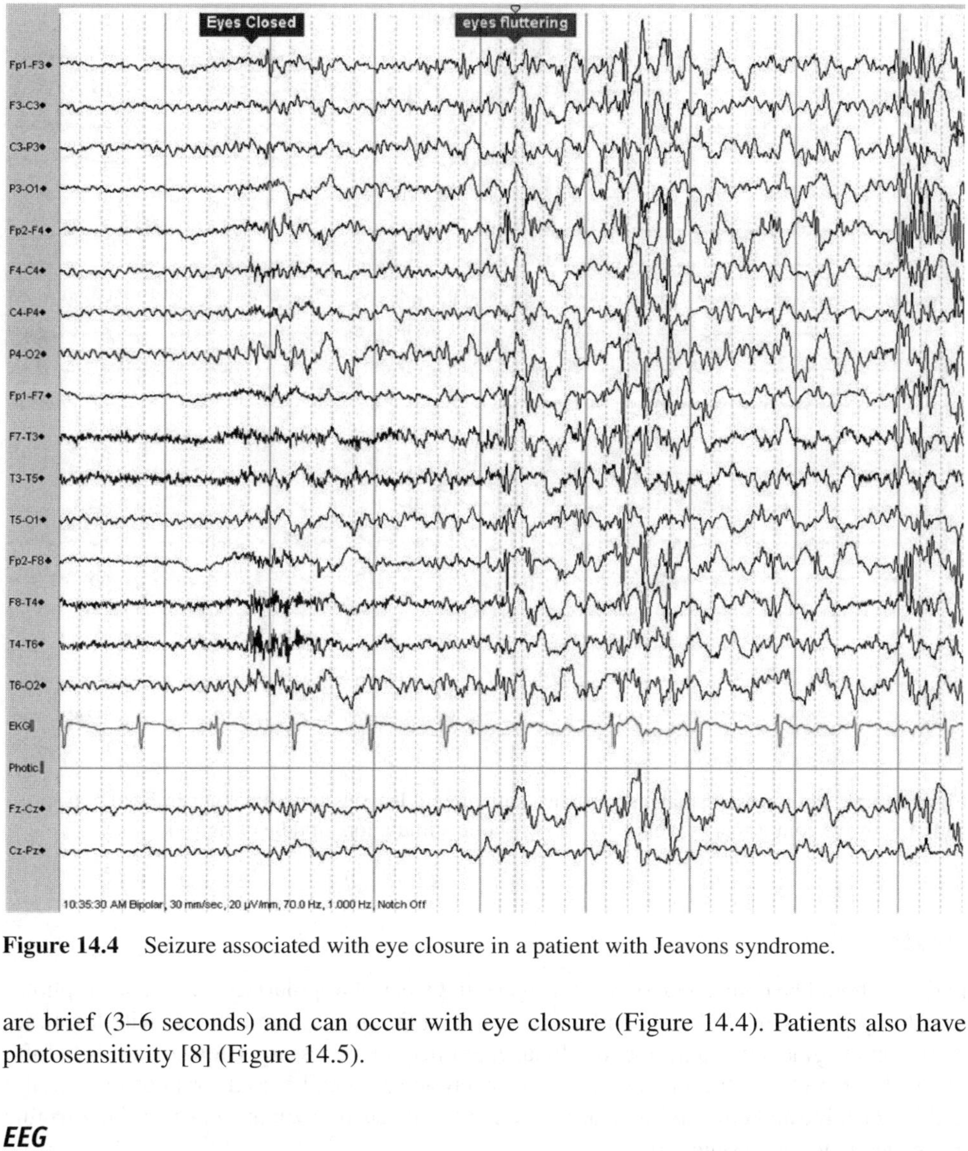

Figure 14.4 Seizure associated with eye closure in a patient with Jeavons syndrome.

are brief (3–6 seconds) and can occur with eye closure (Figure 14.4). Patients also have photosensitivity [8] (Figure 14.5).

EEG

Photoparoxysmal responses are seen in untreated children. During seizures, generalized polyspike and slow-wave complexes at 3–6 Hz are seen, especially with eye closure in an illuminated room [47].

Natural history

Studies apart from the EEG are normal [4]. Jeavons syndrome requires lifelong treatment [8]. Seizures are difficult to control. Photosensitivity may improve in middle age, but eyelid myoclonia continues. Men have a better prognosis than women [4].

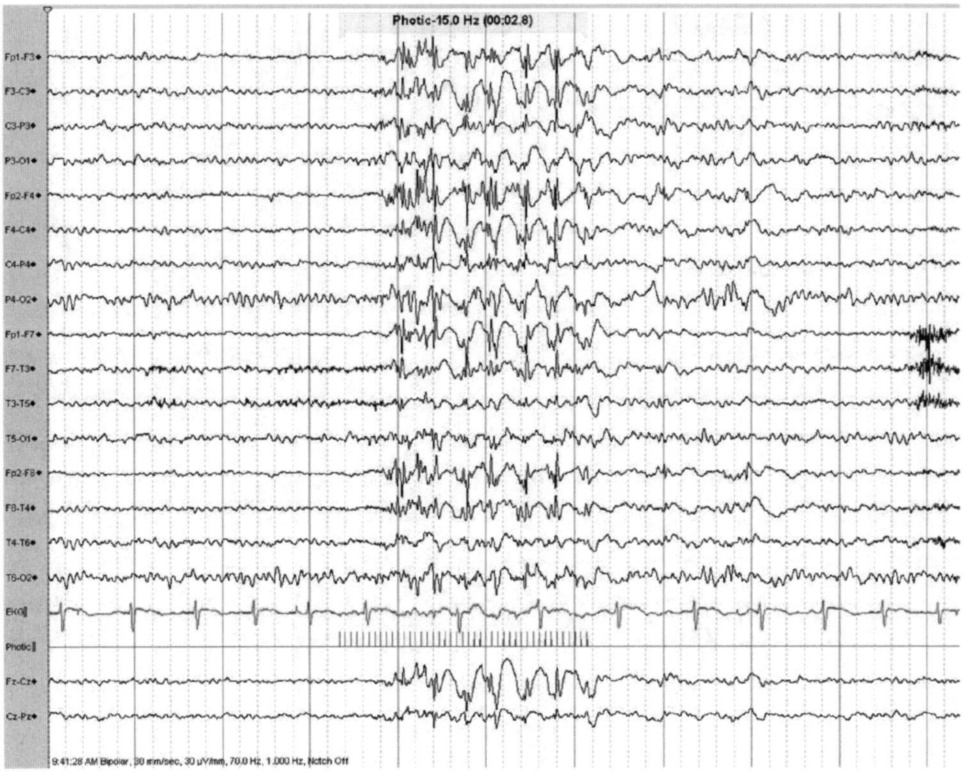

Figure 14.5 Photoparoxysmal response in a patient with Jeavons syndrome (generalized polyspike-and-slow-wave complexes provoked by 15 Hz photic stimulation, middle of figure).

Treatment

Patients should be counseled to avoid triggers and wear blue-polarized sunglasses if photosensitivity is an issue. Valproic acid is a mainstay of treatment. Combination with levetiracetam, lamotrigine, ethosuximide, or clonazepam may be necessary. Clonazepam is helpful for eyelid myoclonia and myoclonic jerks; levetiracetam can be used for photosensitivity; and lamotrigine and ethosuximide are effective for absence seizures. However, lamotrigine can exacerbate myoclonic jerks [4].

14.15 Summary

Idiopathic generalized epilepsies (IGE) present at different ages in childhood and adolescence. Awareness of typical demographic features, age of onset, and EEG features (Tables 14.7 and 14.8; Figure 14.6) will help the clinician determine which IGE the patient has. This is critically important when making decisions regarding further evaluation (including genetic testing) and treatment; and discussions regarding prognosis.

Table 14.7 Comparison of epilepsy syndrome demographic data.

Syndrome	Age of onset	Male to female ratio
MEI	6 months to 3 years	Males > females (2:1 ratio)
CAE	4 to 10 years	Females > males
JAE	10 to 16 years	Females = males
JME	12 to 18 years	Females = males
IGE-GTCs	16.6 to 19.5 years	Males > females (60% are male)
Epilepsy with myoclonic absences	1 to 12 years	Males > females (70% are boys)
Jeavons syndrome/eyelid myoclonia with absences	2 to 14 years	Females > males (2:1 ratio)

CAE, childhood absence epilepsy; IGE-GTCs, epilepsy with generalized tonic-clonic seizures alone; JAE, juvenile absence epilepsy; JME, juvenile myoclonic epilepsy; MEI, myoclonic epilepsy of infancy.

Table 14.8 Comparison of epilepsy syndrome EEG findings.

Epilepsy syndrome	EEG findings
MEI	3–4 Hz GSWD [48]
CAE	3 Hz GSWD
JAE	3.5–4 Hz GSWD
JME	4–6 Hz GPSWD
IGE-GTCs	>3 Hz GSWD
Epilepsy with myoclonic absences	3 Hz GPSWD
Eyelid myoclonia with absences	3–6 Hz GPSWD

CAE, childhood absence epilepsy; GSWD, generalized spike-and-wave discharges; GPSWD, generalized polyspike-and-wave discharges; IGE-GTCs, epilepsy with generalized tonic-clonic seizures alone; JAE, juvenile absence epilepsy; JME, juvenile myoclonic epilepsy; MEI, myoclonic epilepsy of infancy.

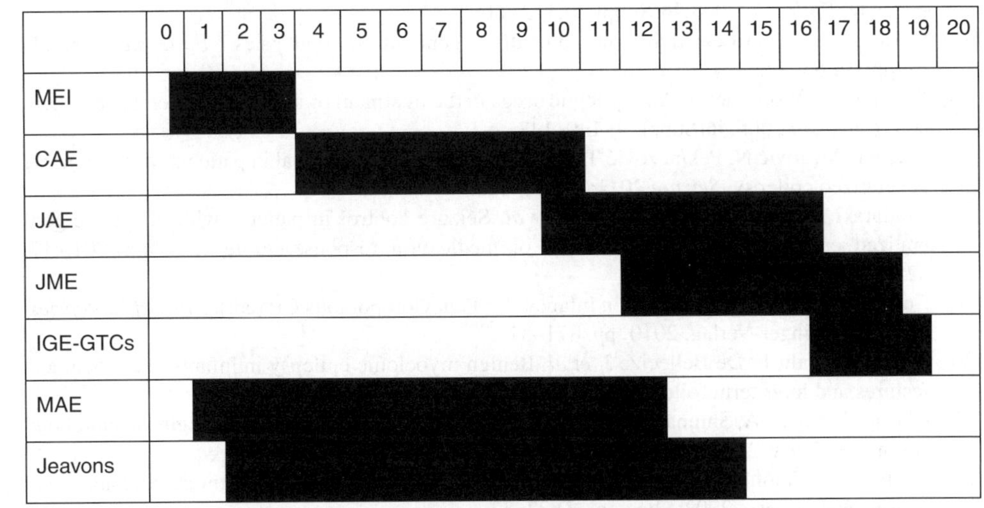

Figure 14.6 Age of onset of epilepsy syndromes (in years). CAE, childhood absence epilepsy; IGE-GTCs, epilepsy with generalized tonic-clonic seizures alone; JAE, juvenile absence epilepsy; JME, juvenile myoclonic epilepsy; MAE, epilepsy with myoclonic absences; MEI, myoclonic epilepsy of infancy.

References

[1] Commission on Classification and Terminology of the International League Against Epilepsy. Proposal for revised classification of epilepsies and epileptic syndromes. *Epilepsia* 1989;**30**: 389.

[2] Jallon P, Latour P. Epidemiology of idiopathic generalized epilepsies. *Epilepsia* 2005;**46**(Suppl. 9):10–14.

[3] Berg AT, Berkovic SF, Brodie MJ, *et al.* Revised terminology and concepts for organization of seizures and epilepsies: report of the ILAE Commission on Classification and Terminology, 2005–2009. *Epilepsia* 2010;**51**:676–685.

[4] Panayiotopoulos CP. *A Clinical Guide to Epileptic Syndromes and their Treatment*. Springer Healthcare Ltd, 2010.

[5] Beghi M, Beghi E, Cornaggia CM, Gobbi G. Idiopathic epilepsies of adolescence. *Epilepsia* 2006;**47**(Suppl. 2):107–110.

[6] Bhise V, Burack G, Mandelbaum D. Baseline cognition, behavior, and motor skills in children with new-onset, idiopathic epilepsy. *Dev Med Child Neurol* 2010;**52**:22–26.

[7] Conant LL, Wilfong A, Inglese C, *et al.* Dysfunction of executive and related processes in childhood absence epilepsy. *Epilepsy Behav* 2010;**18**:414–423.

[8] Panayiotopoulos CP. Typical absence seizures and related epileptic syndromes: Assessment of current state and directions for research. *Epilepsia* 2008;**49**:2131–2147.

[9] Wong M. Too much inhibition leads to excitation in absence epilepsy. *Epilepsy Curr* 2010;**10**:131–132.

[10] Beenhakker MP, Huguenard JR. Neurons that fire together also conspire together: is normal sleep circuitry hijacked to generate epilepsy? *Neuron* 2009;**62**:612–632.

[11] Benbadis SR. Practical management issues for idiopathic generalized epilepsies. *Epilepsia* 2005;**46**(Suppl. 9):125–132.

[12] Online Mendelian Inheritance in Man, OMIM®. Baltimore, MD: McKusick-Nathans Institute of Genetic Medicine, Johns Hopkins University (http://omim.org/).

[13] Lu Y, Wang X. Genes associated with idiopathic epilepsies: a current overview. *Neurol Res* 2009;**31**:135–143.

[14] Camfield C, Camfield P. Management guidelines for children with idiopathic generalized epilepsy. *Epilepsia* 2005;**46**(Suppl. 9):112–116.

[15] Covanis A. Photosensitivity in idiopathic generalized epilepsies. *Epilepsia* 2005;**46** (Suppl. 9):67–72.

[16] Patsalos PN. Properties of Antiepileptic drugs in the treatment of idiopathic generalized epilepsies. *Epilepsia* 2005;**46**(Suppl. 9):140–148.

[17] Pavlović M, Jović N, Pekmezović T. Antiepileptic drugs withdrawal in patients with idiopathic generalized epilepsy. *Seizure* 2011;**20**:520–525.

[18] Szaflarski JP, Lindsell CJ, Zakaria T, *et al.* Seizure control in patients with idiopathic generalized epilepsies: EEG determinants of medication response. *Epilepsy Behav* 2010;**17**: 525–530.

[19] Covanis A. Myoclonic epilepsy in infancy. In: Panayiotopoulous CP (ed.), *Atlas of Epilepsies*. London: Springer-Verlag, 2010; pp. 871–877.

[20] Auvin S, Pandit F, De Bellecize J, *et al.* Benign myoclonic epilepsy in infants: electroclinical features and long-term follow-up of 34 patients. *Epilepsia* 2006;**47**:387–393.

[21] Glauser T, Cnaan A, Shinnar S, *et al.* Ethosuximide, valproic acid, and lamotrigine in childhood absence epilepsy. *N Engl J Med* 2010;**362**:790–799.

[22] Camfield P, Camfield C. Epileptic syndromes in childhood: clinical features, outcomes, and treatment. *Epilepsia* 2002;**43**(Suppl. 3):27–32.

[23] Vega C, Vestal M, DeSalvo M, *et al.* Differentiation of attention-related problems in childhood absence epilepsy. *Epilepsy Behav* 2010;**19**:82–85.

[24] Pearl PL, Holmes GL. Childhood absence epilepsies. In: Pellock JM, Bourgeois BFD, Dodson WE (eds), *Pediatric Epilepsy*, 3rd edn. New York: Demos Medical Publishing, 2008; pp. 323–334.
[25] Wirrell EC, Camfield CS, Camfield PR, *et al.* Long-term prognosis of typical childhood absence epilepsy: remission or progression to juvenile myoclonic epilepsy. *Neurology* 1996;**47**: 912–918.
[26] Glauser T, Ben-Menachem E, Bourgeois B, *et al.* ILAE Treatment guidelines: evidence-based analysis of antiepileptic drug efficacy and effectiveness as initial monotherapy for epileptic seizures and syndromes. *Epilepsia* 2006;**47**:1094–1120.
[27] Kanner AM, Glauser TA, Morita DA. Ethosuximide. In: Wyllie E (ed.), *Wyllie's Treatment of Epilepsy: Principles and Practice*, 5th edn. Philadelphia: Lippincott Williams & Willkins, (2011; pp. 657–667.
[28] Roulet-Perez E, Ballhausen D, Bonafe L, *et al.* Glut-1 deficiency syndrome masquerading as idiopathic generalized epilepsy. *Epilepsia* 2008;**49**:1955–1958.
[29] Byrne S, Kearns J, Carolan R, *et al.* Refractory absence epilepsy associated with GLUT-1 deficiency syndrome. *Epilepsia* 2011;**52**:1021–1024.
[30] Mullen SA, Suls A, De Jonghe P, *et al.* Absence epilepsies with widely variable onset are a key feature of familial GLUT1 deficiency. *Neurology* 2010;**75**:432–440.
[31] Giordano L, Vignoli A, Accorsi P, *et al.* A clinical and genetic study of 33 new cases with early-onset absence epilepsy. *Epilepsy Res* 2011;**95**:221–226.
[32] Wheless JW, Kim HL. Adolescent seizures and epilepsy syndromes. *Epilepsia* 2002;**43**(Suppl. 3):33–52.
[33] Thomas P. Juvenile absence epilepsy. In: Panayiotopoulous CP (ed.), *Atlas of Epilepsies*. London: Springer-Verlag, 2010; pp. 1029–1032.
[34] Grünewald RA. Juvenile Myoclonic epilepsy. In: Panayiotopoulous CP (ed.), *Atlas of Epilepsies*. London: Springer-Verlag, 2010; pp. 1033–1040.
[35] Roebling R, Scheerer N, Uttner I, *et al.* Evaluation of cognition, structural, and functional MRI in juvenile myoclonic epilepsy. *Epilepsia* 2009;**50**:2456–2465.
[36] Mantoan L, Walker M. Treatment options in juvenile myoclonic epilepsy. *Curr Treat Options Neurol* 2011;**13**:355–370.
[37] Engel J. A proposed diagnostic scheme for people with epileptic seizures and with epilepsy: report of the ILAE Task Force on Classification and Terminology. *Epilepsia* 2001;**42**: 796–803.
[38] Iris U, Gerhard B, Eugen T. Epilepsy with generalized tonic-clonic seizures only. In: Panayiotopoulous CP (ed.), *Atlas of Epilepsies*. London: Springer-Verlag, 2010; pp. 1041–1049.
[39] Koutroumanidis M, Aggelakis K, Panayiotopoulos CP. Idiopathic epilepsy with generalized tonic-clonic seizures only versus idiopathic epilepsy with phantom absences and generalized tonic-clonic seizures: One or two syndromes? *Epilepsia* 2008;**49**:2050–2062.
[40] Camfield P, Camfield C. Idiopathic generalized epilepsy with generalized tonic-clonic seizures (IGE-GTC): a population-based cohort with >20 year follow up for medical and social outcome. *Epilepsy Behav* 2010;**18**:61–63.
[41] Karceski S, Morrell MJ, Carpenter D. Treatment of epilepsy in adults: expert opinion, 2005. *Epilepsy Behav* 2005;**7**(Suppl. 1):S1–S64.
[42] Rosenfeld WE, Benbadis S, Edrich P, *et al.* Levetiracetam as add-on therapy for idiopathic generalized epilepsy syndromes with onset during adolescence: analysis of two randomized, double-blind, placebo-controlled studies. *Epilepsy Res* 2009;**85**:72–80.
[43] Covanis A. Epilepsy with myoclonic absences. In: Panayiotopoulous CP (ed.), *Atlas of Epilepsies*. London: Springer-Verlag, 2010; pp. 1025–1028.
[44] Scheffer IE, Berkovic SF. Generalized epilepsy with febrile seizures plus. A genetic disorder with heterogeneous clinical phenotypes. *Brain* 1997;**120**:479–490.

[45] Nordli DR. Generalized epilepsy with febrile seizure plus (GEFS+). In: Panayiotopoulous CP (ed.), *Atlas of Epilepsies*. London: Springer-Verlag, 2010; pp.861–864.
[46] Covanis A. Jeavons syndrome. In: Panayiotopoulous CP (ed.), *Atlas of Epilepsies*. London: Springer-Verlag, 2010; pp.1081–1091.
[47] Hirsch E, Valenti M. Other probable syndromes of idiopathic generalized epilepsies. In: Panayiotopoulous CP (ed.), *Atlas of Epilepsies*. London: Springer-Verlag, 2010; pp.1055–1061.
[48] Korff CM, Nordli DR. Epilepsy with myoclonic-astatic seizures. In: Panayiotopoulous CP (ed.), *Atlas of Epilepsies*. London: Springer-Verlag, 2010; pp.1007–1011.

15 Cryptogenic and symptomatic generalized epilepsies: epilepsies with encephalopathy

Karen Keough
'Specially For Children', Austin, Texas, USA

In April 2010, the International League Against Epilepsy (ILAE) Commission on Classification and Terminology published new recommendations for classifying seizures and epilepsy syndromes [1]. The new definitions and flexible organizational structure allows a coherent grouping of the most refractory types of epilepsy syndromes. Initially conceived as a chapter reviewing symptomatic generalized epilepsy, this chapter originally included several diagnoses that fell outside the historical borders of this heading. The syndromes included in this chapter share the following features:

1. Seizures of one or multiple types, often including both seizures with onset in one hemisphere and seizures with bilateral network involvement from onset.
2. Characteristic EEG abnormalities displayed in most if not all patients within the syndrome, usually including both focal and generalized epileptiform abnormalities.
3. Associated cognitive comorbidity occurring in most patients, to varying degrees. The cognitive features are non-progressive or only slowly progressive, and often fluctuate in proportion to seizure control.

Epilepsy in Children and Adolescents, First Edition. Edited by James W. Wheless.

Box 15.1 Epilepsies with encephalopathy [1,2]

Neonatal onset

- Early myoclonic encephalopathy (EME)
- Early infantile epileptic encephalopathy (EIEE, or Ohtahara syndrome)

Infantile onset

- Infantile spasms
- Migrating partial epilepsy of infancy
- Dravet syndrome*

Childhood onset

- Epilepsy with myoclonic-atonic seizures (Doose syndrome)*
- Lennox–Gastaut syndrome
- Landau–Kleffner syndrome
- Epileptic encephalopathy with continuous spike-and-wave during sleep (CSWS)

*Classified as "genetic epilepsies" in the International League Against Epilepsy (ILAE) 2010 classification [1].

Arranged based on usual age of onset these disorders include:

- neonatal-onset syndromes of early myoclonic encephalopathy (EME) and early infantile epileptic encephalopathy (EIEE, or Ohtahara syndrome);
- infantile-onset syndromes include infantile spasms, migrating partial epilepsy of infancy, and Dravet syndrome;
- childhood-onset syndromes including epilepsy with myoclonic-atonic seizures (Doose syndrome), Lennox–Gastaut syndrome, Landau–Kleffner syndrome, and epileptic encephalopathy with continuous spike-and-wave during sleep (CSWS) (Box 15.1).

Classifying a patient into an epilepsy syndrome requires an understanding of the following: seizure semiology, age of onset, EEG features, imaging results, and neurological findings on examination, especially cognition. The recognition of a specific syndrome guides therapeutic decisions and allows some prognostication, and may also clarify possible etiologies. Many epilepsy patients will not neatly fit within a specific syndrome. These patients should be considered to belong to a non-specific subgroup awaiting further classification as we build our understanding of epilepsy's mechanisms, pathophysiology, and etiologies.

15.1 Neonatal-onset epilepsies with encephalopathy

Table 15.1 compares the clinical features of the two classic syndromes with onset in the earliest stage of life: early myoclonic encephalopathy (EME) and early infantile epileptic

Table 15.1 Comparison of epilepsies with encephalopathy of neonatal or infantile onset [2–4,6].

	Early infantile epileptic encephalopathy (Ohtahara syndrome)	Early myoclonic encephalopathy of infancy	West syndrome
Onset	Earliest, often at birth, prior to 3 months	Days to weeks after birth, prior to 3 months	3–12 months old in most cases, peak around 5 months
Primary seizure type	Tonic seizures often in clusters during wakefulness and sleep	Myoclonic seizures – multifocal, sometimes continuous	Epileptic spasms in clusters often on awakening
Other seizure types	Partial seizures	Partial seizures, tonic seizures	Partial seizures, especially if lesional
Clinical course	Usually evolves to infantile spasms and/or Lennox–Gastaut syndrome	Rarely evolves to infantile spasms	Often self-limited, may evolve to Lennox–Gastaut or other epilepsy types
EEG	Pseudo-rhythmic burst-suppression during both sleep and wakefulness, evolving to hypsarrhythmia	Burst-suppression during deep sleep, may lag clinical onset and may evolve to hypsarrhythmia	Hypsarrhythmia
Etiology (when known)	Structural lesions common	Inborn errors of metabolism common	Either metabolic or structural disorders

encephalopathy (EIEE, or Ohtahara syndrome). EME begins in the first 3 months of life, often in the first days or weeks, but usually later than EIEE. Seizures consist initially of myoclonus often involving various muscle groups, and may be nearly continuous. The prominent myoclonus distinguishes EME from EIEE and most cases of West syndrome. Focal seizures develop later and include any variety of neonatal seizure types including eye deviation, autonomic dysregulation, and partial clonic seizures, and frequently tonic seizures with truncal contraction. Many cases evolve to include infantile spasms. Encephalopathy often manifests as lack of reactivity to environmental stimuli, and may coexist with hypotonia and poor visual function. EEG shows burst-suppression that often evolves to hypsarrhythmia. Many metabolic disorders have been associated with EME, so metabolic screening is essential, including cerebrospinal fluid (CSF) neurotransmitters, urine organic acids, and serum and CSF amino acids. By contrast, imaging often yields normal or non-specific findings such as atrophy. Common etiologies include non-ketotic hypoglycinemia, organic acidurias, and peroxisomal disorders. Pyridoxine dependency has been described. Familial cases are common, reflecting the prevalence of inborn errors of metabolism. Seizures are quite treatment resistant including poor response to adrenocorticotropic hormone (ACTH), and prognosis is dismal. Severe neurodevelopmental impairment and early death are common [2,3].

EIEE (Ohtahara syndrome) also begins shortly after birth, and nearly always prior to 3 months of age, characteristically presenting with tonic seizures. These events may cluster, as with infantile spasms, but very early onset suggests EIEE. Focal clonic and hemiconvulsive seizures occur rarely. The variety of seizures generally remains more restricted than in EME, and myoclonus occurs only rarely. As with EME, EEG also shows burst-suppression. Imaging may reveal a structural lesion, including porencephaly, hemimegaloencephaly, Aicardi syndrome, and other forms of dysgenesis. In contrast to EME, metabolic errors are exceptional diagnoses. Patients are notoriously resistant to treatment, including ACTH, with rare responsiveness to conventional anticonvulsants, and often suffer an early death or progression to infantile spasms and/or Lennox–Gastaut syndrome [4]. Some patients with focal cortical lesions may improve with surgical resection [5].

15.2 Infantile-onset epilepsies with encephalopathy

West syndrome and infantile spasms

In recognition of their occasional onset or persistence in older patients, the term "epileptic spasms" has been introduced as a descriptor for a distinctive type of seizure formerly thought to occur exclusively in infants and very young children [6]. The vast majority of cases do have onset in infancy, usually between 3 and 7 months, and 85% begin before 1 year of age. Much less often they may begin in older children, and rare cases of adult onset have been described. Spasms occur in 2–5 of 10 000 live births, with a slight male predominance (60%). West syndrome comprises a subset of infantile-onset patients who exhibit the triad of spasms, hypsarrhythmia, and psychomotor retardation with or without regression. A working group of experts (the Infantile Spasms Working Group, or ISWG) recently published a thorough review of the current body of knowledge regarding diagnosis, treatment, and prognosis of infantile spasms (IS) [7].

Box 15.2 describes the clinical features of epileptic spasms. Although the semiology of individual spasms often varies between patients, clustering of events and a predilection for occurrence on awakening are distinctive features.

Box 15.2 Clinical features of epileptic spasms [2,6]

1. Individual spasms:
   - Sudden and briefly sustained movements of the trunk
   - Flexor, extensor, or mixed
   - Typically symmetric, sometimes asymmetric
2. Clustering (90% of infantile spasm patients):
   - Each individual spasm lasts up to 10 seconds separated by 5–30 seconds
   - Phasic jerk followed by tonic contraction lasting 2–10 seconds
   - Clusters may last a few or up to 30 minutes in sequence
   - Commonly exhibit "crescendo-decrescendo" evolution through the course of the cluster, becoming stronger and closer together then weaker and farther spaced
   - Commonly occur on awakening, rarely during sleep
   - May cause exhaustion or increased alertness after cluster
3. Other seizure types:
   - Occur in 12–42% of patients
   - Tonic seizures may precede or follow a cluster of spasms
   - Independent myoclonic, clonic, or akinetic seizures often coexist

Psychomotor retardation occurs in many but not all patients with epileptic spasms. Regression may be unidentifiable in patients with impairment prior to onset. Less frequently, normal development may continue after onset of spasms either temporarily or persistently, therefore some patients with infantile spasms may not fall into a diagnostic category of West syndrome. EEG abnormalities may also lag the clinical onset of spasms, especially if only a waking record is captured.

Differential diagnosis of infantile spasms

Atypical movements from non-neurological conditions may mimic spasms, including Sandifer syndrome (dystonic movements due to gastroesophageal reflux), colic, or posturing. These conditions lack the stereotyped repetitive nature of spasms and should not occur in clusters. Conversely, many cases are falsely attributed to these causes before spasms are diagnosed. Neurological mimics of spasms include benign myoclonus of infancy, benign myoclonic epilepsy of infancy, and hyperekplexia. In benign myoclonus of infancy, video EEG reveals a normal EEG even during events. Seizures resulting from benign myoclonic epilepsy of infancy may cluster; however, the background EEG does not show hypsarrhythmia, and video EEG recording shows generalized spike-and-wave discharges during events. Hyperekplexia is a rare familial disease manifested as hypertonia that can be episodic and associated at times with apnea when infants are handled. The triggered nature of the events is characteristic, and the EEG is normal.

Box 15.3 reviews the diverse range of etiologies for spasms. Every case mandates a thorough etiological evaluation since some metabolic disorders may have disease-specific dietary or medical therapies. Some structural lesions may be surgically amenable, including focal cortical dysplasias, Sturge–Weber syndrome, arteriovenous malformations, or tuberous sclerosis that fails medication therapy. Five to thirty percent of patients who lack any abnormal findings with extensive imaging and laboratory testing and who retain normal developmental progress fall into a category of idiopathic infantile spasms [2].

Treatment of infantile spasms (IS)

A joint practice parameter from the American Academy of Neurology (AAN) and the Child Neurology Society (CNS) reviews evidenced-based recommendations for therapy (Box 15.4) [8].

Adrenocorticotropic hormone therapy controls spasms with a 50–75% response rate. A wide range of dose regimens exists, each with variable duration of 2 weeks to 6 months. Oral steroids may also be used but limited data exist comparing these to ACTH. Relapses after initial response are common (33–56%), and may be addressed with a second course of ACTH treatment. Side effects of ACTH include common but manageable complications such as irritability, insomnia, apathy, hypertension, gastroesophageal reflux, and electrolyte abnormalities, but serious or even fatal (mortality 2–5%) complications also occur including infection, renal failure, nephrocalcinosis, and cardiomyopathy. The AAN Practice Parameter states that ACTH is probably effective [8], and the ISWG recommends ACTH as first-line therapy for the treatment of IS. Although there is insufficient evidence to recommend an optimum dosage strategy, short-term treatment with early assessment of therapeutic response is considered preferable [7]. Oral steroids carry a lower morbidity but include many similar adverse effects; however, the AAN Practice Parameter deemed the evidence insufficient to declare oral corticosteroids effective in the treatment of IS, and the

Box 15.3 Identifiable etiologies of infantile spasms [2,6]

Structural lesions

Imaging is abnormal in 61–90% of cases. These can be categorized as follows:

1. Cerebral malformations:
   - Cortical dysgenesis: septo-optic dysplasia, focal dysplasias, lissencephaly, hemimegaloencephaly, holoprosencephaly, schizencephaly, corpus callosum anomalies, porencephaly
   - Leukoencephalopathies
   - Neurocutaneous syndromes, most commonly tuberous sclerosis
   - Aicardi syndrome
2. Vascular disorders: AVM, Sturge–Weber syndrome, strokes
3. Perinatal brain injury (up to one-third of cases)
4. Postnatal insults: hypoxic, infectious, traumatic
5. Tumors (rare)

Metabolic disorders (rare)

- Krabbe disease
- Adrenoleukodystrophy
- Leigh syndrome
- Biotinidase and pyridoxine deficiency
- Non-ketotic hyperglycinemia
- Phenylketonuria (PKU)
- Pyruvate dehydrogenase complex (PDHC) deficiency
- Glucose transporter deficiency syndrome
- Maple syrup urine disease
- Menkes kinky hair disease
- Hyperammonemic disorders

Down syndrome

Three percent develop IS.

Familial cases

These represent 3–6% of cases [2].

ISWG did not reach consensus regarding whether oral steroids should be considered first-line therapy, nor did they recommend a specific dosage strategy [7,8]. Numerous studies of vigabatrin demonstrate rapid control of spasms within days of treatment; complete cessation occurs in 43–60% [9,10]. Several studies suggest a higher response rate in tuberous sclerosis [11]. The AAN Practice Parameter considers the evidence adequate to declare vigabatrin possibly effective for treatment of IS, and the ISWG recommends vigabatrin

Box 15.4 American Academy of Neurology (AAN) and Child Neurology Society (CNS) Practice Parameter 2004 recommendations for medical treatment of infantile spasms [7]

1. ACTH is probably effective but optimum dosage and duration not adequately studied.
2. There is insufficient evidence for efficacy with oral steroids.
3. Vigabatrin
   (a) "Possibly effective" for epileptic spasms, and possibly also for West syndrome in tuberous sclerosis.
   (b) Ophthalmological screening is required but recommendations regarding type of screening and frequency not made due to lack of evidence.
4. Insufficient evidence exists to recommend any other therapies, including other anticonvulsants, pyridoxine, the ketogenic diet, or novel therapies such as intravenous immunoglobulin (IVIG).

as first-line therapy, particularly in patients with tuberous sclerosis [7,8]. Mild side effects include somnolence, insomnia, irritability, and hypotonia. Unfortunately, vigabatrin can cause direct retinal toxicity leading to constriction of peripheral visual fields, a difficult complication to monitor in non-verbal and pre-verbal children. This impairment occurs in 16–44% of testable patients treated long term, but often remains asymptomatic [12,13]. In the United States, the Food and Drug Administration (FDA) mandates patient counseling, consent, and monitoring of ongoing ophthalmological follow-up. No clear methodology has emerged as an effective monitoring strategy for detection of retinal toxicity in infants on vigabatrin. Pyridoxine treatment has had reported success in both deficient and non-deficient cases, with a 10–30% response rate noted in Japan [14]. Published case series describe favorable response to treatment with valproate, topiramate, zonisamide, and the ketogenic diet [15–18]. Although each of these treatments harbors specific potential adverse effects, most are safer than the systemic risks of steroid therapy and lack the potentially irreversible visual risk of vigabatrin. The AAN Practice Parameter and the ISWG agree that lack of adequate evidence for efficacy prevents a recommendation for use of pyridoxine, conventional antiepileptic drugs (AEDs) or the ketogenic diet for first-line agents in the treatment of spasms [7,8]; however, these treatment options may be appropriate considerations in spasm patients with severe structural or metabolic disorders where their etiology impacts prognosis more potently than does their response to treatment. Surgical intervention has shown benefit for patients with focal lesions including cases with normal magnetic resonance imaging (MRI) scans but asymmetric metabolic activity by positron emission tomography (PET) imaging [19].

Prognosis

Most cases of infantile spasms eventually remit regardless of treatment, but duration varies from a few weeks (6–15%) to months or years. Long-term studies report resolution by 1 year of age in 28%, and by 5 years in 72–99% [20]. Spasms patients have a high mortality (6–30% by age 3 years) depending on underlying pathology. Over months the EEG gradually

Box 15.5 Criteria for the diagnosis of idiopathic West syndrome. Children fulfilling these criteria reportedly universally experience a remission of spasms and a normal developmental outcome [17,18]

Basic criteria

1. Normal development before, during and after the seizure period, including visual function.
2. Normal functional and structural brain imaging and absence of genetic or metabolic etiologies.
3. Symmetrical epileptic spasms and hypsarrhythmia on EEG.

Possible additional features

1. Positive family history of other forms of idiopathic epilepsy or febrile seizures.
2. Benign genetic markers on EEG such as generalized spike/wave, rolandic spikes, or photoparoxysmal responses.
3. Normal sleep structures despite hypsarrhythmia.
4. Absence of focal interictal EEG slow waves even after intravenous diazepam.

improves but often remains abnormal. Many patients evolve to other forms of epilepsy, with or without a seizure-free interval. Forty to sixty percent eventually develop Lennox–Gastaut syndrome. Mental retardation occurs in 70–90%, and is severe in one-half of those cases [17]. Neuropsychological comorbidities commonly develop, most often manifest as autism and attention-deficit/hyperactivity disorder (ADHD). Etiology strongly affects prognosis. For example, one-third of tuberous sclerosis patients who have spasms will have a normal cognitive outcome [21]. Children who fulfill strict criteria for idiopathic spasms (Box 15.5) experienced full remission and normal developmental outcome according to two published series [22,23].

Migrating focal seizures of infancy

This rare syndrome manifests in early infancy with multiple types of partial seizures, involving both hemispheres independently. Motor seizures, either tonic or clonic, may progress to secondarily generalized convulsions, often with prominent autonomic features. Most patients do not exhibit infantile spasms. The seizures worsen progressively over weeks and often cluster. No defined etiology has been identified, no reports of familial cases have been recorded, imaging is usually normal, and post-mortem pathology in two reported cases was non-specific. The interictal EEG predictably reflects bilateral independent spikes that increase in coincidence with worsening seizures. Developmental regression with associated motor dysfunction and spasticity uniformly occur, and most patients die within a year. Only transient response to anticonvulsant therapy has been reported [24].

15.3 Epilepsies with encephalopathy with onset later in infancy

Severe myoclonic epilepsy of infancy (SMEI), or Dravet syndrome

Severe myoclonic epilepsy of infancy reliably begins before 1 year of age, often initially manifest as prolonged febrile seizures, which may be unilateral rather than generalized. A history of prolonged febrile seizures in an older child with severe epilepsy should prompt consideration of SMEI. Intercurrent illnesses remain a strong trigger for exacerbation of seizure activity throughout childhood, and status epilepticus occurs commonly. Other seizure triggers include photic stimulation, eye-closure and fixation on patterns, and exogenous body temperature elevation.

Multiple seizure types usually evolve to accompany the frequent focal and secondarily generalized seizures. Myoclonic seizures occur in the majority of SMEI patients, and sometimes precede the onset of febrile convulsions. Myoclonus may be focal and subtle, or intense and generalized, sometimes leading to falls, and may disappear with age. Atypical absence seizures occur in most cases. These differ from typical absence seizures in that they usually last longer, with gradual onset and ending, and have more subtle decreases in responsiveness, but more prominent physical correlates including loss of truncal tone, head control, or myoclonus. Persistent postictal impairment, absent in typical absence seizures, may occur in atypical events. The generalized spike-and-wave correlate of atypical events by definition involves slower frequencies (<2.5 Hz) than seen in typical events (>2.5 Hz). Atypical absence seizures in SMEI usually remain brief (5–10 seconds), but atypical absence status can occur. Tonic seizures occur only rarely, and if present, often occur nocturnally. Incomplete forms of Dravet syndrome may lack myoclonus and atypical absence seizures. The EEG background eventually declines from normal frequencies to 5–6 Hz dominant rhythms; photosensitivity by EEG is an early and distinctive feature [2,25].

Etiology

Imaging may reveal mild cerebral or cerebellar atrophy; metabolic evaluations are uniformly normal. Family history often reveals multiple relatives with febrile seizures. Mutations in the sodium channel gene *SCN1A*, originally implicated in the generalized epilepsy with febrile seizures plus (GEFS+) syndrome of epilepsy, account for many cases (35–100% based on various published series). Most cases result from new mutations, but some may be inherited from asymptomatic parental carriers. Inherited cases tend to have less severe clinical involvement. Variation in clinical severity among people sharing the same mutation suggests a more complex genetic mechanism, requiring input from another or perhaps several other as yet unidentified genes. Clinical diagnosis remains vital since many patients who fulfill clinical criteria for Dravet syndrome lack a diagnostic *SCN1A* mutation. Conversely, identification of an *SCN1A* mutation does not necessarily confirm Dravet syndrome since other types of epilepsy share this genetic etiology [26].

Differential diagnosis

Table 15.2 contrasts Lennox–Gastaut syndrome, myoclonic-astatic epilepsy (Doose syndrome), and Dravet syndrome, three conditions with overlapping clinical features.

Table 15.2 Comparison of later-onset epilepsies with encephalopathy and multiple seizure types [2,25,30].

	Myoclonic-astatic epilepsy (Doose syndrome)	Lennox–Gastaut syndrome	Severe myoclonic epilepsy of infancy (Dravet syndrome)
Heralded by febrile seizures	Sometimes	Never	Majority
Age at onset	Late infancy through early childhood	Varies, usually recognized between ages 2 and 8 years	Late infancy, rarely over 1 year old
Main seizures	Myoclonic-astatic	Tonic, atonic, and atypical absence	Focal seizures with and without generalization often triggered by temperature or visual stimuli
Myoclonic seizures	Always present, symmetric	May be focal	Usually present, focal or generalized, may remit
Atypical absence seizures	May occur	Always present	Often present, usually brief
Development prior to onset	Normal	Delayed	Usually normal
Tonic seizures	Generally absent, ?exclusionary	Common, may lead to drops	Exceptional
Etiology	Presumed genetic, *SCN1A* mutation in some	Many underlying etiologies, not always identifiable	Presumed genetic, *SCN1A* is most common identified mutation
Development from West syndrome	Never	Often	Never
EEG background	May be normal at onset, generalized spike and wave 2–4 Hz, sometimes polyspikes	Slow spike and wave (<2.5 Hz), often with generalized fast (>10 Hz) activity in sleep	Slow background rhythm; multifocal and generalized spikes; photosensitivity common
Developmental prognosis	Frequently normal or mildly impaired	Virtually always severely impaired	Significant regression with eventual plateau
Seizure prognosis	Often treatment responsive, may be self-limited	Uniformly treatment-refractory	Treatment-refractory; eventual improvement but not remission

Early stages of some forms of progressive myoclonic epilepsy could appear similar to Dravet syndrome.

Treatment

Treatment produces incomplete seizure reduction in most patients. Valproate, benzodiazepines, ethosuximide, topiramate, levetiracetam, zonisamide, and phenobarbital and the ketogenic diet have all shown efficacy. Carbamazepine, phenytoin, and lamotrigine are contraindicated. Most patients also require developmental therapy and educational accommodations.

Course and outlook

Developmental decline is severe and seems to correspond to seizure burden. Despite normal early development, most patients eventually become moderately to severely retarded, and often develop motor involvement such as dysarthria, ataxia, and pyramidal signs. Cognitive and motor dysfunction plateau around adolescence, with a decrease but not remission of seizures, which remain susceptible to triggering by febrile illnesses. Myoclonia and atypical absence tend to improve more than convulsive seizures.

15.4 Epilepsies with encephalopathy with onset after infancy

Myoclonic-astatic epilepsy (MAE), or Doose syndrome

Classification of Doose syndrome has engendered some controversy. The 1989 ILAE classification listed MAE as a symptomatic generalized epilepsy [27]. Because many cases showed benign developmental outcomes, reassessment in 2001 shifted the categorization of MAE to an idiopathic category [28]. We include MAE in this chapter because mild to moderate encephalopathy occurs in some cases, creating clinical overlap between these MAE patients and mild to moderate cases of SMEI or Lennox–Gastaut syndrome (LGS).

All MAE patients have normal development prior to onset of seizures, which may begin in late infancy although peak incidence occurs between 2 and 4 years. The classic seizure type consists of a generalized, symmetric myoclonic jerk followed by loss of muscle tone resulting in a fall (hence myoclonic-astatic epilepsy, although more recent taxonomy reclassifies astatic as atonic seizures). Febrile or afebrile generalized seizures may precede the onset of atonic seizures. Drops frequently result in injury. They may occur without a preceding myoclonic jerk, and myoclonus may occur without a drop. Other seizure types include atypical absence seizures. Tonic seizures usually do not occur, and some authors consider them exclusionary for MAE [2,25].

Non-convulsive status epilepticus occurs commonly, presenting as stupor with interspersed subtle myoclonic fragments. Prolonged status episodes have been associated with more severe developmental impairment. Overall, however, most children fare better with MAE than with other subtypes of epilepsy with encephalopathy. Up to 58% in one series had normal IQs, and an additional 20% had only mild mental retardation [29].

EEG findings help distinguish MAE from other types of epileptic encephalopathy. Interictal 3 Hz generalized spike-and-wave runs occur commonly, but may range from 2 to

4 Hz and may include polyspikes. Patients frequently report a family history of epilepsy, and several MAE pedigrees link to *SCN1A* mutations.

Various treatments provide benefit, especially valproate, ethosuximide, and in some cases lamotrigine, topiramate, levetiracetam, and the ketogenic diet. Carbamazepine, phenytoin, and vigabatrin are contraindicated. Intravenous benzodiazepines may terminate an occurrence of convulsive status epilepticus but have been reported to precipitate tonic status epilepticus [25].

Lennox–Gastaut syndrome

Typically diagnosed in young children, Lennox–Gastaut syndrome evolves from other forms of epilepsy, especially West syndrome. Most cases are recognized between 2 and 8 years of age, but later onset would not exclude the diagnosis. A mixture of multiple seizure types is mandatory, most typically tonic seizures, often predominantly or exclusively during sleep. Tonic seizures consist of steady, usually symmetric contraction of proximal muscle groups, or the face and eyes. They may be subtle or severe and diffuse enough to cause a fall. The clinical criteria of LGS vary but generally include requirements for at least two seizure types, one of which must be tonic seizures. Other common seizure types include atypical absence, atonic, and less commonly myoclonic, complex partial, and generalized clonic or tonic-clonic seizures. Atonic seizures may be small, causing only a subtle head drop, or large enough to cause a fall, a frequent cause of injury. Most are very brief, but limpness may persist up to a minute after the fall. Various forms of status epilepticus may develop, involving nearly every seizure type including classic convulsive status, absence status (confusional states), tonic or myoclonic status, or a combination of all these seizures types [30].

EEG findings generally clarify a suspected clinical diagnosis of LGS. The interictal background rhythms are slow and poorly organized. Multifocal and generalized epileptiform activity occurs rhythmically at slow frequencies (1.5–2.5 Hz). Most criteria require the occurrence of episodic fast activity (>10 Hz), most prominently during sleep. Intellectual impairment is nearly universal but not necessarily required for diagnosis.

Identifiable causes of LGS include both diffuse and focal conditions. Since many cases of LGS evolve from West syndrome, they share many etiologies. Structural brain malformations are often identified, but about one-third of cases remain unexplained.

Despite partial response to many anticonvulsant medications, seizure control is rarely complete. Valproate, benzodiazepines, topiramate, and felbamate offer evidence for efficacy. Ethosuximide often proves uniquely effective for atypical absence seizures. Lamotrigine can contribute to seizure control, but may exacerbate myoclonus. Most of the newer generation of anticonvulsants have a role in treatment of LGS, but honeymoon responses occur commonly. Clobazam and rufinamide recently gained FDA approval specifically for atonic seizures in LGS. Non-medical interventions such as the ketogenic diet and vagus nerve stimulation may substantially reduce seizure activity, and are especially attractive in patients who experience limiting toxicities from medications. ACTH or oral steroid therapy may provide short-term benefit in exceptional periods of seizure activity or status epilepticus. Cortical resections rarely prove feasible since most patients have diffuse or multifocal pathology, but corpus callosotomy can minimize or eliminate injury by preventing drops from tonic and atonic seizures.

15.5 Continuous spike wave of sleep (CSWS) and Landau–Kleffner syndrome (LKS)

These two syndromes historically were classified separately, but more recent consensus considers LKS to be a specific subset of CSWS [31]. The clinical and electrophysiological features overlap substantially, as illustrated in Table 15.3.

The hallmark of both disorders requires the marked increase in prevalence of epileptiform activity on EEG during sleep as compared to wakefulness. Although poorly understood, the presumed pathophysiological mechanism invokes a disruption of cognitive function during sleep that prevents normal consolidation of learning and appropriate language, cognitive function, and behavior while awake. The correspondence of onset and resolution of symptoms with EEG abnormalities supports this hypothesis.

Landau–Kleffner syndrome, also known as acquired epileptic aphasia, usually begins with an abrupt or subacute regression of language skills in early childhood (range 2–8 years old), primarily loss of receptive and subsequently expressive language that may progress to fluent aphasia or mutism. Occasionally seizures predate language dysfunction. Behavioral problems coexist in many cases, with hyperactivity, impulsivity, aggression, and rarely psychosis. Despite the typical presence of seizures and florid EEG abnormalities, seizures tend to be rare and responsive to medication, and eventually remit. Seizures are usually convulsive, either generalized or focal, but atypical absence, atonic and non-convulsive seizures with automatisms are also described. Structural imaging is typically normal; however, PET scans often show decreased activity in the temporal lobes [32].

Table 15.3 Continuous spike wave of sleep (CSWS) and Landau–Kleffner syndrome (LKS) [2,31].

		Distinctive features	
	Shared features	LKS	CSWS
EEG features			
EEG during sleep	Always worse than wakefulness	80% have CSWS (not required)	100% have CSWS (required)
Spike localization		Temporal	Frontal more often than temporal
Imaging		Decreased temporal lobe activity by PET	One-third abnormal MRI
Clinical features			
Seizure prevalence	Most or all have seizures	Infrequent and mild, may be absent	Always occur, may be frequent
Impairment	Uniformly present	Verbal auditory agnosia required	Aphasia, OR other cognitive deficits, OR both
Behavioral problems	Hyperactivity, impulsivity, aggression	Common (half)	Almost universal
Prognosis for reasonable recovery		50% near-normal	25% near-normal

CSWS always begins in childhood, with onset peaking at age 8 years. Convulsive seizures begin as infrequent, usually nocturnal events. They increase in frequency coincident with the onset of cognitive and behavioral symptoms, eventually leading to discovery of CSWS during a sleep EEG. Multiple seizure types (except tonic seizures) can occur and tend to be more difficult to control than in LKS. Progression of neuropsychological impairment is gradual in most cases but becomes quite marked and may be associated with motor abnormalities including ataxia, hemiparesis, and dyspraxia, along with drooling and dysarthria from oral motor involvement. Decline of function includes global abilities and expressive language beyond the primarily language-based dysfunction of LKS. Only one-third of MRI scans yield a structural lesion. Behavioral dysfunction including hyperactivity, impulsivity, and aggression tend to be more prominent and more prevalent.

Treatment

Management approaches for both disorders include anticonvulsant management, behavioral intervention with or without psychoactive medications, and steroid therapy. Traditional anticonvulsants and behavioral medications can control seizures and mitigate behavioral symptoms but do not impact language impairment. The most promising medications based on case series include valproate, benzodiazepines, ethosuximide, and possibly levetiracetam. No controlled trials of pharmaceutical treatment confirm the efficacy of immunotherapy, but case series report temporary, or less often, lasting improvements in response to ACTH or high-dose, long-duration oral steroid regimens. Because of the rarity of the condition, and because the natural history of aphasia in LKS can include fluctuations, certain proof of therapeutic responses will require large-scale controlled trials. Even fewer case reports document improvement following IVIG therapy or multiple sub-pial transections, a rarely utilized surgical intervention involving superficial vertical cuts across epileptically active cortical regions.

Prognosis

Eventual remission of seizures can be expected, but incomplete neuropsychological recovery occurs in most. One-half of LKS cases retain language and cognitive impairments despite cessation of seizures. For CSWS, a near-normal level of function eventually develops in only about 25% of cases.

References

[1] Berg AT, Berkovic SF, Brodie MJ, *et al.* Revised terminology and concepts for organization of seizures and epilepsies: report of the ILAE Commission on Classification and Terminology, 2005-2009. *Epilepsia* 2010;**51**:676–685.

[2] Panayiotopoulos CP. Epileptic encephalopathies in infancy and early childhood. In: *The Epilepsies: Seizures, Syndromes and Management*. Bladon Medical Publishing, 2005; pp. 137–197.

[3] Guerrini R, Aicardi J. Epileptic encephalopathies with myoclonic seizures in infants and children (severe myoclonic epilepsy and myoclonic-astatic epilepsy). *J Clin Neurophysiol* 2003;**20**:449–461.

[4] Ohtahara S, Yamatogi Y. Epileptic encephalopathies in early infancy with suppression-burst. *J. Clin. Neurophysiol* 2003;**20**:398–407.

[5] Komaki H, Sugai K, Maehara T, Shimizu H. Surgical treatment of early-infantile epileptic encephalopathy with suppression-burst associated with focal cortical dysplasia. *Brain Dev* 2001;**23**:727–731.

[6] Shields WD, Koh S. Epileptic spasms. In: Wyllie E, Gupta A, Lachhwani D (eds), *The Treatment of Epilepsy Principle & Practice*, 4th edn. Lippincott Williams & Wilkins, 2006; pp. 333–343.

[7] Pellock JM, Hrachovy R, Shinnar S, *et al.* Infantile spasms: A U.S. consensus report. *Epilepsia* 2010;**51**:2175–2189.

[8] Mackay MT, Weiss SK, Adams-Webber T, *et al.* Practice parameter: Medical Treatment of Infantile Spasms. Report of the American Academy of Neurology and the Child Neurology Society. *Neurology* 2004;**62**:1668–1681.

[9] Appleton RE, Peters AC, Mumford JP, Shaw DE. Randomized Prospective Controlled Study of Vigabatrin as first line therapy for infantile spasms. *Epilepsia* 1999;**40**:1627–1633.

[10] Elterman RD, Shields WD, Mansfield KA, Nakagawa J. US Infantile Spasms Vigabatrin Study Group. Randomized trial of vigabatrin in patients with infantile spasms. *Neurology* 2001;**57**:1416–1421.

[11] Hancock E, Osbourne JP. Vigabatrin in the treatment of infantile spasms in tuberous sclerosis: literature review. *J Child Neurol* 1999;**14**:71–74.

[12] Maguire MJ, Hemming K, Wild JM, *et al.* Prevalence of visual field loss following exposure to vigabatrin therapy: a systematic review. *Epilepsia* 2010;**51**:2423–2431.

[13] Sergott RC, Bittman RM, Christen EM, Sagar SM. Vigabatrin-induced peripheral visual field defects in patients with refractory partial epilepsy. *Epilepsy Res* 2010;**92**:170–176.

[14] Watanabe K. Medical treatment of West syndrome in Japan. *J Child Neurology* 1995;**10**:143–147.

[15] Glauser TA, Clark PO, McGee K. Long-term response to topiramate in patients with West syndrome. *Epilepsia* 2000;**41**(Suppl. 1):S91–S94.

[16] Lotze TE, Wilfong AA. Zonisamide treatment for symptomatic infantile spasms. *Neurology* 2004;**62**:296–298.

[17] Siemes H, Brandl U, Spohr HL, Völger S, Weschke B. Therapy of infantile spasms with valproate: results of a prospective study. *Epilepsia* 1998;**29**:553–560.

[18] Kossoff EH, Pyzik PL, McGrogan JR, *et al.* Efficacy of the ketogenic diet for infantile spasms. *Pediatrics* 2002;**109**:780–783.

[19] Chugani HT, Shewmon DA, Shields WD, *et al.* Surgery for intractable infantile spasms: neuroimaging perspectives. *Epilepsia* 1993;**34**:764–771.

[20] Jeavons PM, Harper JR, Bower BD. Long term prognosis in infantile spasms: follow-up of 112 cases. *Dev Med Child Neurol* 1970;**12**:413–421.

[21] Goh S, Kwiatkowski DJ, Dorer DJ, Thiele EA. Infantile spasms and intellectual outcomes in children with tuberous sclerosis complex. *Neurology* 2005;**65**:235–238.

[22] Dulac O, Plouin P, Jambaqué I. Predicting favorable outcome in idiopathic West syndrome. *Epilepsia* 1993;**3**:747–756.

[23] Vigevano F, Fusco L, Cusmai R, Claps D, Ricci S, Milani L. The idiopathic form of West syndrome. *Epilepsia* 1993;**34**:743–746.

[24] Coppola G, Plouin P, Chiron C, Robain O, Dulac O. Migrating partial seizures in infancy: a malignant disorder with developmental arrest. *Epilepsia* 1995;**36**:1017–1024.

[25] Guerrini R, Bonanni P, Marini C, Parmeggiani L. The myoclonic epilepsies. In: Wyllie E, Gupta A, Lachhwani D (eds), *The Treatment of Epilepsy Principle & Practice*, 4th edn. Lippincott Williams & Wilkins, 2006; pp. 411–414.

[26] Scheffer IE, Wallace R, Mulley JC, Berkovic SF. Clinical and molecular genetics of myoclonic-astatic epilepsy and severe myoclonic epilepsy in infancy (Dravet syndrome). *Brain Dev* 2001;**23**:732–735.

[27] Commission on Classification and Terminology of the ILAE. Proposal for revised classification of epilepsies and epileptic syndromes. *Epilepsia* 1989;**30**:389–399.

[28] Engel J Jr. A proposed diagnostic scheme for people with epileptic seizures and with epilepsy: Report of the ILAE Task Force on Classification and Terminology. *Epilepsia* 2001;**42**:796–803.
[29] Oguni H, Tanaka T, Hayashi K. Treatment and long-term prognosis of myoclonic-astatic epilepsy of early childhood. *Neuropadiatrie* 2002;**33**:122–132.
[30] Farrell K, Tatum WO. Encephalopathic generalized epilepsy and Lennox–Gastaut syndrome. In: Wyllie E, Gupta A, Lachhwani D (eds), *The Treatment of Epilepsy Principle & Practice*, 4th edn. Lippincott Williams & Wilkins, 2006; pp. 429–438.
[31] Neville B, Cross JH. Continuous spike wave of slow sleep and Landau–Kleffner syndrome. In: Wyllie E, Gupta A, Lachhwani D (eds), *The Treatment of Epilepsy Principle & Practice*, 4th edn. Lippincott Williams & Wilkins, 2006; 455–460.
[32] daSilva E, Chugani DC, Muzik O, Chugani HT. Landau–Kleffner syndrome: metabolic abnormalities in temporal lobe are a common feature. *J Child Neurol* 1997;**12**:489–495.

Section 5

Partial-onset seizures and localization-related epilepsy syndromes

James W. Wheless

16 Idiopathic partial epilepsies

Freedom F. Perkins Jr

Seton Healthcare and Dell Children's Hospital, Austin, TX, USA

The primary purpose of this chapter is to explore and explain the idiopathic partial epilepsies. However, the International League Against Epilepsy (ILAE) is in the process of redefining and reclassifying epilepsy syndromes [1–3]. The first classification scheme for characterization and classification by the ILAE was published in 1960 and last officially updated in 1981. Epilepsies were also likewise classified most recently in 1989.

These schemes are largely based on clinical descriptions and electroclinical features that have been observed over much of the nineteenth and twentieth centuries. Modern neuroimaging and molecular technology, however, have necessitated a significant revision of seizure and epilepsy classification and terminology [1].

Partial-onset seizures (now commonly referred to as focal seizures) have traditionally been characterized as such based on the initial clinical and electroencephalographic changes attributed to the activation of neurons limited to one part of one cerebral hemisphere. Under the new proposed classification scheme, focal seizures are conceptualized as originating from networks limited to one hemisphere. Likewise, focal seizures have traditionally been subdivided into three general categories: idiopathic, symptomatic, and cryptogenic. The idiopathic focal seizures were those focal seizures in which no underlying cause other than

Epilepsy in Children and Adolescents, First Edition. Edited by James W. Wheless.

a possible hereditary predisposition could be attributed. Symptomatic focal seizures were those seizures occurring as a sequela of a known or suspected disorder of the central nervous system. Finally, cryptogenic focal seizures referred to those seizures caused by an unknown or occult cause. Furthermore, cryptogenic epilepsies were presumed to be symptomatic. Under the proposed classification scheme the idiopathic focal epilepsies are now regarded as genetic. Specifically these epilepsies are known or presumed to have a genetic defect at their root and must be supported by specific evidence [2].

While this is a necessary and laudable endeavor, it is still work in progress. With that in mind we will continue to use the existing nomenclature [4].

For this chapter, idiopathic partial-onset epilepsies are categorized as follows:

- benign infantile seizures;
- benign childhood epilepsy with centrotemporal spikes;
- early-onset benign childhood occipital epilepsy (Panayiotopoulos syndrome);
- late-onset childhood occipital epilepsy (Gastaut type).

16.1 Benign infantile seizures

The ILAE initially recognized two forms of benign infantile seizures: familial and non-familial types [5,6]. In reality, both of these entities refer to an age-related, benign, idiopathic syndrome of infancy. Family history is the only factor differentiating the familial form from the non-familial form. The seizures have a focal onset and the infants develop normally.

Demographics

Seizure onset occurs between 3 and 20 months of life and peaks at around 5–6 months in the sporadic form but starts between 4 and 7 months in the familial form. Also, cases appear equally distributed in the sporadic form whereas females have been identified more frequently in familial cases.

Clinical features

Seizures are focal in onset and more common when the infant is awake. They often occur in clusters (up to several in a row) over 1–3 days and may be quiescent for up to 3 months. Up to one-third of cases will have a single seizure several days prior to the onset of seizure clusters.

The seizures are characterized by:

- poor responsiveness;
- arrest of movement;
- staring;
- head and eye deviation;
- unilateral clonic twitching.

Simple, repetitive motor automatisms are often observed. Motor movements during the seizures may begin on one side and switch to the other. In some cases, hemiconvulsions or generalized convulsions occur.

Table 16.1 Benign infantile seizures.

Type	Onset	Gender distribution	Seizure onset	Genetic etiology	EEG features
Sporadic type	3–20 months	Equal between males and females	Focal	Unknown	Interictal EEG is normal Ictal EEG shows focal spikes and/or fast activity that spreads within the same or to the contralateral hemisphere
Familial type	4–7 months	More prevalent in females	Focal	Linkage to chromosomes 19q12-13.1, 2q24, and 16p12-q12	

Etiology

Genetic studies in the familial form have found a linkage to chromosomes 19q12-13.1, 2q24, and 16p12-q12 [7]. Also described are *benign familial neonatal-infantile seizures*, which occur between 2 days and 7 months of life [6]. This is autosomal dominant, is characterized by non-febrile focal seizures, and tends to resolve within the first year of life. It is caused by a mutation in the sodium channel subunit gene, *SCN2A*.

There is an association between benign infantile seizures and paroxysmal dyskinesia (also referred to as *infantile convulsions and choreoathetosis*) [8]. Familial hemiplegic migraine and benign familial infantile seizures have also been described in a few families, associated with a missense mutation in the *ATP1A2* Na^+/K^+ ATPase pump gene on chromosome 1q23 [9] (see Table 16.1 for a summary of benign infantile seizures).

Diagnostic workup

Physical examination and routine laboratory examinations are normal. The interictal EEG is also normal. An ictal EEG, however, will show focal epileptiform spikes and mixed fast activity, which typically spreads to other brain regions including the contralateral hemisphere and/or whole brain. The seizure onset can be in any location.

Treatment

Benign infantile seizures have a generally good prognosis. Seizures usually resolve within 2 years of onset. Normal development is preserved. Anticonvulsant therapy has been successful with a variety of agents: carbamazepine, valproic acid, and phenobarbital have all been used successfully.

16.2 Benign childhood epilepsy with centrotemporal spikes

Benign childhood epilepsy with centrotemporal spikes (BCECTS) has also been known by a number of other terms, including rolandic epilepsy, benign rolandic epilepsy of childhood, and sylvian seizures. The terms rolandic and sylvian have been used because of the presence of diphasic epileptiform spike discharges seen over the central and temporal head regions on EEG. It should be noted, however, that children with BCECTS do not have temporal lobe symptoms.

Demographics

Seizure onset is typically between ages 1 and 14 years. Seventy-five percent of cases begin between 7 and 10 years of life, with onset typically peaking at 8 or 9 years, and there is a male predominance of 1.5:1. The prevalence is around 15% in children between 1 and 15 years of life with seizures. The incidence is 10–20 per 100 000 children ages 0 to 15 years [3,10].

Clinical features

According to Panayiotopoulos, children with BCECTS experience infrequent focal seizures characterized by unilateral facial sensorimotor symptoms (tingling sensations and/or unilateral facial twitching) in 30% of cases. They experience oropharyngeal manifestations in 53% of cases, speech arrest in 40% of cases, and hypersalivation in 30%.

The unilateral facial sensorimotor symptoms often involve the lower lip or spread to the ipsilateral hand. The motor component comprises sudden onset of clonic contractions lasting a few seconds to 1 minute. Ipsilateral tonic deviation of the mouth and numbness in the corner of the mouth may also be observed. The patient may be drooling excessively and unable to speak.

The oropharyngeal features usually comprise sensorimotor features including tingling or numbness (paresthesias) involving the soft tissues of the oropharynx or tongue. The patients may also produce sounds such as grunting, gasping, or gargling during a seizure. Hypersalivation is characterized by an acute overproduction of saliva and is not simply frothing at the mouth. In some cases the child may be attempting to speak but be unable to produce clear language while simultaneously preserving appropriate receptive language abilities. Other features such as syncope associated with seizure have been described but are relatively rare. Children will recall and describe their seizures in over half the cases.

Approximately 50% of children with BCECTS will experience a secondarily generalized, tonic-clonic convulsion. Seizures associated with BCECTS are usually short and self-limited. They rarely last more than 3 minutes, and many resolve shortly after 1 minute. The majority of seizures occur during non-rapid eye movement (NREM) sleep – often at sleep onset or just prior to awakening.

Status epilepticus is uncommon and when it occurs may present as focal motor or hemiconvulsive status epilepticus. The overall prognosis of BCECTS, as the name suggests, is quite good.

Etiology

BCECTS has a complex genetic basis. There has been evidence of linkage with chromosome 15q14 [11–13]. Autosomal dominant inheritance has been observed in patients with centrotemporal spikes on EEG without the clinical syndrome of BCECTS [4]. Autosomal dominant genetically heterogeneous variants of rolandic epilepsy and speech disorder have occurred in a multigenerational pedigree. Linkage analysis performed on the subjects excluded loci at 11p, 15q, 16p12, and Xq22 for related phenotypes [14]. Centrotemporal spikes on the EEG in rolandic epilepsy have been linked to the elongator protein complex 4 (*ELP4*) gene on chromosome 11p13 [15].

Diagnostic workup

The diagnosis of BCECTS is clinical in nature and reinforced by the EEG. Neuroimaging is not usually required. The interictal EEG demonstrates a normal background with intermittent diphasic centrotemporal spike discharges. These discharges are maximum in the central and temporal regions. They are typically surface negative at the central and temporal electrodes while demonstrating a surface positivity in the ipsilateral frontal electrodes (this is referred to as a tangential or horizontal dipole). Interictal epileptiform activity is much more common in sleep than wakefulness, and may be ipsilateral or bilateral in nature. Generalized epileptiform discharges have been described in BCECTS but are infrequent. These discharges are most common during the peak years of the disorder (most prevalent between 7 and 10 years of life) but may persist into the second decade of life.

Treatment

Many children with BCECTS do not require anticonvulsant therapy because their seizures are either nocturnal and/or infrequent. Diurnal seizures, however, may be particularly stressful for the child and family. In many cases, these seizures may occur at school thereby increasing the likelihood of transfer to the hospital. Moreover, patients experiencing secondarily generalized seizures are good candidates for anticonvulsant therapy. Traditionally, carbamazepine has been the preferred agent. Valproate has also been used. Both of these drugs have been available in many countries for many years, but have also been associated with side effects in a minority of patients including changes in sensorium, weight gain, and hepatic stress. Newer drugs such as oxcarbazepine, lamotrigine, gabapentin, and levetiracetam have also been used to good effect. In some cases the anticonvulsant may actually exacerbate seizures, and each case should be treated individually. Prolonged seizures may be treated with benzodiazepines such as diazepam (which may be administered rectally in gel form at home or by emergency personnel) or intravenous preparations of diazepam or lorazepam in the emergency department.

16.3 Childhood occipital epilepsy (Panayiotopoulos type)

The ILAE has characterized Panayiotopoulos syndrome (PS) as “early-onset benign childhood occipital epilepsy (Panayiotopoulos type)” [2]. It is considered benign; occurring in early to mid-childhood and characterized by focal-onset seizures with a predominance of autonomic symptoms. It has been hypothesized that Panayiotopoulos syndrome represents an early-onset (cf. rolandic epilepsy is a late-onset) phenotype of maturation-related benign childhood seizure syndrome[16]. Autonomic symptoms are a major feature differentiating PS from other childhood focal seizure disorders. Some experts have taken exception to this classification and proposed that Panayiotopoulos syndrome be classified as an autonomic epilepsy [17].

Demographics

Seizure onset ranges from 1 to 14 years of age. Approximately three-quarters of cases begin between 3 and 6 years of age (peaking between ages 4 to 5). Both sexes are equally affected. Prevalence is around 13% of children between the ages of 3 and 6 with one or more non-febrile seizures, and 6% of children in the age group of 1 to 15. In the general population 2–3 of every 1000 children are affected [4,16,17].

Clinical features

Seizures in Panayiotopoulos syndrome are associated with autonomic features, particularly nausea and emesis. Behavioral changes and unilateral eye deviation have also been described. Seizure occurrence is more common in sleep, especially the early part of sleep whether occurring during a daytime nap or at night. If seizures are occurring during wakefulness, consciousness and speech are usually preserved. Nausea and emesis are usually the heralding symptom, and a child will typically complain of feeling sick. Other autonomic symptoms may occur at seizure onset, including: color changes, often pallor but also flushing or cyanosis; pupillary changes especially mydriasis and less often miosis; coughing, cardiorespiratory, and thermoregulatory changes; as well as urinary or even fecal incontinence.

A triad of nausea, retching, and vomiting occurs in up to 74% of seizures. Emesis is usually the first ictal symptom, and hypersalivation has been reported. Headaches and frequently cephalic aura have also been observed. These latter features have contributed to confusion between Panayiotopoulos syndrome and migraine.

Ictal syncope is a described feature of seizures in Panayiotopoulos syndrome. In at least 20% of seizures, the patient becomes unresponsive and flaccid prior to convulsion [4,18]. It is characterized by a transient loss of responsiveness and postural tone. Other behavioral manifestations may also be witnessed including agitation, fitfulness, fearfulness, or even inactivity.

Ten percent of patients will have pure autonomic seizures or pure autonomic status epilepticus. Their seizures comprise autonomic symptoms only. In the remainder of cases, the autonomic features are followed by conventional seizure symptoms. This is characterized by the autonomic symptoms at onset followed by a period of confusion and unresponsiveness. The impairment of consciousness may be mild to moderate. The patient may retain some ability to respond to verbal commands but may not be able to carry on conversation. Unilateral deviation of the eyes is common but does not usually occur at the beginning of the seizure. This may last only a few minutes, or in cases of status epilepticus persist for several hours. Eye deviation may be continuous or intermittent, and in 10–20% of cases occurs without emesis. Seizures without autonomic features are rare and may be seen in individuals who have seizures with autonomic features as well.

Other less common ictal symptoms include speech arrest, hemifacial spasm, visual hallucinations, oropharyngeal movements, unilateral mouth droop, eyelid jerks, myoclonic jerks, nystagmus, and automatisms. Seizures may conclude with hemiconvulsions or with a jacksonian march. In approximately one-fifth of cases there is secondary generalization. Visual symptoms including hallucinations and transient amaurosis have also been described.

Nearly half of seizures last more than 30 minutes and may persist for several hours. This is observed in autonomic status epilepticus. The remainder of seizures usually last from

1 to 30 minutes and usually resolve after several minutes. Despite the duration of seizures, patients usually recover after sleeping. Residual neurological or cognitive difficulties are not typically seen. Hemiconvulsive or convulsive status epilepticus is very rare. Two-thirds of seizures begin in sleep, and sleep appears to be the only precipitating factor.

Etiology

Panayiotopoulos syndrome is believed to be genetic in origin. Often there is no family history of similar seizures though PS, as well as rolandic epilepsy, can be observed in siblings. Febrile seizures have also been reported in patients with Panayiotopoulos syndrome. A *SCN1A* gene mutation has been reported in a few cases and this is speculated to represent cases with a more severe phenotype [7,19] (see Table 16.2 for comparison of early- and late-onset childhood occipital epilepsy).

Diagnostic workup

Similar to patients with other benign idiopathic partial epilepsy since childhood, patients with Panayiotopoulos syndrome have normal neurological examinations. Likewise, MRI scans are usually normal though other causes of autonomic symptoms related to structural brain lesions may be required [16]. The diagnosis of Panayiotopoulos syndrome is established by history and clinical presentation. EEG, however, is the most helpful diagnostic procedure. In 10% of cases, the initial EEG may be normal [4,16]. In approximately 90% of cases, the EEG will demonstrate multifocal, high-amplitude, sharp- and slow-wave complexes. Spikes may also be present and shift between brain regions or hemispheres. Occipital spikes are frequent and may appear intermittently and independently within the

Table 16.2 Childhood occipital epilepsy.

Type	Onset	Gender distribution	Seizure onset/ features	Genetic etiology	Interictal EEG
Early-onset (Panayiotopoulos type)	1–14 years	Equal between males and females	Focal onset; autonomic symptoms, especially nausea and vomiting are common; unilateral eye deviation	*SCN1A* gene mutation reported in a few cases	Multifocal, high-amplitude, sharp- and slow-wave complexes. Occipital spikes are frequent and may appear intermittently and independently within the same or contralateral hemispheres
Late-onset (Gastaut type)	3–15 years	Equal between males and females	Focal onset; simple visual hallucinations/ transient blindness; head and eye deviation	Believed to be genetic but chromosome/ gene linkage to be determined	*Fixation-off sensitivity*: occipital sharp waves/spikes when not visually fixated on an object

same or contralateral hemispheres. Spike discharges, however, may not be observed in up to one-third of cases. Spikes are usually surface negative (i.e., upward deflections on EEG) but may be surface positive (i.e., downward deflections on EEG) in a minority of cases. Brief generalized spikes in slow-wave complexes have also been observed on occasion but are usually associated with focal discharges as well. Sleep should be acquired during the EEG since interictal epileptiform activity is more prevalent in sleep [4,17,20]. The remainder of the EEG is typically normal though occasional slowing can be observed shortly after a seizure.

Ictal EEG frequently consists of rhythmic, unilateral, slow activity often with admixed low-amplitude spike discharges. These discharges are often occipital in onset but can be seen in other regions as well.

Treatment

Half of the patients with Panayiotopoulos syndrome will have five or fewer seizures. Approximately 25% will have six or more seizures, and in some cases frequent seizures have been noted. Seizures typically remit within one to 2 years of onset of Panayiotopoulos syndrome. Moreover autonomic status epilepticus does not cause residual neurological disabilities. In rare cases Panayiotopoulos syndrome may evolve into absence, atonic, or electrographic status epilepticus in sleep (ESES). Up to one-fifth of children with Panayiotopoulos syndrome go on to develop rolandic or occipital seizures. These also typically resolve by age 16 years. The overall risk of epilepsy in adulthood is no higher than in the general population [4,16]. Most patients will not require anticonvulsant therapy. Guidelines used in the management of febrile seizures provide a framework for treatment of Panayiotopoulos syndrome as well. Education about Panayiotopoulos syndrome remains the mainstay of treatment. Autonomic status epilepticus should be thoroughly evaluated to rule out other causes. Benzodiazepines (rectal or intravenous) have been successfully used to terminate non-convulsive status epilepticus. Caution is advised in aggressive therapy since cardiopulmonary arrest is a risk. In cases with frequent seizures, anticonvulsant therapy may be required. Many investigators have recommended carbamazepine though newer drugs with focal-onset seizure coverage have been used.

16.4 Late-onset childhood occipital epilepsy (Gastaut type)

The ILAE reclassified this disorder as "late onset childhood occipital epilepsy (Gastaut type)" replacing the previous name "childhood epilepsy with occipital paroxysms" [2]. Several other terms have been used over the years, including Gastaut type of childhood occipital epilepsy, late onset child occipital epilepsy (Gastaut type), and childhood epilepsy with occipital paroxysms [4].

Demographics

This disorder is rare, with a prevalence of 0.3% of children presenting with new-onset non-febrile seizures, and 2–7% of those with benign focal childhood seizures [21]. It presents between 3 and 15 years of life (with a mean of 8 years), affects both sexes equally, and comprises 2–7% of benign childhood focal seizures [22].

Clinical findings

Seizures are occipital in nature and evidenced by simple visual hallucinations, transient blindness, or both. They are usually diurnal and may be frequent. Additionally, they tend to be short and last only a few seconds. They may be longer, however, rarely lasting longer than 3 minutes. Nocturnal seizures may also occur and tend to be longer in duration.

Simple (elementary) visual hallucinations are the hallmark of seizures and often the only clinical feature. They usually comprise simple circular patterns of multiple colors. They tend to occur in a peripheral visual field but may migrate to the contralateral field while simultaneously becoming larger. Other occipital symptoms have also been reported and include a sensory illusion of ocular movement, ocular pain, tonic deviation of the eyes, eyelids flutter, or repetitive eyelid closure.

Eye deviation is frequently associated with ipsilateral head deviation and is the most frequently observed non-visual seizure symptom. It typically occurs after the initiation of visual hallucinations. It may be mild but often progresses to a hemiconvulsion or generalized tonic on a convulsion. In 10% of patients a forced eyelid closure and/or eyelid blinking are observed simultaneously when consciousness is impaired. This usually portends a secondary generalized tonic on a convulsion.

Ictal blindness may appear from the beginning of a seizure after other clinical phenomena and last for up to several minutes. Complex visual hallucinations are rare. Ictal headaches or orbital pain may also occur, and if present precede visual symptoms. Consciousness is not usually impaired during the visual symptoms but may become altered or lost during the course of the seizure. This usually occurs before eye deviation.

Etiology

Late-onset idiopathic childhood occipital epilepsy (Gastaut type) is believed to be genetically determined but rare. Between 21% and 37% of patients have a family history of epilepsy, and 9–16% have a family history of migraine. A proposal linking idiopathic childhood occipital epilepsy of Gastaut, rolandic epilepsy, and Panayiotopoulos syndrome into a phenotypic spectrum has been proposed [4,21,22].

Diagnostic workup

All diagnostic studies with the exception of EEG should be normal. MRI scan of the brain should also be performed, however, to rule out the incidence of asymptomatic focal occipital epilepsy with similar electroclinical features.

The interictal EEG may show occipital paroxysms. This is demonstrated by a phenomenon known as fixation-off sensitivity. These patients demonstrate occipital sharp waves or spikes when they are no longer visually fixated on an object. This occurs whether the eyes are open or closed. Otherwise, focal occipital spikes may be seen and are more prevalent in sleep. The remainder of the EEG tends to be normal. It should be noted that occipital spikes are not considered exclusive to this syndrome and may be seen in a variety of conditions including symptomatic focal epilepsies and children with congenital or early-onset visual impairment.

Ictal EEG demonstrates fast rhythmic activity with occipital spike or sharp-wave discharges. These discharges tend to be lower in amplitude than the interictal activities. Simple visual hallucinations have been attributed to fast spike activity while complex visual hallucinations have been correlated with slower discharges. The ictal EEG recorded during transient blindness is noted for a pseudo-periodic slow-wave and spike discharges. These have a different morphology than typically seen ictal visual hallucinations. Postictal slowing is not typically observed.

Treatment

Anticonvulsant therapy is usually required for treatment of idiopathic childhood occipital epilepsy of Gastaut due to the frequency of seizures. As with the other idiopathic focal childhood epilepsies, carbamazepine and valproic acid have been used to good effect. Medication may be weaned at least 2 years after last reported seizure. It should be restarted if visual symptoms recur even in the absence of convulsive activity.

The prognosis of idiopathic childhood occipital epilepsy of Gastaut is uncertain though remission has been reported in 50–60% of children within 2–4 years of onset of seizures. Carbamazepine has been shown to be effective in more than 90% of patients. Up to 50% of patients treated with anticonvulsants continue to have visual seizures and infrequent secondary generalized tonic convulsions. Similar to Panayiotopoulos syndrome, atypical progression to electrographic status epilepticus in sleep (ESES) has been observed. Moreover, children may rarely exhibit absence seizures.

References

[1] Berg AT, Berkovic SF, Brodie MJ, *et al.* Revised terminology and concepts for organization of seizures and epilepsies: report of the ILAE Commission on Classification and Terminology, 2005–2009. *Epilepsia* 2010;**51**:676–685.

[2] Engel J. A proposed diagnostic scheme for people with epileptic seizures and with epilepsy: report of the ILAE Task Force on Classification and Terminology. *Epilepsia* 2001;**42**:796–803.

[3] Berg, AT, Scheffer IE. New concepts in classification of the epilepsies: entering the 21st century. *Epilepsia* 2011;**52**:1058–1062.

[4] Panayiotopoulos CP. *A Clinical Guide to Epileptic Syndromes and Their Treatment*. London: Springer-Verlag, 2010.

[5] Specchio N, Vigevano F. The spectrum of benign infantile seizures. *Epilepsy Res* 2006; **70**(Suppl. 1):S156–167.

[6] Vigevano F. Benign familial infantile seizures. *Brain Dev* 2005;**27**:172–177.

[7] Grosso S, Orrico A, Galli L, *et al.* SCN1A mutation associated with atypical Panayiotopoulos syndrome. *Neurology* 2007;**69**:609–611.

[8] Espeche A, Cersosimo R, Caraballo RH. Benign infantile seizures and paroxysmal dyskinesia: a well-defined familial syndrome. *Seizure* 2011;**20**:686–691.

[9] Vanmolkot KR, Kors EE, Hottenga JJ, *et al.* Novel mutations in the Na^+, K^+-ATPase pump gene ATP1A2 associated with familial hemiplegic migraine and benign familial infantile convulsions. *Ann Neurol* 2003;**54**:360–366.

[10] Bouma PA, Bovenkerk AC, Westendrorp RG, Brouwer OF. The course of benign partial epilepsy of childhood with centrotemporal spikes: a meta-analysis. *Neurology* 1997;**48**:430–437.

[11] Neubauer BA, Fielder B, Himmelein B, *et al.* Centrotemporal spikes in families with rolandic epilepsy: linkage to chromosome 15q14. *Neurology* 1998;**51**:1608–1612.

[12] Ottman R. Progress in the genetics of the partial epilepsies. *Epilepsia* 2001;**42**(Suppl. 5):24–30.

[13] Helbig I, Mefford HS, Sharp, AJ, *et al.* 15q13.3 microdeletions increase risk of idiopathic generalized epilepsy. *Nat Genet* 2009;**41**:160–162.

[14] Kugler SL, Bali B, Lieberman P, *et al.* An autosomal dominant genetically heterogeneous variant of rolandic epilepsy and speech disorder. *Epilepsia* 2008;**49**:1086–1090.

[15] Strug LJ, Clarke T, Chiang T, *et al.* Centrotemporal sharp wave EEG trait in rolandic epilepsy maps to Elongator Protein Complex 4 (ELP4). *Eur J Hum Genet* 2009;**17**:1171–1181.

[16] Covanis A. Panayiotopoulos syndrome: a benign childhood autonomic epilepsy frequently imitating encephalitis, syncope, migraine, sleep disorder, or gastroenteritis. *Pediatrics* 2006;**118**: e1237–1243.

[17] Ferrie C, Caraballo R, Covanis A, *et al.* Panayiotopoulos syndrome: a consensus view. *Dev Med Child Neurol* 2006;**48**:236–240.

[18] Panayiotopoulos CP. Autonomic seizures and autonomic status epilepticus peculiar to childhood: diagnosis and management. *Epilepsy Behav* 2004;**5**:286–295.

[19] Livingston JH, Cross JH, Mclellan A, *et al.* A novel inherited mutation in the voltage sensor region of SCN1A is associated with Panayiotopoulos syndrome in siblings and generalized epilepsy with febrile seizures plus. *J Child Neurol* 2009;**24**:503–508.

[20] Michael M, Tsatsou K, Ferrie CD. Panayiotopoulos syndrome: an important childhood autonomic epilepsy to be differentiated from occipital epilepsy and acute non-epileptic disorders. *Brain Dev* 2010;**32**:4–9.

[21] Caraballo R, Koutroumanidis M, Panayiotopoulos CP, Fejerman N. Idiopathic childhood occipital epilepsy of Gastaut: a review and differentiation from migraine and other epilepsies. *J Child Neurol* 2009;**24**:1536–1542.

[22] Panayiotopoulos CP, Michael M, Sanders S, *et al.* Benign childhood focal epilepsies: assessment of established and newly recognized syndromes. *Brain* 2008;**131**:2264–2286.

17 Cryptogenic and symptomatic partial epilepsies

Stephen Fulton

Department of Neurology and Pediatrics, University of Tennessee Health Science Center; LeBonheur Comprehensive Epilepsy Program, Le Bonheur Children's Hospital, Memphis, TN, USA

The International Classification of Epilepsies and Epilepsy Syndromes divides epilepsy, first, on the basis of whether the seizures are partial (localization-related epilepsies) or generalized; and, second, by etiology (idiopathic, symptomatic, or cryptogenic). (The idiopathic partial seizures are discussed in Chapter 16). Symptomatic epilepsies comprise syndromes based on anatomical localization and are considered to be the consequence of a known or suspected disorder of the central nervous system. Cryptogenic epilepsies are presumed to be symptomatic, but the etiology is not clear.

17.1 Etiology

By definition, partial seizures imply the presence of a focal abnormality in one cerebral hemisphere. A definite etiological factor can often be identified by magnetic resonance imaging (MRI). These factors include birth asphyxia, intrauterine infections, congenital brain structural abnormalities, head trauma, meningitis, viral encephalitis, parasitic infections, neoplasms, arteriovenous malformations, stroke, and neurocutaneous diseases (e.g., tuberous sclerosis complex, hypomelanosis of Ito, neurofibromatosis).

Epilepsy in Children and Adolescents, First Edition. Edited by James W. Wheless.

17.2 Seizure phenomena

The symptomatology of partial seizures depends greatly on the location of the seizure focus within the cerebral cortex. Although a given symptom may occur with seizures arising from different locations, the combined information from seizure symptomatology and electroencephalogram (EEG) findings enables one to determine the location of the seizure focus.

Classifying seizures on the basis of the anatomical lobe of the brain implicated as the seizure focus is challenging at times. Seizures can begin in a clinically silent region of one lobe with rapid spread to another lobe, with the first clinical symptoms occurring after this spread has occurred. Additionally, functional circuits can include more than one lobe, so seizures arising from different lobes can have similar semiologies.

Most surgical series and population studies find that temporal lobe epilepsies are the most common, followed by frontal lobe epilepsies. Occipital epilepsies are less common, with parietal lobe epilepsies being the least common. In this chapter, I discuss the cryptogenic/symptomatic localization-related epilepsies according to the region of the brain implicated in a seizure.

17.3 Temporal lobe epilepsy

Temporal lobe epilepsy, which is practically a field of study unto itself, was originally described by John Hughlings-Jackson in 1876 [1]. He described the clinical histories of several patients 12 years later and added observations of other cases of this "Reminiscence" state that we now refer to more commonly as *déjà vu*, or the feeling that one has already experienced one's current situation [2]. Hughlings-Jackson includes other sensations in his description, including symptoms of altered smell and taste, strange epigastric sensations, automatisms, chewing and lip-smacking, along with varying degrees of alteration of consciousness [2]. He also finally had clinicopathological correlation for what he termed the "discharging lesion" of his dreamy state to the medial temporal area, for what he designated the "Uncinate Group of Fits" [1]. When reviewing his findings with our current experience, this concise summary of mesial temporal lobe epilepsy is apparent.

When electroencephalography (EEG) came into use in the twentieth century, temporal lobe epilepsy was further characterized, and the neuropathological abnormalities seen in mesial temporal sclerosis in patients with mesial temporal lobe epilepsy followed. Later, in the early 1940s, temporal sharp waves localized to the hippocampus were linked with psychomotor seizures [3]. With surgical advances came more definitive association of mesial temporal sclerosis with mesial temporal lobe epilepsy. It was clear with pathological study of specimens from surgical resection that not only was mesial temporal sclerosis a common occurrence, but its presence in these specimens portended a good outcome for these patients [3].

Mesial temporal lobe epilepsy with mesial temporal sclerosis has been further defined with time. The features of mesial temporal sclerosis – prolonged febrile seizures often in the first year life, partial-onset seizures without fever occurring later in adolescence or young adult years, and inadequate response of these patients to various antiepileptic medications – have become well recognized.

Febrile seizures have an incidence in the general population that varies from 3% to 5%, though retrospective correlations of patients with partial-onset seizures with mesial temporal sclerosis found an incidence in that population up to 40–50%. Typically febrile seizures in this population were more prolonged and recurred more frequently in these patients. With the discovery of a positive family history of mesial temporal sclerosis in many patients, a postulate of genetic susceptibility is reasonable. It is also not entirely clear whether febrile seizures lead to mesial temporal sclerosis and later intractable seizures, or whether those febrile seizures simply signify an underlying increased tendency toward epileptic seizures. Familial mesial temporal sclerosis has also been described [4].

The typical onset of these partial-onset seizures without fever is often delayed until adolescence. These cases are often initially responsive to therapy, but later become refractory to therapy with multiple agents. They are often characterized by brief auras (<60 seconds) of fear or a "rising sensation" in the epigastrium, and more occasionally associated with *déjà vu*. Autonomic symptoms of sweating, tachycardia, and pallor are often seen, and oral-buccal-lingual automatisms occur frequently. Localizing signs are often seen during the ictal period, such as passive head turning that is ipsilateral to the side of onset, and dystonic posturing of the upper extremity, which is contralateral to the side of onset, as opposed to more active automatisms in the upper extremity, which are often ipsilateral.

During these events, some activities that the patient was attempting prior to the onset of the seizure can be continued throughout the ictal period and persist into the postictal state. One example would be a patient who continues to dress (if they had started prior to the onset of the event) despite having had a seizure.

When pathological specimens from patients with mesial temporal sclerosis were analyzed histologically, neuronal loss and gliosis were seen throughout the mesial temporal region. The hippocampal CA1, subiculum, and CA4 areas appeared more susceptible, while CA2 and the dentate gyrus were often incompletely spared from the pathological abnormalities [3].

Temporal epileptiform discharges are the most common interictal EEG abnormality seen in adults with partial epilepsy. The amplitude is typically seen maximally over the anterior regions of the temporal lobe, and is much more commonly seen in sleep as opposed to awake recordings [5–7]. The scalp EEG during a temporal lobe seizure usually has diffuse onset over the entire lobe. The activity is often lateralized paroxysmal higher-amplitude rhythmic discharges, which may evolve into more diffuse rhythmic slowing seen more over the side of seizure onset. Postictal recordings often demonstrate focal temporal or diffuse slow waves. Frequently, there is increased interictal temporal lobe epileptiform activity visualized after cessation of the seizure [2].

The localization value of scalp EEG in partial seizures with origin in the temporal lobe is not absolute, with reports varying widely from 40% to 90% [8,9]. Sphenoidal electrodes can record from the mediobasal limbic region to assist in presurgical localization [8], though they are often not well tolerated, and their sensitivity and specificity are no greater than inferior lateral temporal scalp electrodes [10].

In the subset of patients with anterior temporal lobe epilepsy, however, ictal EEG can show temporal, diffuse hemispheric, or even generalized epileptiform activity [11,12].

ILAE classification

In 1981, the International League Against Epilepsy (ILAE) classified partial-onset seizures into three distinct groups: simple partial, complex partial, and partial-onset with secondary generalized tonic-clonic seizures [13]. Temporal lobe epilepsies can occur with characteristics of any of the above groups.

Later, in 1989, the ILAE was more specific in its classification of temporal lobe epilepsy [14]. They further subdivided temporal lobe epilepsy into medial and lateral syndromes with different electroencephalographic onset in the limbic (medial) and neocortical (lateral) areas. These were separated by their initial structures involved on intracranial EEG recordings, as well as their clinical semiology. There have subsequently been several studies that tried to define the electroclinical syndromes of medial and lateral temporal lobe epilepsy [15].

Medial and lateral temporal lobe epilepsy

When looking at ictal scalp recordings, an early, prominent, lateralized anterior temporal rhythmic discharge greater than 5 Hz was very predictive of medial temporal lobe epilepsy, while the same temporal rhythmic discharge, if less than 5 Hz, was more commonly seen with onset over the lateral temporal lobe. If lateralized theta-frequency rhythmic patterns were seen later in the course of a seizure, the onset was more likely to be in the neocortex [15].

Wieser looked at clinical semiologies of events using stereotactic intracranial EEG, comparing the clinical episode with neuroanatomical patterns of progression [16]. He organized his findings into five typical subsets:

1. The "temporobasal limbic" pattern, with hippocampal and often amygdala involvement. These episodes had alteration of consciousness, nausea, "cephalic" aura, pallor, flushing, "warm" sensation, fear/sadness, and one-sided motor manifestations.
2. "Temporopolar" pattern with the cortex in the medial and lateral temporal pole involved. These episodes often had increasing alterations of consciousness, abnormal respiration/heart rate, staring, orobuccolingual automatisms (OBLs), and psychic phenomena.
3. Posterior neocortical localization. These episodes often had aphasia, staring or expression change, vestibular hallucinations, visual illusion/hallucination, and gestural automatisms of the upper limb.
4. Opercular type (likely involving the insula). These episodes often had auditory hallucinations, nausea and cephalic aura, aphasia, and "intact-warning" changes in consciousness.
5. Frontobasal-cingulate type. These episodes had gesticulatory complex automatisms, severe confusion and abrupt loss of consciousness, staring or changes in facial expression, and bilateral automatisms usually in the lower limbs (walking) and trunk (up and down).

When looking at the anatomical connections between the limbic portion and the neocortex of the temporal lobe, there are three distinct subtypes of temporal lobe seizures that were characterized by stereotactic electrodes as having distinct progression patterns depending on the site of onset.

- The medial subtype is the most frequently encountered and usually has onset with an epigastric sensation, fear, "dream state," or a warm ascending sensation. Typically, medial-onset seizures have a longer duration, usually intact sensorium in the initial period, and delayed oral-buccal-lingual or upper limb automatisms. This type of temporal lobe seizure is often seen at a younger age and these children have often had a history of febrile seizures earlier in life. The ictal discharge is seen only in the medial structures with no neocortical involvement.

- The lateral subtype often has an initial auditory hallucination or sensory manifestation, along with early "loss of contact." It usually has a short duration relative to the medial type, often secondarily generalizes, and is typically seen in older children. These lateral-onset seizures will not infrequently have a neocortical lesion as compared to the other subtypes. The ictal discharge is seen over the lateral temporal neocortex.
- The medial-lateral subtype is often initially similar to the medial subtype, with a longer duration and similar onset phenomena, with the exception of early loss of contact and oral-buccal-lingual automatisms that occur earlier in the course of the seizure. The ictal discharge is seen over limbic and neocortical areas simultaneously.

Familial syndromes

There are several types of temporal lobe epilepsy with familial patterns. Based on seizure characteristics, genetic linkage, and MRI findings, one can arrange them into familial mesial temporal lobe epilepsy (with a benign familial mesial temporal lobe epilepsy subtype) and familial lateral temporal lobe epilepsy.

Benign familial mesial temporal lobe epilepsy usually presents with a mild clinical history, without any history of febrile seizures, no MRI evidence of mesial temporal sclerosis, and onset delayed until the second to fourth decades. This subgroup seems to have a significantly higher percentage of people with *déjà vu* and *jamais vu* than the other groups.

Familial mesial temporal lobe epilepsy with mesial temporal sclerosis has typical mesial characteristics for their events with a rising epigastric sensation and psychic phenomena. Complex partial events are common, with oral-buccal-lingual automatisms, and significant postictal confusion. Some individuals go on to have secondarily generalized tonic-clonic seizures, usually early in the course. This group usually has onset of seizures before age 30, with a mean age of 10 years. Obvious mesial temporal sclerosis is seen in both asymptomatic and symptomatic family members, which gives evidence to the fact that abnormalities in the hippocampus itself do not guarantee epilepsy. The seizures in these patients can be refractory in almost one-third of patients. Despite the fact that there are unaffected family members with mesial temporal sclerosis, there are many with refractory seizures who have surgical resection and become seizure free. Therefore, while the mesial temporal sclerosis appears similar in both affected and unaffected individuals, there is another unknown factor that predisposes some to epilepsy, while allowing others to simply have structural changes in that region.

Familial lateral temporal lobe epilepsy is a benign syndrome that is dominated by auditory auras. It usually has onset between 10 and 20 years of age. The auras usually manifest as sound distortion, buzzing, motor or electronic equipment noise, or even distinct words. Other symptoms can include psychic auras, cephalic sensation, and motor and sensory phenomena, but these pale in comparison to the frequency of the auditory aura. Occasional aphasia and visual changes can occur during the ictal period. MRI imaging has no signs of any mesial abnormalities, but in almost one-half of individuals there is an abnormality seen in the lateral portion of the temporal lobe. Strangely, the left temporal lobes of affected individuals are often disproportionately larger compared with unaffected individuals. Moreover, sometimes there is an "encephalocele-like" protrusion laterally, whose significance is unknown. The EEG is usually normal, but occasionally epileptiform discharges are seen in the posterior portion of the temporal lobe. Gene mutations in *LGI1* have been found in 50% of these families, though their significance is also uncertain.

Pathophysiology

Temporal lobe epilepsy has both local and distant effects on brain function through neuronal networks and interconnected areas of the brain.

In patients with longstanding temporal lobe epilepsy, interictal changes are seen in various areas on MRI, positron emission tomography (PET), single photon emission computed tomography (SPECT), and functional MRI (fMRI), which support the involvement of these neuronal networks. Intracranial EEG has shown regional involvement electrographically in structures around the temporal lobe [16]. These are likely secondary to propagation of seizures through these neuronal networks. Intracranial EEG does have a significant limitation in being isolated to certain locations, leaving other parts of the brain unmonitored. With recent progress in functional imaging, we are able to look more at global brain changes during ictal activity. Ictal SPECT has contributed significantly with evidence of broad areas of both inhibition and activation during partial seizures, specifically temporal lobe seizures. The corpus striatum, insula, and anterior and medial temporal lobe have all shown activation during temporal lobe seizures on ictal SPECT. Distant inhibition is also rather important in the understanding of temporal lobe seizures. Association cortex is inhibited bilaterally in temporal lobe seizures after initial spread to midline subcortical areas.

Clinical semiology is also being illuminated more by ictal SPECT. For example, ictal dystonia, which localizes to the contralateral hemisphere, shows hyperperfusion in the contralateral basal ganglia [17].

A small number of patients have preserved responsiveness during temporal lobe seizures, and have the ability to respond to simple questions during their events, and these individuals have right temporal lobe onset. When looking at SPECT studies in patients with seizures that seem clinically similar, those with left temporal lobe epilepsy have a 60-fold increased probability of having hyperperfusion in the brainstem tegmentum relative to those with right temporal lobe seizures [17]. This area is significant in regulation of consciousness and awareness and may help explain why these patients have less derangement in their ability to respond.

The electrographic involvement of nearby structures outside the temporal lobe during temporal lobe seizures can add insight to the various symptoms, both positive and negative, that are visible during these events. Both network inhibition and activation play a role in many semiological changes. Depth electrodes have shown conclusive involvement of the insula in many patients with temporal lobe epilepsy, and this involvement clearly plays a role in the ictal semiology of temporal lobe epilepsy.

Neuroimaging classifications

MRI has proven invaluable in temporal lobe epilepsy diagnosis and classification. In patients with a clinical history of seizures suspicious for temporal lobe onset, a measurable difference in the left and right hippocampal volumes can be predictive of favorable surgical outcomes [3]. Patients with temporal lobe epilepsy who do not have an obvious lesion on MRI and who are medically refractory have evidence of hippocampal volume loss two-thirds of the time. This leaves one-third of patients with medically refractory temporal lobe epilepsy with normal MRI evaluations.

Positron emission tomography scanning with fluorodeoxyglucose (FDG-PET) has been found to be the most sensitive functional interictal imaging technique for the purposes of identifying a focal functional deficit associated with mesial temporal sclerosis. FDG-PET can show abnormalities in non-lesional temporal lobe epilepsy patients. Typically, the affected temporal lobe has significant hypometabolism on imaging, and this often includes other ipsilateral structures such as the basal ganglia and thalamus. Some patients will also have hypometabolism seen in adjacent frontal and parietal neocortex. The metabolic abnormalities themselves still do not have a known cause. This hypometabolism is a phenomenon seen more commonly in patients with intractable temporal lobe epilepsy than in well-controlled patients with epilepsy. Another striking feature is that the hypometabolism has been partially reversible after successful surgical intervention. And postoperative seizure control is significantly better in those patients who had a comparatively more significant level of hypometabolism in the surgically resected area, regardless of pathology.

In the study of patients with temporal lobe epilepsy who have pathological findings on PET imaging, obvious differences have been seen in those with and without MRI evidence of mesial temporal sclerosis. Typically, those without mesial temporal sclerosis on MRI who are also without any hippocampal asymmetry often have lateralized, widespread temporal hypometabolism on FDG-PET. These patients represent their own subset of epilepsy patients with PET-positive, MRI-negative temporal lobe epilepsy. These patients, compared to typical mesial temporal sclerosis patients, have less frequent histories of febrile seizures, less chance of having histopathological mesial temporal sclerosis, and slower ictal EEG onset rhythm patterns, but have comparable postsurgical outcomes, even with hippocampal-sparing procedures. In the groups of patients with and without loss of hippocampal volume on neuroimaging by MRI, the histopathological abnormalities of these groups were quite different. When looking at patients with negative MRIs with temporal lobe epilepsy, they should no longer be considered "camouflaged" mesial temporal sclerosis patients or ones with bilateral sclerosis. Those with PET-positive lesions with negative MRIs should be considered as a separate category with a surgically amenable syndrome.

Continuing in the neuroimaging distinguishable patients, ictal SPECT has clearly separable patterns in different subsets of temporal lobe epilepsy patients [18]. Patients with ictal foci in their mesial temporal lobes often show ipsilateral hyperperfusion in both the mesial and lateral temporal regions. However, those with ictal foci in the lateral temporal region have hyperperfusion in bilateral temporal lobes.

In patients with unrevealing pathology of their temporal lobe specimens who had successful surgical treatment of their epilepsy, ictal SPECT typically shows hyperperfusion, seen mostly in the anteromesial temporal region. In an attempt to explain this phenomenon, the neuroanatomy must be considered. The structures in the mesial temporal lobe have projections to most of the ipsilateral temporal neocortex, especially in the pole and superior temporal gyrus, which fits with the mesial hyperperfusion described above. The amygdala, on the other hand, has anterior commissural projections from the contralateral temporal neocortex, but not the contralateral amygdala. The bilateral temporal lobe hyperperfusion seen in lateral temporal lobe seizures is supported when considering these anatomicAL connections.

Epilepsy surgery in temporal lobe epilepsy

In the initial randomized trial of surgery for temporal lobe epilepsy, surgery was found to be superior to medical therapy in several areas in patients with poorly controlled temporal lobe epilepsy: control of the seizures themselves, quality of life, rates of employment, and rates of school attendance. At 1-year follow-up, 58% of the surgical group were no longer having seizures with impairment of consciousness as compared to 8% of the medically treated group [19].

Typically, epilepsy surgery is deemed a reasonable option when seizures are not controlled with the correct antiepileptic medications , and when they interfere with quality of life. Usually affected individuals with mesial temporal sclerosis do not have more than two seizures per week, but the seizures themselves, both in character and in daily timing, are not often predictable. Surgical management of focal epilepsies is based on the idea that resection of the region of the brain that is generating the patient's seizures will cause cessation of seizures.

17.4 Extratemporal epilepsy

Frontal lobe epilepsy

Seizures that arise from the frontal lobe are more commonly brief, frequent, nocturnal, and usually have a very brief postictal state, or none at all (Table 17.1). They are characterized by a sudden onset of excessive motor activity. Typically, the ictal EEG does not show any seizure activity as abundant muscle and movement artifacts cloud the recording, as well as the fact that much of the frontal lobe cortex is not easily accessible to scalp recording [20].

The ILAE subdivides frontal lobe epilepsy into seven different anatomical regions. These can go on to involve other regions or secondarily generalize [21]. Given the odd character and sudden onset, frontal lobe seizures are often mistaken for non-epileptic events.

Table 17.1 Differentiating features of frontal versus temporal lobe complex partial seizures.

	Frontal	Temporal
Duration	Brief, <30 seconds	60–90 seconds
Time of day	Sleep > wake	Wake > sleep
Clusters	Common	Uncommon
Automatisms	Proximal and coarse; bicycling movements, pelvic thrusting	Distal and discrete; oroalimentary, manual, gestural, mimetic, ictal speech, ictal vomiting, perseverative
Aura	General body sensation, cephalic aura	Epigastric, psychic
Motor posturing	Bilateral, asymmetric tonic	Contralateral dystonic posturing, often with automastisms on the opposite side
Vocalizations	Prominent	Less common
Partial loss of consciousness	Noted early in the seizure	Noted later in the seizure
Version	Ipsilateral head deviation followed by contralateral version before secondary generalization	Contralateral version precedes generalization

Supplementary sensorimotor area seizures

Seizures that originate in the supplementary sensorimotor area are usually nocturnal and occur in clusters. Typically seizures are consistent within the individual, but vary across different patients. As stated before, they typically have an abrupt onset and termination, and typically occur as multiple brief events, usually less than 30 seconds in duration. Seizures arising in the supplementary sensorimotor area usually have an aura with somatosensory symptoms or a "difficult to describe" sensation. They often begin with bizarre movements and posturing that are usually asymmetric and bilateral, though unilateral movements can be seen on occasion.

There are events with prominent motor activity but without posturing, called "hyperkinetic" or "hypermotor" seizures, which arise from the supplementary sensorimotor area and in other areas in the frontal lobes. In these events, vocalizations and/or speech arrest are frequently seen. Importantly, seizures in this area can have *preserved* consciousness even with bilateral motor involvement. This is yet another reason why these can be mistaken for non-epileptic events. As stated earlier, postictal states are not often seen.

A characteristic, but infrequently seen feature of supplementary sensorimotor seizures, is the "fencer" posture: the contralateral arm is elevated, externally rotated, and flexed at the elbow; the ipsilateral arm is extended at the elbow; the head turns toward the contralateral arm.

With the scalp EEG not having a clear change with onset, along with the odd physical movements of this seizure type, these seizures are frequently misdiagnosed as non-epileptic events. One way to increase the usefulness of the scalp EEG is to review the event in the transverse montage, as abnormalities are more frequently seen from the supplementary sensorimotor area in this arrangement.

Dorsolateral frontal lobe epilepsy

Head/eye version, aphasia, speech arrest, tonic or clonic movements contralateral to the seizure focus, and automatisms often characterize seizures with onset in the dorsolateral frontal lobe. These are not uncommonly preceded by an aura of fear, epigastric sensation, cephalic sensation, or visual change. These patients often have preserved consciousness during the event. As compared to more medial onset seizures, these *do not* have bilateral posturing or somatosensory auras associated.

Opercular area epilepsy

Seizures with onset from the opercular area are fairly rare. Of those reported, chewing, swallowing, speech arrest, salivation, laryngeal symptoms, and autonomic changes are typical symptoms. Clonic activity is common and often involves the face or limbs, and can be bilateral or contralateral. Cases of ipsilateral clonic facial movements have also been reported. Epigastric and gustatory sensations as well as fear can be seen. Typically, consciousness is preserved past at least the onset of clonic activity. If the onset was in the opercular area of the dominant hemisphere, postictal language deficits are seen.

Cingulate gyrus epilepsy

Seizures arising in the cingulate gyrus often have features similar to those with onset in the mesial temporal lobe, secondary to the connections of the cingulate gyrus and the temporal lobe. Changes in affect, including aggressive behavior, profound fear, and screaming, are seen. Autonomic disturbances including pallor, sweating, tachypnea, and tachycardia are also not infrequently seen. Patients can exhibit facial and hand automatic behaviors, and loss of awareness, and clonic movements of both the face and limbs can be present. "Absence-like" seizures with staring, head nodding, and unresponsiveness have been reported.

Anterior frontopolar epilepsy

Seizures arising from the anterior frontopolar region often are characterized by associated loss of contact with the environment, focal clonic movements, falls, head and eye version, autonomic signs, and forced thinking. Seizures from this area can often be misinterpreted as absence seizures from their clinical description with staring and unresponsiveness, and they can even have 3 Hz generalized spike-wave apparent EEG tracings.

Orbitofrontal epilepsy

Seizures that arise from the orbitofrontal area can show semiology that resembles mesial temporal lobes seizures, secondary to the significant number of connections with the limbic system. These events consist of face and hand automatisms, staring, head and eye version, and loss of awareness. They not infrequently have autonomic symptoms such as sweating, sensations of hunger and thirst, piloerection, fear, and epigastric sensations. Less commonly, olfactory hallucinations, screaming, laughing, pelvic thrusting, sexual automatisms, and urinary incontinence occur.

Motor area epilepsy

Motor area seizures typically have tonic or clonic motor activity depending on the portion of the motor strip that is affected. These often start as simple partial seizures and spread to adjacent areas along the motor cortex prior to secondarily generalizing. Statistically speaking, the spread of the seizure most commonly occurs from distal to proximal. They can affect different regions of the homunculus sequentially; for example, going from the face to the ipsilateral hand. The term "jacksonian march" was coined in honor of the British neurologist John Hughlings Jackson, as he first reported this phenomenon in 1868 [22]. This report is important as it first described the somatotopic representation of the body in the nervous system.

As an example, seizure activity in the inferior lateral aspect of the motor cortex will be associated with tonic or clonic activity in the contralateral face, at times along with vocalizations or arrest of speech. If the superior motor strip that maps to the upper extremity is involved, the clonic activity most frequently starts in the contralateral fingers and spreads to the more proximal arm as the seizure propagates. If the superior and mesial regions of the motor strip are affected, then clonic activity of the contralateral lower extremity begins and can lead to ipsilateral tonic activity in the leg if the ipsilateral supplementary motor cortex becomes involved.

Often, seizures that involve the motor cortex are followed by hemiplegia or hemiparesis in the postictal period, termed "Todd's paralysis." The affected body part(s) corresponds to the section of the motor strip involved during the seizure. Seizures in this area have the possibility to progress into simple partial status epilepticus, or epilepsia partialis continua (EPC). Rasmussen encephalitis can present with focal motor seizures or EPC. Kojewnikow syndrome, characterized by repetitive focal motor seizures, myoclonus, and EPC, can occur with a perirolandic lesion.

17.5 Occipital lobe epilepsy

Seizures from the occipital lobe are less frequent than either frontal or temporal lobe seizures. Rapid spread to the temporal lobe is a frequent occurrence, as are visual disturbances, which are varied and intricate.

Elementary visual hallucinations are sensations of light, be it white light or colors, or even a mixture of colors. These can be in various shapes and sizes. The hallucinations can vary remarkably. They move, pulsate, rotate, and on occasion, remain still. They often appear in blind or defective visual fields. In instances of status epilepticus, repeated elementary visual hallucinations are seen. Twinkling lights or pulsations are seen with epileptic discharges over the lateral convexity of the occipital cortex. These visual hallucinations can arise from lesions in the parietal lobe, occipital lobes, optic chiasm, or even the calcarine area. If the visual hallucinations are isolated to one visual hemifield, they do assist in localizing to the contralateral hemisphere.

Complex visual hallucinations can occur as a release phenomenon in non-epileptic events such as migraines, or can occur as an ictal event. These can occur in combination with the aforementioned elementary visual hallucinations or separately. The events can be short-lived or prolonged, and this can help distinguish between ictal and non-ictal phenomena. Typically those with seizures last from seconds to minutes, whereas those related to non-ictal phenomena last longer on average. These hallucinations can be restricted or seen over the entire visual field, and can manifest as discrete objects, letters, numbers, and even more extensive scenes and images. They can stay motionless in the field, move laterally or medially, or even move closer or farther in the visual field of the person having the event. They can vary in size, color, relative proportions, and in some individuals can even appear lifelike. These hallucinations are often seen with seizures in patients with parieto-occipital lesions and occasionally with temporal lobe lesions. A rare manifestation of complex visual hallucinations seen in patients with lesions in the temporoparieto-occipital junction is autoscopia, in which affected individuals see mirror images of themselves.

Visual illusions are also encountered during occipital lobe seizures. They differ from the hallucinations mentioned earlier in that they are actual distortions of sensory perception, in contrast to hallucinations, which are in fact a perception in the absence of stimuli. Visual illusions are varied and can include metamorphopsia (distortions of color, speed, size, or proportion); micropsia (objects appear smaller than their actual size); and macropsia (objects appear larger than their actual size). Palinopsia can be due to ictal activity or as a release phenomenon in the absence of ictal activity. Palinopsia is a visual illusion in which the visual image persists or recurs in the absence of the original stimulus that produced the image. These illusions are linked to lesions adjacent to the optic radiations or visual cortex, especially in the non-dominant occipital lobe. However, they can also be seen with temporal and parieto-occipital discharges.

Pulling or moving sensations in the eyes with actual eye movement, ictal nystagmus, and rapid bilateral eye blinking have been associated with occipital lobe seizures. Horizontal nystagmus can be seen in association with a seizure in the temporoparieto-occipital junction, and has its fast phase and gaze deviation away from the seizure focus [23]. Distortions of visuospatial perception such as loss of stereoscopic vision have been reported in association with lesions of the parieto-occipital lobe.

Ictal amaurosis, which is blurring or loss of vision secondary to seizure activity, can engulf the entire visual field, or simply portions of it. This is typically seen with lesions in the visual association cortex, but also can be associated with headache and seizures in benign occipital epilepsy. Actual postictal blindness occurs in relation to seizures in the occipital cortex.

17.6 Parietal lobe epilepsy

Seizures originating in the parietal lobe tend to be the least common when separating by lobes, and usually evoke sensory alterations, apraxias, and visuospatial disorientation. Sensory alterations do not exclusively occur in parietal lobe seizures, and can be seen in association with temporal and occipital lobe seizures, though to a lesser degree. Negative or positive sensory abnormalities can be present, and typically multiple sensory modalities are altered over the entire course of the seizure. Unilateral sensory disturbances would seem to logically occur most often in relation to contralateral seizure activity. However, if the seizure activity occurs in parasagittal regions, supplementary motor cortex, or in the second sensory area (on the suprasylvian border) it can evoke bilateral sensory symptoms. And specifically, those associated with the suprasylvian border can give *ipsilateral* sensory symptoms.

Paresthesias or numbness can be frequently seen with seizures arising from or involving the primary sensory cortex. Often the sensory symptoms will march along the homunculus as well, typically distal to proximal. Associated clonic activity is also commonly seen. One of the rare instances of painful seizure activity can be seen with ictal activity in the contralateral rolandic region and in temporal lobe epilepsy. Temperature sensations, both hot and cold, can be seen with suprasylvian region seizure activity near the second sensory area.

Vertigo without nystagmus has been reported in association with seizures involving the temporoparietal junction, the occipital lobe, and the suprasylvian border around the central sulcus.

Idiomotor apraxia, which is the feeling of being unable to move a part of the body without any sense of weakness, has been shown to be related to lesions in the parietal, central, and parasylvian regions in either the left or right hemispheres.

Unilateral sensations in the genital regions have been correlated to seizure activity in the contralateral parietal sensory cortex (possibly the mesial paracentral parietal lobule). These sensations are usually unpleasant or painful, in contrast to sensations in the genital area from temporal lobe seizures, which have been reported as pleasurable.

Abnormalities in the perception of body image can be seen with ictal events that involve the inferior parietal lobule and the superior postcentral gyrus, most commonly in the non-dominant hemisphere. This can include the illusion of movement of a single limb, or even the entire body with a sensation of "floating." Odd sensations including shortening, elongating, enlarging, and shrinking of the limb can occur. Asomatognosia (the sensation that a body part is absent) or a phantom limb has been reported. Illusions of eye movement are associated with ictal activity from the occipital lobe.

17.7 Hypothalamic hamartoma

The hypothalamic hamartoma is a very rare congenital malformation that can lead to intractable epilepsy with unique manifestations. It is by far the best example of epileptogenesis from the subcortical region. These are congenital malformations of tumor-like masses of neuronal tissue in an ectopic area, and there are two main types. The first is the pedunculated lesion that attaches to the inferior surface of the hypothalamus and typically presents with precocious puberty. These typically respond well to gonadotropin-releasing hormone agonists. The second type is a sessile lesion that has a broad base of attachment and is typically associated with intractable epilepsy. Hypothalamic hamartoma with epilepsy in children only occurs in 1 in 200 000 children.

In classic descriptions, hypothalamic hamartomas are associated with laughing (gelastic) seizures as a common type, though there are usually multiple seizure types in each patient with this entity. These types include tonic, tonic-clonic, and complex partial seizure. The earliest presenting seizures typically are the gelastic seizures, though they often begin with a brief ictal laugh or smile, which often goes unnoticed, which can delay the diagnosis by months or years, until other seizure types manifest. Fear and anxiety can also be associated with gelastic seizures. There are theories that the gelastic seizures arise from the hamartoma itself and that the other seizures have their onset in the cerebral cortex.

Examination of the routine scalp EEG in patients with hypothalamic hamartomas has varied findings. It can frequently be normal, or have diffuse or focal slowing, and at times it will have epileptiform abnormalities. The epileptiform changes can be focal in any region of the brain, multifocal, or generalized. In ictal recordings, the EEG can also be normal, or have false localizing signs, including temporal or extratemporal discharges as opposed to midline abnormalities.

Gelastic seizures, and other seizures, associated with hypothalamic hamartomas are usually refractory to medical treatment. Even with significantly high doses of multiple antiepileptic medications, significant seizure reduction or seizure freedom is rare. Transcallosal or endoscopic resection can achieve 50% seizure freedom in affected patients, and 90% will have a 50% reduction in their seizure frequency [24]. Gamma knife and stereotactically implanted radioactive iodine-125 seeds can be used alternatively for hypothalamic hamartomas. Usually with destruction or resection of the hamartoma, immediate relief from the gelastic seizure type follows, as well as later improvement in the other seizure types over the next several months.

17.8 Other localizing and lateralizing signs

Ictal eye closure can be highly predictive of psychogenic non-epileptic spells, with a positive predictive value (PPV) of 99%, whereas ictal eye opening is highly predictive of epileptic seizures (PPV 94%). Pelvic thrusting, bicycling movements of the legs, and back arching can be seen in both psychogenic non-epileptic events as well as frontal lobe seizures.

Other physical manifestations can be helpful in lateralization. Unilateral clonic activity is almost exclusively contralateral to the seizure focus. Unilateral tonic stiffening is contralateral to the ictal focus in 90% of patients with frontal lobe epilepsy, but is much less helpful if the patient has temporal lobe epilepsy. The figure-of-four sign (which is asymmetric tonic posturing), which consists of rigid extension of one arm usually with a clenched fist and flexion of the elbow of the contralateral arm, typically has the ictal focus contralateral to the extended arm between 70% and 94% of the time [25]. Unilateral postictal paralysis is always contralateral to the seizure focus [25]. Version (forced head and eye deviation) is contralateral to the seizure focus in over 90% of cases when it comes before a generalized seizure [25]. Unilateral dystonic posturing is contralateral to the seizure focus over 95% of the time [25].

References

[1] Hogan RE, Kaoboriboon K. The "dreamy state": John Hughlings-Jackson's ideas of epilepsy and consciousness. *Am J Psychiatry* 2003;**160**:1740–1747.

[2] Hughlings-Jackson J. On a particular variety of epilepsy ("intellectual aura"), one case with symptoms of organic brain disease. *Brain* 1888;**11**:179–207.

[3] Hogan RE. Mesial temporal sclerosis: clinicopathological correlations. *Arch Neurol* 2001;**58**:1484–1486.

[4] Andermann F, Kobayashi E, Andermann E. Genetic focal epilepsies: state of the art and paths to the future. *Epilepsia* 2005;**46**(Suppl. 10):61–67.

[5] Wieser HG, Engel J, Williamson, PD, *et al.* Surgically remediable temporal lobe syndromes. In: Engel J (ed.), *Surgical Treatment of the Epilepsies.* New York: Raven Press, 1993; pp. 49–63.

[6] Wesmoreland BF. The electroencephalogram in patients with epilepsy. In: Aminoff MJ (ed.), *Neurology Clinics.* Philadelphia: WB Saunders, 1985; pp. 599–613.

[7] Gotman J, Marciani MG. Electroencephalographic spiking activity, drug levels, and seizure occurrence in epileptic patients. *Ann Neurol* 1985;**17**:597–603.

[8] Quesney LF. Extracranial EEG evaluation. In: Engel J Jr (ed.), *Surgical Treatment of the Epilepsies.* New York: Raven Press, 1987; pp. 129–166.

[9] Wyllie E, Luders H, Morris HH, *et al.* Clinical outcome after complex or partial resection of intractable partial epilepsy. *Neurology* 1987;**33**:1634–1641.

[10] Sharbrough FW. Commentary: extracranial EEG monitoring. In: Engel J Jr (ed.), *Surgical Treatment of the Epilepsies.* New York: Raven Press, 1987; pp. 167–171.

[11] Engel J Jr. Epileptic seizures. In: Engel J Jr (ed.), *Seizures and Epilepsy.* Philadelphia: FA Davis, 1989; pp. 137–138.

[12] Sharbrough FW. Complex partial seizures. In: Luders H, Lesser RP (eds), *Epilepsy: Electroclinical Syndromes.* Berlin: Springer-Verlag, 1987; pp. 279–302.

[13] Proposal for revised clinical and electroencephalographic classification of epileptic seizures. From the Commission on Classification and Terminology of the International League Against Epilepsy. *Epilepsia* 1981;**22**:489–501.

[14] Proposal for revised classification of epilepsies and epileptic syndromes. Commission on Classification and Terminology of the International League Against Epilepsy. *Epilepsia* 1989;**30**:389–399.

[15] Maillard L, Vignal JP, Gavaret M, *et al.* Semiologic and electrophysiologic correlations in temporal lobe seizures subtypes. *Epilepsia* 2004;**45**:1590–1599.

[16] Wieser HG. *Part 3. Electroclinical features of the psychomotor seizure.* London: Butterworths, 1983; pp. 177–235.

[17] Hogan RE, Kaiboriboon K, Bertrand ME, *et al.* Composite SISCOM perfusion patterns in right and left temporal seizures. *Arch Neurol* 2006;**63**:1419–1426.

[18] Ho SS, Berkovic SF, McKay WJ, *et al.* Temporal lobe epilepsy subtypes: differential patterns of cerebral perfusion on ictal single photon emission computed tomography. *Epilepsia* 1996;**37**:788–795.

[19] Wiebe S, Blume WT, Girvin JP, Eliasziw M. A randomized controlled trial of surgery for temporal-lobe epilepsy. *N Engl J Med* 2001;**345**:311–318.

[20] Foldvary-Schaefer N. Symptomatic focal epilepsies. In: Wyllie E (ed.), *Treatment of Epilepsy: Principles and Practice*, $th edn. Philadelphia: Lippincott Williams & Wilkins, 2006; pp. 365–372.

[21] Williamson PD, Spencer DD, Spencer SS, *et al.* Complex partial seizures of frontal lobe origin. *Ann Neurol* 1985;**18**:497–504.

[22] Hughlings Jackson J. Notes on the physiology and pathology of the nervous system. *Med Times Gaz* 1868,**ii**:696.

[23] Commission on Classification and Terminology of the International League Against Epilepsy. Proposal for revised classification of epilepsies and epileptic syndromes. *Epilepsia* 1989;**30**: 389–399.
[24] Ng YT, Rekate HL, Prenger EC, *et al.* Endoscopic resection of hypothalamic hamartomas for refractory symptomatic epilepsy. *Neurology* 2008;**70**:1543–1548.
[25] Loddenkemper T, Kotagal P. Lateralizing signs during seizures in focal epilepsy. *Epilepsy Behav* 2005;**7**:1–17.

Section 6

Epilepsies relative to age, etiology, or duration

Yu-Tze Ng

18 Neonatal seizures

Eric V. Hastriter
Mayo Clinic Hospital, Phoenix, AZ, USA

Neonatal seizures are common in the first 28 days of life, otherwise known as the neonatal period, and can present in many forms. They occur at any time around birth, including *in utero*, and at any gestational age. They can be associated with acute neonatal encephalopathies, causing significant morbidity and mortality. The interesting aspect of neonatal seizures is their presentation and pathophysiology, which differ from those of all other ages. The differences are thought to be in the mechanisms of epileptogenesis and in the relatively greater importance of non-epileptic mechanisms of seizure generation in this age. This chapter is intended to help clinicians recognize seizures presenting during the neonatal period, to appreciate their epidemiology, and to recognize common etiologies of neonatal seizures. It will also discuss the pathophysiology of neonatal seizures, help clinicians make informed decisions on when to treat and when not to treat, and discuss commonly used therapeutic agents.

18.1 Significance of neonatal seizures

The incidence of seizures in the first 28 days of life ranges from 1% to 5%. It is one of the highest risk periods for seizures in humans. A review of the literature reveals that

Epilepsy in Children and Adolescents, First Edition. Edited by James W. Wheless.

seizures occur during this period at a rate of 1.5–5.5 per 1000 neonates [1]. Most of these occur during the first week of life. Of course, risk factors that predispose neonates to have seizures may influence the incidence. When looking at all neonates with seizures, Lanska *et al.* reported the incidence to be 3.5 per 1000 [2]. However, when stratifying this for birthweight among very low birthweight (<1500 g), low birthweight (1500–2499 g), and normal birthweight (>2500 g), the incidence of neonatal seizure was very different. Very-low-birthweight neonates had an incidence of 57.5 out of 1000. Low-birthweight neonates had an incidence of 4.4 out of 1000. Normal-birthweight neonates had an incidence of 2.8 out of 1000. Looking at maturity, Scher and colleagues demonstrated that 3.9% of neonates with conceptual age less than 30 weeks had seizures, while 1.5% of neonates greater than 30 week had neonatal seizures [3].

The neonatal brain has not fully matured, and maturational changes continue to occur throughout development. Its resulting plasticity is greater than that of fully mature adult brains, and the molecular infrastructure is different, both of which make it more susceptible to seizures. Finally, the neonatal brain is vulnerable to a wide range of toxic or metabolic conditions. These include sepsis/meningitis, hypoxic ischemic encephalopathy (HIE), hypoglycemia, and other metabolic derangements. It is imperative for clinicians to discern seizures and to determine their etiology as some are reversible, making timely treatment crucial. There are some situations where seizures in the neonatal period cannot be eliminated and are treated in order to minimize developmental delay, and to maximize the potential for development in that particular neonate.

The neonatal brain, compared with the mature adult brain, may be especially prone to seizures when injured. One proposed explanation is that there is an imbalance between inhibition and excitation. There is delayed maturation of inhibitory circuitry in the neonatal brain compared to that of adults, in contrast to a more developed excitatory circuitry, which is needed for the process of learning and development. This, however, can lead to easier potentiation of electrical activity in the neonatal brain causing seizures that present with different manifestations [4]. Moreover, studies in the neonatal rat have shown that gamma-aminobutyric acid (GABA), the major inhibitory neurotransmitter in the mature brain, may exert paradoxically excitatory effects in early central nervous system (CNS) development [5].

18.2 Pathophysiology of neonatal seizures

In the developing brain a significant electrophysiological change in cotransporters of chloride occurs. Depending on the age of the neonate the balance between intracellular and extracellular chloride concentration differs according to the expression of these chloride cotransporters. This can lead to hyperpolarization or depolarization depending on the concentration of these cotransporters, and therefore inhibition versus excitation.

Developmental changes in intracellular chloride concentration are due to changes in the expression of the two major chloride cotransporters, NKCC2 and NKCC1. Early in development the NKCC1 transporter predominates and actively transports chloride into the neuron, while NKCC2, a cationic chloride cotransporter, which is developmentally dependent, extrudes chloride into the extracellular space. NKCC2 reaches full maturity in the rat hippocampus after the third postnatal week. After the development of NKCC2, there is a switch in the cotransporter concentration, the intracellular chloride level is kept low, and activation of the $GABA_A$ receptor allows chloride to run down its electrochemical gradient into the neuron, hyperpolarizing and allowing for the inhibitory action of the receptor [6]. This occurs in the rat hippocampus at the end of postnatal week 2, which is approximately equivalent to that of a human toddler [7]. Therefore, when the ligand-gated $GABA_A$ receptor is activated in the immature rat, the extracellular chloride follows its electrochemical gradient out of the neuron and paradoxically depolarizes it. During the neonatal period this imbalance favors depolarization and excitation and places neonates at increased risk for seizures.

This excitatory effect of GABA during the neonatal period contributes to the refractoriness of neonatal seizures to phenobarbital and benzodiazepines. In some animal models of induced neonatal seizures, inhibition of the NKKC1 transporter with bumetanide alters chloride transport and significantly enhances the anticonvulsant effects of phenobarbital in the neonatal rat hippocampus [8]. The application of this observation to the treatment of neonatal seizures in humans is not clear at this time (studies are ongoing).

Glutamatergic receptors also undergo developmental changes in the neonatal period and may contribute to the propensity for neonates to have seizures. Glutamate receptors are classified according to their ligand sensitivity: *N*-methyl-D-aspartate (NMDA), α-amino-3-hydroxy-5-methyl-4-isoxazolepropionic acid (AMPA), and kainate. These receptors can have various functional properties based on their subunit composition changes during development. NMDA receptors in immature neurons express primarily the NR2B subunit that prolongs the duration of the excitatory postsynaptic potential. Increased expression of the NR2C, NR2D, and NR3A subunits confers a reduced sensitivity to blockade by magnesium, resulting in increased excitability [9].

Neonatal seizures are powerful prognostic indicators of mortality and neurological morbidity. In the literature over the past 50 years, mortality has been reported as between 40% and 16%. The general trend is downward, and some of this improvement is attributable to improved obstetrical and neonatal care for these patients. Survivors of neonatal seizures face neurological morbidity, for example, cerebral palsy, mental retardation, and chronic epilepsy. Even after neonatal seizures, children may appear normal, but have impaired neurological function [10].

Comparative studies of the prognosis after neonatal seizures have been done and included infants who have had electroencephalographically confirmed seizures. Outcome was assessed in terms of survival, neurological disability, developmental delay, and postnatal epilepsy. Ortibus and colleagues reported that 28% died, 22% of survivors were neurologically normal at an average of 17 months of age, 14% had mild abnormalities, and 36% had severe abnormalities [11].

The Neonatal Seizures Clinical Research Center collected data from 1992 to 1997. Two hundred-and-seven full-term infants were followed with video-EEG confirmed seizures, 28% of whom died. Two-year follow-up data were available for 122 of the remaining infants, or 86% of the survivors. Abnormal neurological findings were present in 42%, a Mental Developmental Index (MDI) score below 80 in 55%, a Psychomotor Developmental Index (PDI) score of less than 80 was present in 50%, and chronic postnatal epilepsy was seen in 26% [12].

Are seizures harmful to the developing brain, or is it the amount of seizure burden that is a better predictor of future outcome? Some infants have brief infrequent seizures with relatively good outcome, but those with prolonged seizures often do not have good outcomes. Studies of neonates with EEG-confirmed seizures have attempted to describe features of prognostic significance. Overall, neurological outcome was more favorable with fewer than two seizures per hour. If asphyxia was the etiology of seizure, cerebral palsy was seen in follow up if neonate experienced five or more seizures per hour [13].

Prolonged, repetitive neonatal seizures may be intrinsically harmful to the developing brain. If neonates have prolonged seizures, it is usually due to an underlying cause, such as acute brain injury, which perhaps is the reason why the neurological outcome is poor, not the seizures themselves causing poor outcome. Neonatal brains are more resistant to damage related to seizures than are adult brains; however, despite this fact, neonates that are exposed to seizures have impaired visuospatial memory and a reduced seizure threshold as well as altered brain neurogenesis, synaptogenesis, synaptic pruning, neuronal migration, and sequential expression of genes including neurotransmitter receptors and transporters. This was described by Holmes and colleagues, who documented impaired spatial learning and memory, decreased activity levels, significantly lower threshold to induced seizures, and sprouting of CA3 mossy fibers in adult rats, after recurrent neonatal seizures, compared to the rats that had not experienced recurrent neonatal seizures [14].

Neonatal seizures are most frequently seen in the setting of hypoxic ischemic encephalopathy in both the term and preterm neonate. A decrease in GluR2 receptor expression, as shown in a rodent study, allows an influx of calcium that may contribute to the chronic epileptogenic effects of hypoxia-induced neonatal seizures. In neonatal rodents experiencing hypoxic ischemic seizures, it was shown that treatment with AMPA receptor antagonists, but not NMDA receptor or $GABA_A$ receptor antagonists, reduced their susceptibility to seizures and seizure-induced injuries later in life [15]. Topiramate, which acts by blocking AMPA/kainate receptors, exerts anticonvulsant activity against perinatal hypoxic ischemic-induced seizures in animal models. This observation has led to the suggestion of the potential utility of topiramate in treating neonatal seizures secondary to hypoxic ischemic insults, but the lack of an intravenous formulation makes treating critically ill neonates challenging [16].

Neonatal seizures in rodent models show an alteration in the composition of $GABA_A$ receptors. Each receptor is composed of five subunits that are assembled into a functional ligand-gated receptor. The specific composition of each receptor depends on the developmental age. Rat models that experience more neonatal seizures had substantially higher proportion of α_1 $GABA_A$ subunits compared to control rodents. This particular subunit may provide a protective role in decreased severity and frequency of seizures later in life [17].

18.3 Classification and clinical features of neonatal seizures

Neonatal seizures can be classified by clinical manifestations, relationship between clinical seizure and electrical activity on electroencephalogram, and the seizure pathophysiology. The International League Against Epilepsy (ILAE) has specified five neonatal syndromes, including benign neonatal convulsions (BNC), benign familial neonatal convulsions (BFNC), early myoclonic encephalopathy (EME), early infantile epileptic encephalopathy (EIEE), and migrating partial seizures of infancy.

Early classification of neonatal seizures by their clinical manifestations focused on clinical differences between seizures in neonates compared to older children. Neonatal seizures were reported to be clonic or tonic, but not tonic-clonic. When they were focal they were either unifocal or multifocal. Later in classification schemes, myoclonic features were included. Another feature of neonatal seizures, described as "subtle," included oral-buccal movements like sucking or chewing; bicycling movements of the legs, swimming movements of the arms, or random eye movements. These movements were initially thought to be epileptic in origin but later deemed to be exaggerated reflex behaviors called "brainstem-release phenomena" or "motor automatisms." A current classification scheme based on clinical features is seen in Table 18.1, which can be applied with thorough observation.

18.4 Electrographic seizures

An electrographic seizure is a discrete clinical event of at least 10 seconds in duration with a definite beginning, middle, and end accompanied by an electroencephalographic seizure. A typical neonatal seizure begins as low-amplitude, rhythmic, or sinusoidal waveforms, or spike or sharp waves [18]. As it evolves the amplitude increases, while frequency decreases. Rhythmic activity of any frequency (delta, theta, alpha, or beta) can compose ictal patterns measured at the scalp surface.

Some clinical neonatal seizures may not have electrographic evidence of seizure activity, while some electroencephalographic (EEG) or occult seizures occur in the absence of any clinical events. Some neonatal seizures are clearly epileptic with close EEG correlation of seizure activity. The increase in cellular and synaptic excitation and a tendency to enhance propagation of an epileptic discharge are two properties of the developing brain that allow seizure initiation, maintenance, and propagation. Clinical events that are most clearly epileptic in origin include focal tonic, focal clonic, some types of myoclonic, and rarely spasm (Table 18.1). Electrical-only seizures by definition are epileptic.

Non-epileptic seizures are events that occur in the absence of electrical seizure activity but have clinical characteristics resembling reflex behaviors. These events can be suppressed or altered by restraining or repositioning the neonate. Some types of myoclonic events, generalized tonic posturing, and motor automatisms can be classified as non-epileptic (Table 18.1).

Paroxysmal changes in the autonomic nervous system, including stereotyped episodic alterations in heart rate, respirations, and blood pressure, may also signal seizures. Skin flushing, apnea, salivation, and pupillary dilation may be autonomic signs of seizures but are usually associated with other clinical manifestations, except in therapeutically paralyzed infants [19].

18.5 Monitoring and recording

Visual observation is critical in evaluation of neonatal seizures. However, the EEG offers an important means of confirmation and characterization. Normal background activity is much less likely to be seen in neonates who are having seizures or who are likely to develop neonatal seizures. An extremely abnormal background, for example, burst suppression or isoelectric state, self-evidently signifies profound disruption and forecasts a high risk for death or adverse neurological outcome, while a nearly normal interictal background suggests relatively preserved neurological health despite a clinically observed seizure [20].

The background can also guide the clinician to the etiology of the seizure. For example, persistent focal sharp waves may suggest a geographically focal injury such as subarachnoid hemorrhage, stroke, or contusion, while multifocal sharp waves suggest diffuse dysfunction. Electrolyte abnormalities such as hypocalcemia can have well-maintained background features but with excessive bilateral central spikes. Some inborn errors of metabolism, like

Table 18.1 Classification, characteristics, and presumed pathophysiology of neonatal seizures.

Classification	Characteristics	Pathophysiological basis
Focal clonic	Repetitive rhythmic contraction of muscle groups of limbs, face, or trunk Unifocal or multifocal Synchronous or asynchronous in muscle groups on one side of body Simultaneous, asynchronous on both sides Cannot be suppressed by restraint	Epileptic
Focal tonic	Sustained posturing of single limb Sustained asymmetric posturing of trunk Sustained eye deviation Cannot be provoked by stimulation or suppressed by restraint	Epileptic
Spasms	May be flexor, extensor, or mixed May occur in clusters Cannot be provoked by stimulation or suppressed by restraint	Epileptic
Myoclonic	Random, single, rapid contractions of muscle groups of limbs, face or trunk Typically not repetitive or may recur at a slow rate May be generalized, focal, or fragmentary May be provoked by stimulation	Epileptic or non-epileptic
Generalized tonic	Sustained posturing of limbs, trunk, and neck May be flexor, extensor, or mixed May be provoked/intensified by stimulation May be suppressed by restraint/repositioning	Presumed non-epileptic
Motor automatisms	Random, roving eye movements or nystagmus (distinct from tonic eye deviation) May be provoked by tactile stimulation	Non-epileptic
Oral-buccal-lingual	Sucking, chewing, tongue protrusions May be provoked/intensified by stimulation	Non-epileptic
Progression movements	Rowing or swimming movements Pedaling/bicycling movements of legs May be provoked/intensified by stimulation May be suppressed by restraint/repositioning	Non-epileptic
Complex purposeless	Sudden arousal with transient increased random activity of limbs May be provoked/intensified by stimulation	Non-epileptic

maple-syrup urine disease, can be associated with specific EEG abnormalities (vertex and wicket spikes). In herpes simplex encephalitis, periodic lateralizing epileptiform discharges can be seen. If acquired diseases are excluded and the EEG is still grossly abnormal, the cause may be cerebral dysgenesis. Interictal EEG spikes have uncertain diagnostic significance; for instance, interictal focal sharp waves and spikes are not typically considered epileptogenic the same way as they are in older children and adults. Only a few neonates with confirmed seizures exhibit interictal characteristics seen in older infants and children, and many show no excessive spikes or sharp waves.

The epileptic process is characterized by abnormal, excessive, repetitive electrical firing of neurons. Neurons lose their autonomy and are engulfed by synchronized bursts of repeated electrical discharges. Repetitive action potentials will eventually propagate beyond the site of origin resulting in seizure. At its conclusion inhibitory influences stop the electrophysiological cascade and terminate the seizure.

Despite the difference between term and pre-term neonatal brains, the variety of types of electrographic seizures does not differ between them [21]. Neonatal brains lack the structural and functional organization that is necessary for motor manifestation seen in older children; hence, generalized seizures that appear simultaneously, synchronously, and symmetrically in both hemispheres are not seen. Individual seizures in neonates always arise focally and migrate to adjacent areas and can finally engage the entire hemisphere, and may migrate from one hemisphere to the other [22]. Occasionally simultaneous focal seizures may act independently and spread to all brain regions and masquerade as a generalized seizure; however, the ictal pattern is usually not composed of spike or polyspike slow-wave discharges. Encephalopathies caused by meningitis, hypoglycemia, or hypoxia-ischemia would be expected to generate generalized seizures, but in the neonatal brain each seizure instead arises from a restricted area of cortex. Multifocal onset seizures are multiple seizures that each originate from different scalp regions.

Most electrographic neonatal seizures do not provoke distinct clinical signs, and if the neonate is paralyzed clinical recognition is impossible. The number of recorded electrographic seizures varies widely, in similar situations. The duration of electrographic seizures also varies. In order to describe the "burden" of electrographic seizures, a percentage of time in which seizure activity is present in any brain region is described. There is only modest correlation between seizure counts and the percentage of the EEG recordings showing seizure activity. The most detailed measure of seizure burden incorporates knowledge of their spatial distribution. Electrographic seizures may remain confined to their area of origin or may spread substantially to other regions, but this varies considerably among individual neonates.

Typically electrographic neonatal seizures last 1–2 minutes and are followed by interictal periods of various lengths. Single prolonged electrographic seizures in neonates are rare, while repetitive brief seizures are much more characteristic. Few studies describe the natural history of electrographic seizures during continuous monitoring from the onset of acute neurologic illness. The electroencephalogram in Figure 18.1 is a sequential neonatal seizure showing a fairly typical focal (fronto-temporal) evolution with rhythmic changes. The initial high-voltage burst of diffuse activity was part of the encephalopathic burst-suppression background (Figure 18.1).

Electrical seizures of the depressed neonatal brain are long, low in voltage, and highly localized. They may be unifocal or multifocal and show little tendency to spread or modulate. They occur when the EEG background is depressed and undifferentiated, and suggest a poor

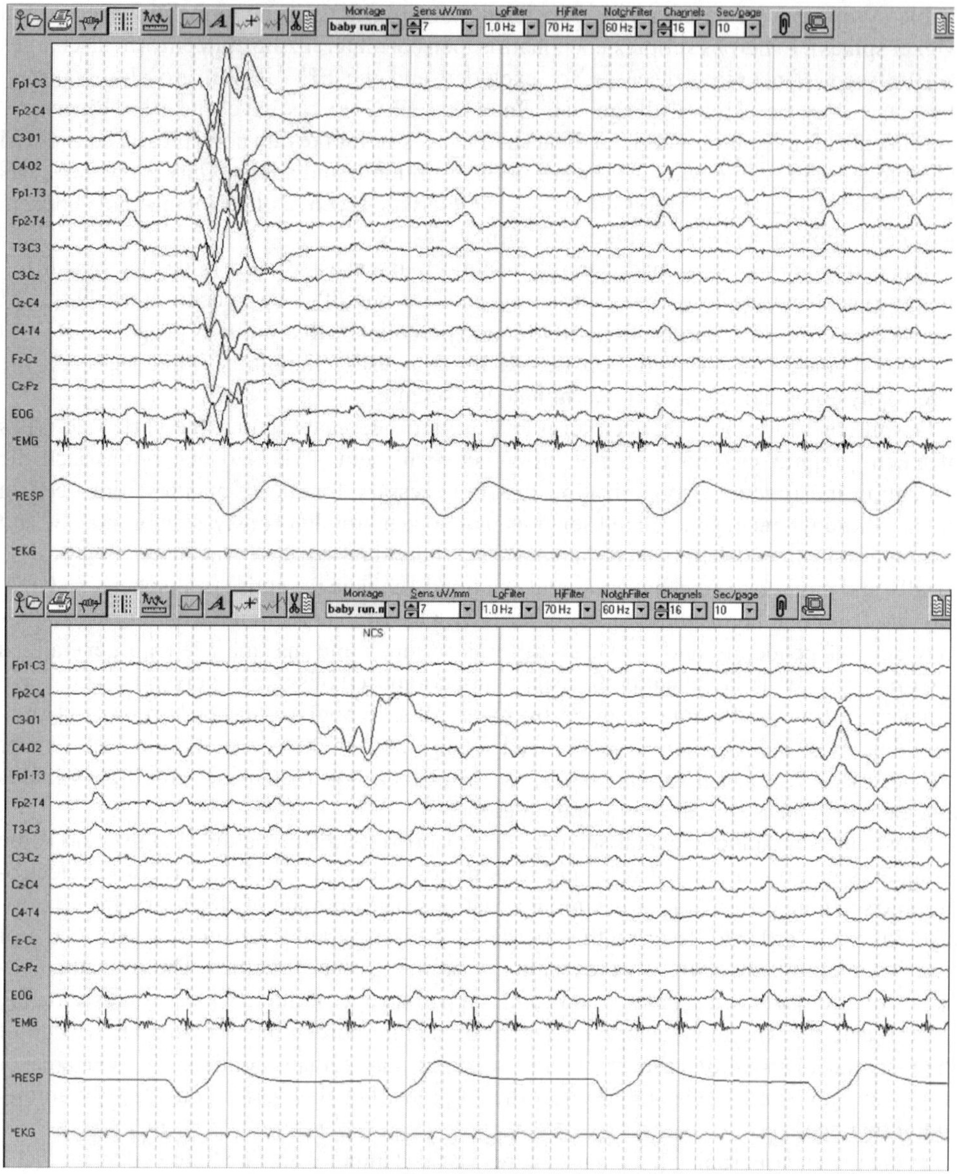

Figure 18.1 Neonatal electroencephalogram. Sequential transverse montage showing a neonatal seizure with a fairly typical fronto-temporal evolution and rhythmic changes. Courtesy of Dr Kevin Chapman.

prognosis. Alpha-frequency seizure activity is characterized by sudden, transient, rhythmic activity in the alpha range (8–12 Hz) in the temporal or central region, unaccompanied by clinical events [23]. An alpha discharge usually indicates a severe encephalopathy and is associated with a poor prognosis.

Video-EEG monitoring has been the basis of clinical investigations into classification, therapy, and prognosis of neonatal seizures, but unfortunately is not widely available for routine use [24]. The conventional way of monitoring newborns with seizures is attended EEG with simultaneous observation by trained electroneurodiagnostic technologists.

Amplitude-integrated EEG (aEEG) is increasingly used in neonatal intensive care units for bedside evaluation of cerebral activity. Two electrodes are commonly used to acquire data, which are then processed and compressed to provide a simple trend of background EEG activity in those areas. Widespread availability, ease of application, and lack of dependence on specially trained neurophysiologists are advantages of aEEG over conventional EEG. The compressed data provide a background EEG that can be used for prognostic purposes, for example, in therapeutic neuroprotection such as head cooling. On aEEG, neonatal seizures are detected as sudden elevations of the margins of the background tracings. Clearly aEEG is not as detailed as conventional EEG and cannot replace it, but can provide very useful complementary information that may guide decision-making at the bedside in real time.

Measurement of the proportion of time with electrographic seizure does not take into consideration the spatial distribution of the seizures. One way to overcome this is to reduce the entire neonatal EEG into five non-overlapping areas of interest including left and right frontotemporal areas, left and right centro-occipital areas, and one midline region. Summating the percent of time in each of those areas gives the most comprehensive evaluation of electrographic seizure burden [25].

18.6 Etiology of neonatal seizures

Acute or chronic conditions can give rise to seizures. Table 18.2 lists potential causes of neonatal seizures.

The most common cause of neonatal seizures is acute neonatal encephalopathy characterized by lethargy or coma (depressed mental status), seizure, hypotonia – either axial or appendicular – with overall decrease in motor movement, and clear bulbar dysfunction with poor sucking, swallowing, and inexpressive face. This is typically due to a hypoxic ischemic event, but can be caused by other entities such as inborn errors of metabolism, pyridoxine dependency, stroke, coagulopathies, sinovenous thrombosis, as well as fetal sepsis syndrome secondary to sepsis or associated with chorioamnionitis.

The diagnosis of a hypoxic ischemic event relies on criteria set out by the American College of Obstetricians and Gynecologists Task Force on Neonatal Encephalopathy and Cerebral Palsy, which includes: (i) fetal umbilical cord evidence of metabolic acidosis obtained at delivery (pH <7, and base deficit >12 mmol/L); (ii) early onset of severe or moderate neonatal encephalopathy in infants born at 34 weeks or after; (iii) subsequent cerebral palsy of either the spastic quadriplegic or dyskinetic type; and (iv) exclusion of all other causes such as infectious conditions, coagulopathies, trauma, or genetic disorders. These four criteria occur with a hypoxic event before or during labor including uterine rupture, placental abruption, or umbilical cord prolapse, with associated sudden fetal bradycardia that is sustained, or absent heart rate variability, or persistent late or variable decelerations [26]. Most have low Apgar scores and have multisystem involvement within 72 hours, including acute renal tubular necrosis, elevated liver function tests, necrotizing enterocolitis, and thrombocytopenia secondary to ischemic bone marrow. Acute diffuse cerebral abnormalities consistent with hypoxic ischemia should be seen on neuroimaging.

Perinatal stroke is another cause for neonatal seizures, and is defined as a cerebrovascular event that occurs between 28 weeks of gestation and 7 days of life. It occurs 1 in 4000

Table 18.2 Etiologies of neonatal seizures.

Acute
Acute neonatal encephalopathy (classic hypoxic-ischemic encephalopathy, ante/intrapartum)
Arterial ischemic stroke
Sinovenous thrombosis
Extracorporeal membrane oxygenation
Congenital heart disease
Vein of Galen malformation
Giant arteriovenous malformation
Hypertensive encephalopathy
Intracranial hemorrhage (subdural, subarachnoid, intraventricular, intraparenchymal)
Trauma (intrapartum and non-accidental)
Infections (sepsis, meningitis, encephalitis)
Transient, simple, metabolic disorders
Inborn errors of metabolism (including pyridoxine-dependent seizures)
Intoxication
Chronic
Isolated cerebral dysgenesis (lissencephaly, hemimegaloencephaly)
Cerebral dysgenesis associated with inborn errors of metabolism
Chronic infection (TORCH – toxoplasmosis, other infections, rubella, cytomegalovirus, and herpes)
Neurocutaneous syndromes:
incontinentia pigmenti
hypomelanosis of Ito
Sturge–Weber syndrome
tuberous sclerosis
linear sebaceous nevus (epidermal nevus syndrome)
Genetic conditions:
22q11 microdeletion
ARX (aristaless-related homeobox) mutations
Specific very early onset epilepsy syndromes:
Fifth day fits (benign neonatal convulsions, BNC)
Benign familial neonatal convulsions (BFNC)
Early myoclonic encephalopathy (EME)
Early infantile epileptic encephalopathy (EIEE)
Migrating partial seizures of infancy

live births, and has two clinical presentations. One presentation is an acute appearance of neonatal seizures, hypotonia, feeding difficulties, and rarely hemiparesis, while the other presentation is discovered through the gradual appearance of congenital hemiparesis, or the onset of a partial seizure disorder in an infant who was previously healthy at birth. Factors that increase risk for perinatal stroke include congenital heart defects, lipid and blood disorders, infections, placental disorders, trauma, vasculopathy, dehydration, and use of extracorporeal membrane oxygenation (ECMO) [27].

Intracranial sinovenous thrombosis may cause neonatal seizures. It occurs in 0.67 of 100 000 children per year in neonates and older children. The neonatal presentation most frequently includes seizures (57–71%) and lethargy (35–58%). Risk factors in mothers include pre-eclampsia, gestational diabetes, meconium-stained placenta, and meconium aspiration. Sagittal and transverse sinuses are most commonly involved; however, multiple sinus thromboses can occur. Mortality data vary between 2% and 13%. Follow-up on these neonates showed that 21% had normal development, 60% had cognitive impairment, 64% had motor impairment, and 40% had epilepsy [28].

Congenital heart disease increases the risk for neonatal seizures, either preoperatively or postoperatively. These infants often have difficult times transitioning from intrauterine life into extrauterine life, with difficult deliveries, depressed Apgar scores, and persistent hypoxia, which can lead to hypotension, acidosis, and multisystem failure including encephalopathy with seizures. Congenital heart disease may also be associated with central nervous system cerebral dysgenesis. Strokes may occur from multiple mechanisms such as right-to-left shunting, or embolization during cardiac catheterization [29]. If the patient has DiGeorge syndrome, the accompanying hypocalcemia may trigger seizures. Seizures can arise after congenital heart surgery, and are influenced by suspected or confirmed genetic disorders, need for prolonged deep hypothermic circulatory arrest, or aortic arch obstruction. The ability to provide neuroprotection preoperatively in this patient population to prevent seizure is the subject of ongoing investigation [30].

18.7 Metabolic causes for neonatal seizures

Changes in electrolytes can be the cause of neonatal seizures. Hypoglycemia, hyponatremia, hypernatremia, hypocalcemia, hypomagnesemia, and acute hyperbilirubinemia can all be associated with neonatal seizures, and are easily screened by laboratory tests. Hypoglycemia itself may inflict brain damage independent of seizures, and can be caused by prematurity, infections, maternal diabetes, galactosemia, defects in gluconeogenesis , respiratory chain defects, and glycogen storage diseases. Glucose transporter deficiency (GLUT1 deficiency) is associated with infantile seizures usually between 6 and 12 weeks of life, developmental delay, ataxia, and progressive microcephaly, and affected newborns may appear completely normal at birth [31]. Neonatal seizures may occur, initially rarely but increasing in frequency as developmental delay becomes evident. Diagnostically, glucose is unable to cross the blood–brain barrier and has low concentrations in the brain and cerebrospinal fluid. There are several point mutations that cause GLUT1 transporter deficiency syndrome. Fortunately, treatment with the ketogenic diet supplies the brain with an alternative source of energy, decreasing seizures.

18.8 Inborn errors of metabolism

Inborn errors of metabolism that may lead to neonatal seizure are numerous. Common examples are maple-syrup urine disease, ketotic and non-ketotic hyperglycinemia, and urea acid cycle disorders, which are all potential causes of acute neonatal encephalopathy associated with neonatal seizures.

Maple-syrup urine disease is a defect in the decarboxylation of branched-chain amino acids such as leucine, isoleucine, and valine, which manifests after a protein load such as milk. Neonates will often develop a shrill cry, hypotonia punctuated with episodic posturing, progressive obtundation, and seizures. Hypoglycemia may be associated with this entity, and urine may be tested for 2,4-dinitrophenylhydrazine (DNPH), which makes the sweet maple syrup smell characteristic of the urine in this entity.

Non-ketotic hyperglycinemia presents catastrophically with intractable seizures, coma, hiccups, apnea, pupil-sparing ophthalmoparesis, spontaneous and stimulus-induced myoclonus, and burst-suppression pattern on EEG. Glycine levels are elevated in serum and cerebrospinal fluid. This entity is due to the inability to cleave glycine, an important inhibitory as well as excitatory neurotransmitter. Treatment with an NMDA antagonist, magnesium, sodium benzoate, and dextromethorphan has been used with limited success. Ketotic hyperglycinemias, including propionic and methylmalonic acidemias, present with multisystem failure and dehydration along with ketoacidosis and fulminant CNS signs such as seizures, vomiting, and coma. Serum amino acids and measurement of specific enzymes can confirm the diagnosis.

Urea cycle disorders, including carbamoylphosphate synthetase deficiency, ornithine carbamyl transferase deficiency, citrullinemia, and arginosuccinic acidemia can cause neonatal seizures in the first days to weeks of life. Coma and bulbar dysfunction, with ophthalmoparesis, fixed pupils, absent gag reflex, poor sucking, and apnea, are seen. Serum ammonia elevation may correlate with EEG background discontinuity [32]. Biotinidase deficiency can produce seizures as early as the first weeks of life, and may produce alopecia, seborrheic dermatitis, developmental delay, hypotonia, and ataxia. Diagnosis can be made by demonstrating a low level of serum biotinidase activity, while treatment with oral replacement of biotin on a daily basis is required.

Pyridoxine-dependent seizures arise usually between birth and 3 months of life, but can occur as late as 3 years of age. It is an autosomal recessive disorder, so a family history of an affected sibling helps in the diagnosis. The neonate usually will present with agitation, irritability, jitteriness, diminished sleep, and intractable clonic seizures. EEG patterns are non-specific, including abnormal backgrounds, multifocal sharp waves, and focal electrographic seizures, which may evolve into a hypsarrythmia pattern during the first year of life. Diagnosis can be made with complete cessation of clinical seizures immediately with resolution of EEG abnormalities within a few hours, after the intravenous administration of 50–100 mg of pyridoxine. Treatment is with lifelong replacement of pyridoxine 50–100 mg/day. Despite early treatment, mental retardation as well as MRI evidence of leukodystrophy may be seen. Mutations in the α-aminoadipic semialdehyde (α-AASA) dehydrogenase (antiquitin) leading to inactivation of pyridoxal phosphate (PLP) have been discovered in patients with pyridoxine-dependent seizures [33]. PLP is an essential cofactor in the formation of GABA as well as multiple other enzymatic reactions. Elevations of α-AASA in the urine can be used as a screening tool for identifying individuals with antiquitin mutations; however, this should not substitute for a pyridoxine trial, especially in the acute setting.

Folinic acid-responsive neonatal seizures were first described in the first hours or days of life in term newborns by Hyland. Intractable seizures develop, associated with severe developmental delay, progressive atrophy on MRI examination, and frequent status epilepticus. Patients usually do not respond to pyridoxine, but have seizure resolution with addition of 2.5 mg folinic acid twice a day. Gene mutations in antiquitin were subsequently discovered, and patients should be given pyridoxine as well as folinic acid if the patient has α-AASA dehydrogenase deficiency, with α-AASA discovered in urine [34].

Molybdenum cofactor is essential for proper functioning of sulfite oxidase and xanthine dehydrogenase. Deficiency of this cofactor and isolated sulfite oxidase deficiency are both autosomal recessive disorders, which produce severe neurological symptoms including poor feeding, high-pitched cry, jitteriness, and intractable seizures. Urine samples demonstrate decreased levels of uric acid with elevated levels of xanthine and hypoxanthine. This chemical malfunction can arise from mutations in three molybdenum cofactors or in gephyrin. Synthesis of this molybdenum cofactor requires activities of at least six gene products, including gephyrin, a polypeptide responsible for the clustering of inhibitory glycine receptors and postsynaptic membranes in the rat model central nervous system [35]. There is no effective treatment, and prognosis for recovery neurologically and survival is poor.

Toxic causes may occasionally need to be considered. Local pudendal anesthesia for delivery may erroneously be injected into the fetal cranium, and the lidocaine, bupivacaine, or mepivacaine can produce seizures in the neonate. Other substances that can cause neonatal seizures include cocaine, heroin, amphetamines, propoxyphen, and theophylline; these can be found in the patient, in the mother, or through the history.

Chronic causes of neonatal seizures can be the result of long-standing disorders such as cerebral dysgenesis, neurocutaneous syndromes, genetic disorders, or early-onset epilepsy.

Cerebral dysgenesis, including lissencephaly, schizencephaly, and hemimegaloencephaly can present with normal birth history and delivery, with no acute cause for seizures, yet the neonate may experience seizures. The use of MRI can identify cerebral dysgenesis as a cause; however, evidence on imaging must not preclude the clinician from seeking evidence of inborn errors of metabolism as both may coexist. Some examples of inborn errors of metabolism that can be associated with a brain malformation include: cytochrome oxidase deficiency, glutaric aciduria types I and II, 3-hydroxyisobutyric aciduria, 3-methylglutaconic aciduria, 3-ketothiolase deficiency; sulfite oxidase deficiency, pyruvate dehydrogenase deficiency, neonatal adrenoleukodystrophy, fumaric aciduria, ketotic hyperglycinemia, and Zellweger syndrome [36].

Evidence of congenital infections, termed TORCH (toxoplasmosis, other infections, rubella, cytomegalovirus, and herpes virus), can be found by thorough physical examination with ophthalmological changes, microcephaly, periventricular calcifications on neuroimaging, and appropriate serological blood tests. Congenital infections that are acquired during the first trimester may cause an acquired form of migrational defect giving rise to a dysgenesis pattern on MRI scanning [37].

Neurocutaneous disorders may also give rise to neonatal seizures, and a careful skin examination of the neonate as well as a family history is imperative. The disorders that may give rise to neonatal seizures include incontinentia pigmenti, tuberous sclerosis, linear sebaceous nevi, and Sturge–Weber syndrome. Familial incontinentia pigmenti, an X-linked dominant disorder, is lethal in males and is characterized by perinatal inflammatory vesicles that are followed by verrucous patches that produce a distinctive pattern of hyperpigmentation with dermal scarring. In contrast to the hyperpigmented familial form, a sporadic form also known as hypomelanosis of Ito exists, with cutaneous lesions appearing as hypopigmented areas.

Tuberous sclerosis is another neurocutaneous disorder that can give rise to neonatal seizures. It can do so in two different ways; first through cortical tubers; and secondly from embolic strokes from intracardiac tumors. The classic neurocutaneous signs often are not visible during the neonatal period; however, under Wood's lamp they are apparent. Linear sebaceous nevi are a group of disorders with raised, waxy, sometime verrucous nevi on the scalp or face that are associated with hemihypertrophy, hemimegaloencephaly, and neonatal seizures [38]. Sturge–Weber syndrome, characterized by a distinctive port-wine stain on the face with an associated vascular anomaly over the cortical surface, can manifest with neonatal seizures and is inherited sporadically.

Early infantile onset epilepsy syndromes have been described in the 1970s, by French neurologists who coined the term "fifth day fits" to describe benign neonatal convulsions [39]. These convulsions unexpectedly arose between the fourth and sixth days of life, usually were partial clonic, often with apnea and status epilepticus. More than half the neonates seen with this diagnosis had distinctive bursts of cerebral activity in the discontinuous part of the record, showing sharply contoured theta waves especially in the central regions, which can also be seen in patients with hypoxic ischemic encephalopathy.

Another early-onset epilepsy syndrome, and the first idiopathic epilepsy syndrome to be caused by a single gene mutation, is benign familial neonatal convulsions (BFNC). By the third day of life, neonates with this disorder have partial seizures. Of these patients, 10–15% will go on to have epilepsy later in life [40]. There are three known genetic defects that are responsible for this syndrome. BNFC type 1 has a defective *KCNQ2* gene at chromosome 20q13.3 with an aberrant alpha-subunit of a voltage-gated potassium channel. BNFC type II has a defective *KCNQ3* gene at chromosome 8q24, which also is responsible for coding an aberrant alpha-subunit of a voltage-gated potassium channel. The third type of BNFC with myokymia has been reported as a separate mutation of *KCNQ2*, also at chromosome 20q13.3 [41]. There are some so-called benign familial neonatal-infantile seizures that typically appear in the first year of life, and present with neonatal seizures. These are associated with an aberrant *SCN2A* gene, located on chromosome 2q24, that encodes a defective alpha-subunit of a voltage-gated sodium channel [42].

Migrating partial seizures of infancy comprise another entity that may be seen in the neonatal period, characterized by unprovoked, alternating electroclinical seizures, and associated with neurodevelopmental devastation [43]. Although multifocal neonatal seizures are not uncommon after infections, metabolic disorders, and hypoxia-ischemia, they can also accompany cerebral dysgenesis and some other neonatal seizure syndromes. In migrating partial seizures of infancy, healthy infants without cerebral dysplasia display multifocal partial seizures that arise independently and sequentially from both hemispheres within the first 6 months of life and progress to become intractable, ultimately leading to severe psychomotor retardation. Prognosis has been described as poor, with 28% mortality and the majority of survivors being profoundly retarded and non-ambulatory.

Early myoclonic epilepsy (EME) is characterized by maternal reports of the fetus repeatedly kicking in rhythmic fashion, with oligohydramnios or polyhydramnios, normal Apgar scores, and seizures appearing anywhere from the first day of life through several months, but typically around age 16 days. Erratic myoclonic activity, massive myoclonia, stimulus-sensitive myoclonia, and partial seizures may be present. The EEG is usually markedly abnormal, with a burst-suppression background. Patients are completely resistant to antiepileptic medications. Progressive decline in head circumference percentiles, bulbar signs (especially apnea), feeding difficulties, cleft or high-arched palate, and severe psychomotor delay may be seen. Progressive cerebral atrophy may be seen on neuroimaging scans [44].

Early infantile epileptic encephalopathy (EIEE), also known as Ohtahara syndrome, is characterized by intractable tonic seizures in the setting of severe encephalopathy and a burst-suppression background on EEG. The EEG findings appear similar to EME, and possibly these two entities represent a spectrum of disease [45]. Many of these patients have overt cerebral dysgenesis or cortical dysplasias. Survivors often have typical infantile spasms with hypsarrythmia, and progress to Lennox–Gastaut syndrome with multifocal spikes on EEG.

18.9 Treatment

Despite decades of neonatal seizure recognition, treatment recommendations rest almost entirely on traditional practices. Antiepileptic medications should be used to treat seizures of epileptic origin, and because of this, initial consideration is given to the clinical presentation and the EEG features of these specific clinical events. Should treatment of all seizures, however brief, be attempted? The answer to this question is not obvious as many neonatal seizures have ended by the time medication is administered. If frequency is low the value of prophylaxis must be weighed against the potential toxicity of the agent. However, epileptic seizures occurring during the neonatal period that are long, frequent, and not self-limiting should be rapidly and aggressively controlled with antiepileptic medications.

To date, studies do not demonstrate unequivocally the efficacy of barbiturates in the prevention of neonatal seizures due to hypoxic ischemic insult. In one study, high doses of phenobarbital given after perinatal asphyxia resulted in a lower rate of recurrent seizures compared with placebo, although the difference between treatment and placebo was not shown to be statistically significant [46]. In contrast, in another smaller study, prophylactic treatment using phenobarbital was evaluated in neonates with seizures secondary to perinatal asphyxia and resulted in a statistically significant decrease in the incidence of neonatal seizures [47]. However, there was a lack of EEG evidence for seizures. In another study of 31 neonates using EEG and clinical evidence of seizure, treatment with phenobarbital resulted in only two infants having complete cessation of EEG and clinical seizures (13 had clinical seizure arrest, but continued having electrographic seizures, while the remainder continued having seizures both clinically and on the EEG) [48].

A comparative efficacy study for the treatment of neonatal seizures using phenobarbital and phenytoin showed that 43% of the neonates given phenobarbital stopped seizing, and 45% of those given phenytoin stopped seizing, but there was no placebo control group to determine absolute efficacy [49]. According to a recent Cochrane review, at the present time anticonvulsant administration in the immediate period following perinatal asphyxia cannot be recommended for routine clinical practice, other than in the treatment of prolonged or frequent clinical seizures, and there is little evidence from randomized controlled trials to support the use of any of the anticonvulsants currently used in the neonatal period [50]. Anecdotal experiences of using intravenous levetiracetam in neonatal intensive care units has been described, and Ng and colleagues showed safety and efficacy down to the 6-month age range [51].

Despite the frequent empirical selection of phenobarbital in clinical practice for the treatment of neonatal seizures, evidence of its efficacy is limited, and animal studies raise the concern that phenobarbital itself may have deleterious effects on the developing nervous system. The National Institutes of Health and the US Food and Drug Administration jointly recommended the development of a newborn drug development initiative, fostering ethical, well-controlled trials of pharmaceutical agents used in neonatal neurology, cardiology, anesthesia, pain management, and related disorders, as they recognized that few drugs have undergone adequately powered, randomized, placebo-controlled investigations to demonstrate safety and efficacy. Drugs with potential for the treatment of neonatal seizures are no exception.

In clinical practice it is common to administer anticonvulsant medication in an effort to reduce or eliminate seizures in the newborn. Studies have been done with a phenobarbital loading dose of 15–20 mg/kg (aiming for serum levels of 15–20 μg/mL), followed by maintenance doses of 3–4 mg/kg/day.

When using fosphenytoin or phenytoin in the neonatal period, a level of 25–30 μg/mL should be the target goal. Phenytoin has complex pharmacokinetics. The enzymatic pathways through which it is metabolized become saturated unpredictably resulting in a switch from zero-order to first-order kinetics. Moreover, there are also variable rates of metabolism in the neonatal period, including decreases in the hepatic metabolism elimination rates during the first weeks of life. It is highly bound to plasma protein and the effective concentration can be affected either through displacement by other agents or by variations in serum albumin concentration. It is a powerful inducer of its own metabolism, and this may be induced by other co-administered drugs, for example, barbiturates. Phenytoin should be given by direct intravenous infusion no faster than 1 mg/kg/min. Excessively rapid administration of high concentrations can result in serious cardiac arrhythmias. Phenytoin is strongly alkaline and may lead to local venous thrombosis. Extravasation can cause severe tissue burn damage. Using fosphenytoin reduces this risk.

While phenobarbital remains first-line therapy for neonatal seizures, there is some debate about second-line therapy. In two surveys of pediatric epileptologists in the United States and Europe, phenobarbital was identified as the treatment of choice, while intravenous benzodiazepines and fosphenytoin or phenytoin were also considered first-line therapy [52]. In a review of five neonatal intensive care units in the United States, phenobarbital was the most common first-line anticonvulsant medication, followed by lorazepam and phenytoin. Second-line therapy after treatment failure to the first was most frequently lorazepam, phenytoin, and phenobarbital.

Benzodiazepines, typically lorazepam (0.15 mg/kg) and diazepam (0.3 mg/kg), can be effective therapies. Side effects of acute administration include hypotension and respiratory depression. Alternative or adjuvant anticonvulsant medications have also been empirically prescribed for refractory neonatal seizures [53]. Clonazepam, lidocaine, and midazolam are administered intravenously. Carbamazepine, primidone, valproate, vigabatrin, and lamotrigine have been given orally [54–59].

Administration of anticonvulsant medications may terminate the clinical manifestations of the seizure while the electrographic discharge continues. This disconnect is termed uncoupling and poses serious concerns for the clinician and researchers in determining response rates for different anticonvulsant medications. Scher and colleagues found that 58% of patients continued to have electrographic seizures after administration of antiepileptic medication had stopped their clinical event [60]. This may be explained by the maturational switch in the neonatal period from NKCC1 to NKCC2, allowing medications to be more effective against brainstem and spinal cord neurons before more rostral structures. The relatively high rates of uncoupling stress the importance of EEG documentation of resolution of neonatal seizures.

18.10 Chronic postnatal epilepsy and the need for long-term treatment

Chronic postnatal epilepsy may occur following neonatal seizures. For many patients, permanent fixed brain injuries, such as resolving stroke, ischemia, or traumatic lesions, serve as the nidus for future epilepsy. Repeated neonatal seizures may have "instructed" the brain how to have future seizures, resulting in a persistent lowering of the seizure threshold and the development of chronic epilepsy. Neonatal seizures may represent the beginning of very early onset epilepsy, which persists. The most common occurrence, however, is epilepsy after neonatal seizures that are triggered by acute neonatal conditions. Approximately 20% of survivors of neonatal seizures experienced one or more seizures up to 7 years of age, nearly two-thirds of the seizures occurred within the first 6 months of life [61]. Other researchers have reported rates ranging from 17% to 30%. Partial and generalized seizures characterize postneonatal epilepsy and do not seem to be preventable by the long-term administration of antiepileptic medication after neonatal seizures. Not all neonates require extended therapy after acute seizures have been controlled, although no criteria for long-term maintenance antiepileptic medication use have been sufficiently studied. For chronic therapy, phenobarbital 3–4 mg/kg/day is given and serum levels are monitored. Reported schedules for discontinuation of maintenance therapy range from 1 week to 12 months after the last seizure, one being withdrawal of antiepileptic medications 2 weeks after the last seizure [62].

18.11 Potential adverse effects of antiepileptic drugs on the immature CNS

Antiepileptic medications prevent or interrupt electrographic seizures by the blockade of voltage-dependent sodium channels and glutamatergic excitatory neurotransmission and enhancment of GABA-mediated inhibition. However, at this critical time of early brain development, suppression of synaptic transmission may have incidental undesirable consequences, because neuronal and synaptic pruning are activity dependent. Since the 1970s, it has been demonstrated in rat models that phenobarbital-treated rats have reductions in brain weight and in total brain cell count. How antiepileptic medications may harm the developing rat brain remains under investigation, but evidence suggests that these drugs may cause apoptotic neurodegeneration in the forebrain and suppress an endogenous neuroprotective system already in place [63]. The clinical impact of these findings is less certain. Most neonates are given phenobarbital to treat seizures, and it is difficult to determine how much of any long-term aftermath is the result of the seizures' underlying etiology, the attacks themselves, or the medications administered to stop or suppress them. Some neonates receive phenobarbital for other reasons, such as to provide sedation or to accelerate hepatic maturity in neonatal hyperbilirubinemia and appear to experience no ill effects. Likewise benzodiazepines are commonly administered for sedation or to reduce agitation, and no obvious adverse effects are associated with their use, although careful studies are currently lacking.

18.12 Conclusion

Neonatal seizures are significant events that occur in the neonatal period. Careful physical examination, thorough history, laboratory testing, and imaging will typically reveal the etiology of seizures, and guide treatment. Seizures can be either acute or chronic, and neonates may or may not benefit from treatment; some may have an early-onset epilepsy syndrome. The data are equivocal on whether or not treatment should be initiated, and this decision rests entirely on length and frequency of the seizures; typically treatment includes phenobarbital or fosphenytoin. However, more studies need to be done regarding treatment, as newer medications have been produced in intravenous formulations but not tested in the neonate. Finally, outcomes for neonates who experience seizures also vary depending on etiology, severity, and frequency.

References

[1] Ronen G, Penney S. The epidemiology of clinical neonatal seizures in Newfoundland, Canada. *Ann Neurol* 1995;**38**:518–519.

[2] Lanska MJ, Lanska DJ, Baumann RJ, *et al.* A population based study of neonatal seizures in Fayette County, Kentucky. *Neurology* 1995;**45**:724–732.

[3] Scher M, Aso K, Beggarly M, *et al.* Electrographic seizures in preterm and full-term neonates: clinical correlates, associated brain lesions and risk for neurologic sequelae. *Pediatrics* 1993;**91**:128–134.

[4] Johnston MV. Selective vulnerability in the neonatal brain. *Ann Neurol* 1998;**44**:155–156.

[5] Zhang G, Hsu FC, Raol YH, *et al.* Selective alterations of GABA A receptor subunit expression and function in hippocampal dentate granule cells after seizures in the developing brain. *Epilepsia* 2001;**42**:224.

[6] Staley K. Enhancement of the excitatory actions of GABA by barbiturates and benzodiazepines. *Neurosci Lett* 1992;**146**:105–107.

[7] Dzhala VI, Talos DM, Sdrulla DA, *et al.* NKCC1 transporter facilitates seizures in the developing brain. *Nat Med* 2005;**11**:1205–1213.

[8] Dzhala VI, Brumback AC, Stale KJ. Bumetanide enhances phenobarbital efficacy in a neonatal seizure model. *Ann Neurol* 2008;**63**:222–235.

[9] Silverstein FS, Jensen FE. Neonatal seizures. *Ann Neurol* 2007;**62**:112–120.

[10] Temple CM, Dennis J, Carney R, *et al.* Neonatal seizures: long-term outcome and cognitive development among "normal" survivors. *Dev Med Child Neurol* 1995;**37**:109–118.

[11] Ortibus EL, Sum JM, Hahn JS. Predictive value of EEG for outcome and epilepsy following neonatal seizures. *Electroencephalogr Clin Neurophysiol* 1996;**98**:175–185.

[12] Mizrahi EM, Clancy R, Dunn JK, *et al.* Neurologic impairment, developmental delay and post-natal seizures two years after video-EEG documented seizures in near-term and full-term neonates: report of the Clinical Research Centers for Neonatal Seizures. [Abstract]. *Epilepsia* 2001;**102**:47.

[13] Legido A, Clancy RR, Berman PH. Neurologic outcome after electroencephalographically proven neonatal seizures. *Pediatrics* 1991;**88**:583–596.

[14] Holmes FL, Gairsa JL, Chevassus-Au-Louis N, *et al.* Consequences of neonatal seizures in the rat: morphological and behavioral effects. *Ann Neurol* 1998;**44**:845–857.

[15] Sanchez RM, Koh S, Rio C, *et al.* Decreased glutamate receptor 2 expression and enhanced epileptogenesis in immature rat hippocampus after perinatal hypoxia-induced seizures. *J Neurosc* 2001;**21**:975–991.

[16] Sankar R, Painter MJ. Neonatal seizures: after all of these years we still love what doesn't work. *Neurology* 2005;**64**:776–777.

[17] Raol YH, Lund IV, Bandyopadhyay S, *et al.* Enhancing GABA A receptor α1 subunit levels in hippocampal dentate gyrus inhibits epilepsy development in an animal model of temporal lobe epilepsy. *J Neurosci* 2006;**26**:11342–11346.

[18] Clancy RR, Legido A. The exact ictal and interictal duration of electroencephalographic neonatal seizures. *Epilepsia* 1987;**28**:537–541.

[19] Watanabe K, Hara K, Miyazaki S. Electroclinical studies of seizures in the newborn. *Folia Psychiatr Neurol Jpn* 1977;**31**:383–392.

[20] Laroia N, Guillet R, Burchfiel J, *et al.* EEG background as predictor of electrographic seizures in high-risk neonates. *Epilepsia* 1998;**39**:545–551.

[21] Clancy R, Bergqvist AC, Dlugos D. Neonatal electroencephalography. *Curr Pract Clin EEG* 2003;160–234.

[22] Mizrahi EM, Kellaway P. *Diagnosis and Management of Neonatal Seizures*. Philadelphia: Lippincott-Raven, 1998.

[23] Knauss T, Carlson C. Neonatal paroxysmal monorhythmic alpha activity. *Arch Neurol* 1978;**35**:104–107.

[24] Mizrahi EM. Neonatal seizures: problems in diagnosis and classification. *Epilepsia* 1987;**28**:546–555.

[25] Bye AM, Flanagan D. Spatial and temporal characteristics of neonatal seizures. *Epilepsia* 1995;**36**:1009–1016.

[26] ACOG Task Force on Neonatal Encephalopathy and Cerebral Palsy. Neonatal Encephalopathy and Cerebral Palsy: Defining the Pathogenesis and Pathophysiology. Washington, DC: American College of Obstetricians and Gynecologists, 2002; pp. 73–80.

[27] DeVeber G, Andrew M, Canadian Pediatric Ischemic Stroke Study Group. Cerebral sinovenous thrombosis in children. *N Engl J Med* 2001;**345**:417–423.

[28] Wasay M, Dai AI, Ansari M, *et al.* Cerebral venous sinus thrombosis in children; a multicenter cohort from the United States. *J Child Neurol* 2008;**23**:23–31.

[29] Clancy R. The neurology of hypoplastic left heart syndrome. In: Rychi J, Wenovsky G (eds), *The Hypoplastic Left Heart Syndrome*. Boston: Kluwer Academic, 2003; pp. 251–273.

[30] Clancy RR, McGaurn S, Wernovsky G, *et al.* Risk of seizures in survivors of newborn heart surgery using deep hypothermic circulatory arrest. *Pediatrics* 2001;**111**:592–601.

[31] Maher F, Vannucci S, Simpson I. Glucose transporter proteins in the brain. *FASEB J* 1994;**8**:1003–1011.

[32] Clancy R, Chung HJ. EEG changes during recovery from acute severe neonatal citrullinemia. *Electroencephalogr Clin Neurophysiol* 1991;**78**:222–227.

[33] Mills PB, Struys E, Jakob C, *et al.* Mutation in antiquitin in individuals with pyridoxine-dependent seizures. *Nat Med* 2006;**12**:307–309.

[34] Gallagher RC, Van Hove JL, Scharer G, *et al.* Folinic-acid responsive seizures are identical to pyridoxine-dependent epilepsy. *Ann Neurol* 2009;**65**:550–556.

[35] Stallmeyer B, Schwartz G, Sculze J, *et al.* The neurotransmitter receptor-anchoring protein gephyrin reconstitutes molybdenum cofactor biosynthesis in bacteria, plants and mammalian cells. *Proc Natl Acad Sci USA* 1998;**96**:1333–1338.

[36] Tharp BR. Neonatal seizures and syndromes. *Epilepsia* 2002;**43**:2–10.

[37] Hayward JC, Titelbaum D, Clancy R, *et al.* Lissencephaly-pachygyria associated with congenital cytomegalovirus infection. *J Child Neurol* 1991;**6**:109.

[38] Clancy R, Kurtz M, Baker D. Neurological manifestations of the organoid nevus syndrome. *Arch Neurol* 1985;**42**:236–240.

[39] Dehan M, Navelet Y, d'Allest AM, *et al.* Quelques precisions sur le syndrome des convulsions du cinquième jour de vie. *Arch Fr Pediatr* 1982;**39**:405–407.

[40] George AJ. Molecular basis of inherited epilepsy. *Arch Neurol* 2004;**61**:473–478.

[41] Dedek K, Kunath B, Kananura C, *et al.* Myokymia and neonatal epilepsy caused by a mutation in the voltage sensor of the KCNQ2 K^+ channel. *Proc Natl Acad Sci USA* 2001;**98**:12272–12277.

[42] Herlenius E, Heron SE, Grinton BE, *et al.* SCN2A mutations and benign familial neonatal-infantile seizures: the phenotypic spectrum. *Epilepsia* 2007;**48**:1138–1142.

[43] Coppola G, Plouin P, Chiron C, *et al.* Migrating partial seizures in infancy: a malignant disorder with developmental arrest. *Epilepsia* 1995;**36**:1017–1024.

[44] Clancy R, Chung HJ, Hayward JC, *et al.* Early myoclonic epileptic encephalopathy. *Ann Neurol* 1990;**28**:472–473.

[45] Djukic A, Lado FA, Shinnar S, *et al.* Are early myoclonic encephalopathy (EME) and the Ohtahara syndrome (EIEE) independent of each other? *Epilepsy Res* 2006;**70**:68–76.

[46] Hall RT, Hall FK, Daily DK. High-dose phenobarbital therapy in term newborn infants with severe perinatal asphyxia: a randomized, prospective study with three-year follow-up. *J Pediatr* 1998;**132**:345–348.

[47] Singh D, Kumar P, Narang A. A randomized controlled trial of phenobarbital in neonates with hypoxic ischemic encephalopathy. *J Matern Fetal Neonatal Med* 2005;**18**:391–395.

[48] Connell J, Oozeer R, de Vries L, *et al.* Clinical and EEG response to anticonvulsants in neonatal seizures. *Arch Dis Child* 1989;**64**:459–464.

[49] Painter MJ, Scher MS, Stein AD, *et al.* Phenobarbital compared with phenytoin for the treatment of neonatal seizures. *N Engl J Med* 1999;**341**:485–489.

[50] Booth D, Evans DJ. Anticonvulsants for neonates with seizures. *Cochrane Database Syst Rev* 2004;(3):CD004218.

[51] Ng YT, Hastriter EV, Cardenas JF, Khoury EM, Chapman KE. Intravenous levetiracetam in children with seizures: a prospective safety study. *J Child Neurol* 2010;**25**:551–555.

[52] Wheless JW, Clarke DF, Carpenter D. Treatment of pediatric epilepsy: expert opinion. *J Child Neurol* 2005;**20**:S1–S56.

[53] Bartha AI, Shen J, Katz KH, *et al.* Neonatal seizures: multicenter variability in current treatment practices. *Pediatr Neurol* 2007;**37**:85–90.

[54] Hellstrom-Westas L, Westgren U, Rosen I, *et al.* Lidocaine for the treatment of severe seizures in newborn infants, I: clinical effects and cerebral electrical activity monitoring. *Acta Paediatr Scand* 1988;**77**:79–84.

[55] Macintosh D, Baird-Lampert J. Is carbamazepine an alternative maintenance therapy for neonatal seizures? *Dev Pharmacol Ther* 1987;**10**:100–106.

[56] Sapin J, Riviello JJ, Grover W. Efficacy of primidone for seizure control in neonates and young infants. *Pediatr Neurol* 1988;**4**:292–295.

[57] Gal P, Otis K, Gilman J, *et al.* Valproic acid efficacy, toxicity and pharmacokinetics in neonates with intractable seizures. *Neurology* 1988;**38**:467–471.

[58] Aicardi J, Mumford J, Dumas C. Vigabatrin as initial therapy for infantile spasms: a European retrospective study. *Epilepsia* 1996;**37**:638–642.

[59] Barr P, Buettiker V, Anthony J. Efficacy of lamotrigine in refractory neonatal seizures. *Pediatr Neurol.* 1999;**20**:161–163.

[60] Scher MS, Alvin J, Gaus L, *et al.* Uncoupling of EEG-clinical neonatal seizures after antiepileptic drug use. *Pediatri Neurol* 2003;**28**:277–280.

[61] Ellenberg JH, Hirtz D, Nelson KB. Age at onset of seizures in young children. *Ann Neurol* 1984;**15**:127–134.

[62] Fenichel G. Paroxysmal disorders. In: *Clinical Pediatric Neurology*, 3rd edn. Philadelphia: WB Saunders, 2001; pp. 1–45.

[63] Bittigau P, Sifringer M, Genz K. Antiepileptic drugs and apoptotic neurodegeneration in the developing brain. *Proc Natl Acad Sci USA* 2002;**99**:15089–15094.

19 Febrile seizures

Marie Francisca Grill

Department of Neurology, University of California San Francisco, San Francisco General Hospital, San Francisco, CA, USA

19.1 Introduction

Febrile seizures represent the most common pediatric seizure disorder and occur in an estimated 2–5% of children [1]. Given their frequency, it is essential for the practitioner to understand the clinical presentation and to be aware of the workup and management recommendations and controversies. Knowledge regarding febrile seizures, like other epilepsy syndromes, has evolved with continuing advancements in the field of genetics as there has been increasing identification of genes linked with febrile seizure syndromes. In this chapter we will discuss febrile seizure etiology, presentation, management, and prognostic implications, in addition to related epilepsy syndromes.

19.2 Definition

According to the International League Against Epilepsy (ILAE), a febrile seizure is defined as "a seizure occurring in childhood after one month of age, associated with a febrile illness not caused by an infection of the central nervous system, without previous neonatal seizures

Epilepsy in Children and Adolescents, First Edition. Edited by James W. Wheless.

or a previous unprovoked seizure, and not meeting criteria for other acute asymptomatic seizures" [2]. This definition does not specify the degree of hyperthermia. Febrile seizures can fall into one of two groups – simple febrile seizures or complex febrile seizures – based on seizure phenotype, duration, and frequency. Simple febrile seizures refer to those febrile seizures that lack any focal features (e.g., are generalized), resolve spontaneously within less than 10 minutes, and do not occur more that once within a 24-hour period [3]. In contrast, complex febrile seizures are those that have evidence of focality, last longer than 10–15 minutes, or are recurrent within a 24-hour period [4]. An estimated 70–75% of febrile seizures are simple whereas 9–35% meet the criteria for a complex febrile seizure [5,6]. The majority of febrile seizures are tonic or tonic-clonic in their semiology, although atonic seizures sometimes occur [7]. However, as we will see throughout this chapter, this simplified dichotomous classification may not tell the whole story as a composition of factors should be considered when deciding how to counsel parents on significance and prognosis.

19.3 Incidence and prevalence

Population studies show that the incidence and prevalence of febrile seizures may vary geographically, with Guam having an estimated cumulative incidence of 14% of children (in contrast to the 2–5% of children in the United States) [8]. In the United States, an estimated 500 000 febrile seizures occur annually [9]. Recent receipt of pediatric vaccinations (such as measles, mumps, and rubella (MMR) and diphtheria-tetanus-whole cell pertussis (DTP)), viral infections (including influenza A, human herpesvirus 6, and metapneumovirus), developmental delay, daycare attendance, and family history of febrile and afebrile seizures have all been associated with the occurrence of an initial febrile seizure [10].

19.4 Pathophysiology

There are multiple theories as to the underlying pathophysiological mechanism of a febrile seizure. An increase in brain temperature itself has been shown to be associated with fevers in children via perturbation of temperature-sensitive ion channels, which subsequently alters neuronal firing resulting in the synchronous neuronal discharge characteristic of a seizure [11]. Interleukin-1β (IL-1β) has also been implicated as this inflammatory cytokine acts as both pyrogen and seizure provocator, in the latter case by acting on both glutamate and GABA (gamma-aminobutyric acid) pathways to increase neuronal excitability. Generation of fever has been shown to result in synthesis of IL-1β specifically within the hippocampus [12,13]. Another postulated mechanism is that hyperthermia-induced brain alkalosis results in neuronal excitability thus leading to seizures in models in which there is a prolonged latency between fever and seizure onset (e.g., 30 minutes), though not all syndromes associated with alkalosis lead to clinical seizures [14]. In addition, genetic factors likely play a significant role in febrile seizure development and are discussed later in the genetics section of this chapter.

19.5 Prognosis

While the majority of febrile seizures occur in isolation, they recur at an estimated rate of 1 in every 3 children, with half of these children going on to have multiple recurrences. The age at which the initial febrile seizure occurs appears to impact recurrence rate as those children whose initial febrile seizure occurs at less than 1 year of age have a recurrence rate as high as 50% [15]. Predictors of recurrent febrile seizures also include family history of febrile seizures, focal and prolonged initial seizure, temperature greater than 40°C at time of seizure, and influenza A viral infection [10]. Recurrence rates can be cited based on number of risk factors, as follows:

- low: 10% recurrence risk over an 18-month period in children with no risk factors;
- intermediate: 25–50% recurrence risk in children with one to two risk factors;
- elevated: 50–100% recurrence risk in those with three or more risk factors [16].

In one cohort study comprising 1706 children with febrile seizures, approximately 8% of those with a simple febrile seizure later developed a complex febrile seizure by the age of 7 years. This risk increased in those with recurrent febrile seizures; for example, the risk of complex seizure increased with each additional febrile recurrence, though the overall risk of any recurrent febrile event was the same whether the initial event was simple or complex [14].

Another study prospectively analyzed 428 children with first febrile seizure to evaluate predictors of recurrent unprovoked seizures. A total of 26 children (6.1%) had at least one unprovoked event: half had only one, the other half had more than one recurrent seizure meeting the criteria for epilepsy. Of these, 8 had partial-onset and 18 had generalized-onset seizures. In this study, the main predictors for recurrence of unprovoked seizures were neurodevelopmental abnormalities, complex febrile seizures (with stronger association when multiple complex features were present in recurrent febrile seizures with no single complex feature more predictive than any other), recurrent febrile seizures (with an increasing risk with increasing frequency of recurrence), and duration of recognized fever, the latter showing an increased risk of unprovoked seizures in those with briefer duration of fever. While a family history of epilepsy and febrile seizures is a recognized risk factor for recurrent febrile events, there was no significant association in this study with subsequent unprovoked events. No consistent association was found between subsequent unprovoked seizures and the degree of temperature elevation, age, gender, or racial background. The study authors made the point of concluding that the role of complex features is not clearly understood and agreeing that unprovoked seizures are still the exception rather than the rule, and that not treating these patients is an appropriate approach given the low incidence of future unprovoked seizures and the lack of evidence demonstrating that preventive treatment with antiepileptic drugs has any effect in altering this risk of subsequent epilepsy [4].

19.6 Initial evaluation and management

Most children with febrile seizures are initially evaluated in the emergency department and are usually not seizing by the time they arrive. As with any seizure or similar emergency, the first steps of evaluation should include checking the ABCs of the child: airway, breathing, and circulation. That being said, since most seizures have ceased prior to arrival, most children do not require airway support with the exception of occasional mild respiratory support during the postictal period. If the child is still seizing upon emergency medical services (EMS) arrival to the home or the emergency department, benzodiazepines are generally used as first-line therapy, frequently by the rectal route. As a general rule, it is agreed that any seizure lasting more than 5 minutes should be treated [17]. Should the seizure persist, increasing amounts of benzodiazepines may be required and respiratory status should be closely monitored. If the seizure still fails to abort and the patient is in status epilepticus, using an operational definition of continuous seizure activity for more than 10 minutes or a cluster of shorter events without returning to baseline in between, then status epilepticus treatment protocol should be followed. Again, the overwhelming majority of febrile seizures will have terminated spontaneously prior to initial evaluation in the emergency department, thus such action is not necessary for the majority of children presenting with a febrile seizure. A thorough history should be taken to include symptoms of febrile illness or symptoms to suggest meningitis/encephalitis, an antecedent toxic or traumatic event that may have triggered the seizure, a history of prior neurological disorder or developmental delay, and any personal or family histories of prior afebrile and febrile seizures. Other historical points of interest include recent immunization, sick contacts, and daycare attendance.

Physical examination should be performed to include evaluation of signs indicative of underlying febrile illness as well as neurological evaluation to look for any localizing signs that would suggest an underlying focal abnormality of the central nervous system. This should specifically include ruling out any evidence of increased cranial pressure (i.e., worsening mental status, papilledema, or cranial nerve palsies) or focal signs such as Todd's paralysis (i.e., asymmetry on motor examination). Examination should also include skin survey to rule out any neurocutaneous stigmata that may suggest an underlying neurological disorder with predisposition for seizures. Any decline in general or neurological examination is suggestive of a more malignant underlying infectious, metabolic, or structural process, and more aggressive workup such as neuroimaging and lumbar puncture is indicated [18].

American Academy of Pediatrics (AAP) practice parameters have been published giving recommendations for the evaluation of a child with a first-time febrile seizure. It should be noted that these guidelines apply only in the case of a simple febrile seizure, if the child is between the ages of 6 months and 5 years, and if the child presents within 12 hours of the seizure. Lumbar puncture should be strongly considered for patients under 12 months of age since there are often few or no clinical signs or symptoms of meningitis on examination in this specific age group. For similar reasons, lumbar puncture should be at least considered in children 12 to 18 months of age. Finally, lumbar puncture is not routinely recommended in children older than 18 months of age unless they exhibit signs of meningeal irritation on examination or have a history or other neurological exam feature suggestive of intracranial infection [19]. That being said, the AAP committee also added that "because this practice parameter is for practitioners with a wide range of training and experience, the committee chose a conservative approach with an emphasis on the value of lumbar puncture in diagnosing meningitis," so the experienced child neurologist may feel more comfortable about ascertaining when a lumbar puncture is or is not necessary. Another special consideration is the child who has received antibiotics prior to seizure presentation; in this case, lumbar puncture should strongly be considered as antibiotic treatment could mask some of the clinical signs and symptoms of meningitis.

Given the lack of published evidence for the therapeutic and prognostic information afforded by obtaining an electroencephalogram (EEG), this electrodiagnostic test is not recommended either on initial evaluation or on follow-up within the subsequent month for an otherwise healthy child presenting with an initial simple febrile seizure. While there is a reported increase in abnormal EEGs if the study is obtained after some delay following the event, there are no data to show that any prognostic value is gained even if abnormalities are detected. In addition, routine use of neuroimaging in the diagnostic workup of patients meeting the criteria for simple febrile seizures is not recommended.

Blood studies such as serum electrolytes, complete blood count (CBC), calcium, phosphorus, magnesium, or blood glucose not be routinely performed in these patients given the lack of evidence showing any benefit in ordering these tests. The consensus is that thorough and careful history-taking and physical examination should guide the practitioner in identifying metabolic perturbations such as dehydration. However, if obtundation persists in the postictal period, a blood glucose test is recommended. Laboratory studies should generally be guided by diagnostic proceedings for the underlying febrile illness rather than being included as a component of a routine workup for a simple febrile seizure. For example, a CBC may be helpful if there are concerns for bacteremia.

The literature regarding the management of complex febrile seizures is much more sparse; thus, those patients who do not meet criteria for the definition of simple febrile seizures frequently undergo a comprehensive evaluation including neuroimaging (magnetic resonance imaging (MRI) of the brain), lumbar puncture, and EEG, in addition to cultures and other related workup to evaluate potential sources of infection. Although in practice EEGs are routinely ordered in patients presenting with complex febrile seizures, there is no evidence that any knowledge is obtained regarding the risk of subsequent development of epilepsy. Similarly, despite lack of evidence showing that neuroimaging changes the management of these patients, computed tomography (CT) and/or MRI of the brain is frequently obtained for these patients.

A recently conducted retrospective cohort review looked specifically at the yield of lumbar puncture in pediatric patients presenting with their first complex febrile seizure. Of the 526 patients evaluated in the emergency department between 1995 and 2008, with a median age of 17 months (range 6 to 60 months), 340 (60%) underwent lumbar puncture to rule out acute bacterial meningitis. Only 14 patients demonstrated a pleocytosis within the cerebrospinal fluid (CSF), and of those, only three had acute bacterial meningitis. The two patients who grew *Streptococcus pneumoniae* in the CSF culture were clinically altered on presentation: one was non-responsive while the other was apneic and had a bulging fontanelle. The third patient was generally well-appearing and had a lumbar puncture "contaminated with blood" from which the CSF culture was ultimately negative, though blood culture was ultimately positive for *S. pneumoniae* so the child was empirically treated for bacterial meningitis for 14 days. Other interesting observations from this study included the fact that 90 children (17%) had a prior history of simple febrile seizures, 384 had one feature of complex febrile seizures (CFS), 122 had two features of CFS, and 10 had three features of CFS. The study authors concluded that "few patients who experienced a CFS had acute bacterial meningitis [ABM] in the absence of other signs or symptoms." Also of interest, 22 of the 28 patients who were intubated were apneic from anticonvulsant medications, while the remaining six were intubated due to respiratory distress from the seizure itself [20].

Antipyretics and other cooling measures have not been shown to be effective in either decreasing the occurrence of an initial febrile seizure or in preventing recurrent febrile seizures [19]. This was found to be the case whether antipyretics were given around the clock (i.e., every 4 hours) or whether given sporadically (i.e., based on when elevated temperature was detected on measurement). The lack of beneficial effect of antipyretic use was also independent of the medication used, for example, whether aspirin or acetaminophen (paracetamol).

Both acetaminophen and ibuprofen are generally considered safe and effective antipyretics, though both are associated with side effects if the recommended weight-based dose is exceeded (including hepatotoxicity or renal failure, respiratory failure, metabolic acidosis, and coma). In summary, antipyretics may be useful in treating a febrile illness but confer no additional benefit in the prevention of febrile seizures.

19.7 Long-term management

Management remains controversial when it comes to febrile seizures. In 1980, a National Institutes of Health (NIH) consensus statement was published regarding long-term management of children with seizures associated with fever. The committee stated that the risk of developing epilepsy was generally low with the exception of a high-risk group for which one study showed a 13% increased risk of epilepsy in patients with two of the following risk factors: family history of afebrile seizures, developmental delay or neurological dysfunction prior to the febrile seizure, and complex features of the febrile seizure. They also added that there was no evidence to support the use of long-term antiepileptic drugs to prevent subsequent development of epilepsy, but that antiepileptic medications *may* be considered in children with seizures lasting longer than 15 minutes, seizures that are focal in nature or followed by neurological abnormalities, and in children with a first-degree family history of afebrile seizures. They found no risk of mental or neurological impairment secondary to febrile seizures. Finally, they stressed the generally excellent prognosis associated with febrile seizures and emphasized parent education and counseling [21].

For those who do meet the aforementioned criteria of simple febrile seizure, the AAP says that given the risks and benefits of antiepileptic drug therapy, no medications, either continuous or intermittent, are recommended [19]. While evidence exists to show that intermittent therapy with diazepam and continuous therapy with anticonvulsants, specifically phenobarbital, primidone, and valproic acid, are effective in decreasing the recurrence of febrile seizures, the identified risks with use of these medications are felt to outweigh the potential benefits.

Based on the literature, the AAP outlines four potential theoretical negative outcomes that may be associated with febrile seizures and may be impacted by the use of antiepileptic medications. The first is intellectual decline, though two studies are cited showing that no difference in learning was observed in children (without prior neurological impairment) who experience febrile seizures compared with controls in children without prior neurological impairment. No studies have shown any behavioral problems, declines in IQ or academic performance, or any inattention that is thought to be secondary to febrile seizures in neurologically normal children. Nelson and Ellenberg reported that the increased risk of intellectual deficit occurred only in those children with febrile seizures who had pre-existing developmental delay or some other neurological disturbance [15]. A second theoretical consideration is the increased risk of epilepsy. For the majority of children who experience a febrile seizure, the risk of developing epilepsy by age 7 years is thought to be no greater than the 1% risk estimated for the general population. Exceptions to this are those children who are less than 1 year old at the time of their initial febrile seizure, those who have a family history of epilepsy, and those with multiple febrile seizures, as they are thought to have a 2.4% increased risk of developing epilepsy by the age of 25 years. A third theoretical consideration of untreated febrile seizures is the increased risk of recurrence. As previously discussed, patients whose initial febrile seizure occurs at an age less than 1 year have a higher risk of recurrence compared to children of other ages. A last consideration is the theoretical risk of death secondary to a seizure, which may be due to cardiac arrhythmia, respiratory failure/aspiration, or severe injury. No reports of death secondary to a simple febrile seizure are reported.

In a large cohort study of 1706 children with febrile seizures, seven (0.4%) developed hemiparesis consistent with postictal Todd's paralysis, and all had clinical resolution within 7 days. Thus, the risk of permanent hemiparesis is not considered to be a significant potential adverse consequence of febrile seizures [15].

Given these potential adverse risks, use of both intermittent and continuous antiepileptic drug prophylactic therapy has been at least considered. Phenobarbital has been reported to be effective in preventing the recurrence of simple febrile seizures as long as it is given daily and the drug level remains in the therapeutic range. Despite these results, an overall benefit of phenobarbital treatment was not appreciated due to high rates of non-compliance in at least one study [22]. Well-recognized adverse effects secondary to phenobarbital include behavioral changes such as lethargy, irritability, hyperactivity, and sleep disturbances, as well as acute hypersensitivity reactions such as Stevens–Johnson syndrome, and liver dysfunction. In addition, there may be a lasting effect on neuropsychological function with use of phenobarbital, which may persist despite discontinuation of the medication. Results of studies investigating the use of primidone and valproic acid showed that while these drugs were effective in reducing the risk of recurrent febrile seizures, they both were also associated with adverse effects, including risks of pancreatitis, gastrointestinal dysfunction, thrombocytopenia, weight disturbances, and fatal hepatitis (particularly in children less than 2 years of age). Both phenytoin and carbamazepine were not found to be effective in reducing the risk of recurrent febrile seizures, while other antiepileptic drugs have not been specifically studied in this population.

Diazepam has been evaluated specifically for intermittent use in the prevention of recurrence of febrile seizures. The literature includes a double-blinded placebo-controlled study in which children who had a prior febrile seizure were given 0.33 mg/kg of oral diazepam every 8 hours for 48 hours or a placebo when fever was detected. A 44% decrease in the risk of recurrent febrile seizures per person-year was detected by intention-to-treat analysis. While the use of diazepam in interrupting simple febrile seizures lasting less than 5 minutes has been found to be effective in the short term at aborting the febrile seizure, no difference has been found in long-term febrile seizure recurrence. Finally, benzodiazepines such as diazepam also have their respective potential adverse effects including drowsiness, ataxia, and respiratory depression. One concern is that use of these benzodiazepines may lead others to incorrectly implicate the medication as the source of subsequent lethargy, therein masking the symptoms of an underlying febrile illness (i.e., meningitis). It also seems that some of the lack of efficacy with this intermittent therapy found in prior studies was due to significant non-compliance, the use of low and presumed ineffective doses of diazepam, and the use of a very-low-risk study sample. Some investigators have concluded that in spite of conflicting evidence in the literature, for those with an increased risk of febrile seizure recurrence, intermittent use of diazepam for prophylaxis may be justified in those children thought to be at higher risk of recurrence. The suggested dose is 0.3–0.5 mg/kg administered orally or rectally whenever the rectal temperature is greater than 38.5°C, with no more than four consecutive doses [7].

After performing a comprehensive review of previously published peer-reviewed literature, it is concluded that except in a select group with a high rate of seizure recurrence, the other events have a low likelihood of occurring thus failing to justify the use of prophylactic medications. The risk of developing epilepsy is thought to be increased relative to the general pediatric population, but this remains low for those patients who have a simple febrile seizure. The practice parameters also state that there are no data to suggest that prophylactic treatment of these children would have an impact on this risk since the risk of future epilepsy is more likely to be genetically based rather than secondary to any structural brain damage resulting from simple febrile seizures themselves [23]. The general consensus is that while febrile seizures are not infrequent events, most children are expected to have an excellent prognosis.

An estimated 3% of children with febrile seizures go on to develop epilepsy [24]. The Rochester study found that the risk of subsequent development of epilepsy was 2.4% for children with simple febrile seizures, 6–8% for children with one complex feature, 17–22% for children with two complex features, and 49% for children with all three features [25]. In the British Child Health and Education Study (CHES) cohort, 13 of 382 children (3.4%) later developed afebrile seizures, while only 1.6% of the total developed an epilepsy syndrome consisting of complex partial seizures. This cohort study paralleled the Rochester study in demonstrating that the subsequent development of epilepsy more often occurred in children fitting diagnostic criteria for a complex febrile seizure (6.3% in this case) compared to those diagnosed with a simple febrile seizure (1.0%). Of those with complex febrile seizures, the children with the highest risk of future epilepsy were specifically those with prolonged seizures (9.4%) and those with focal seizure semiology (29.0%) [24]. Generalized idiopathic epilepsy with tonic-clonic seizures is the most common type in children who do go on to develop epilepsy. Genetic advances have increased awareness regarding syndromes of both febrile and afebrile seizure types, for example, generalized epilepsy with febrile seizures plus (GEFS+). There are also rare reports of recurrent febrile seizures preceding the onset of severe myoclonic epilepsy (Dravet syndrome).

There have been conflicting studies regarding the association of prolonged febrile seizures with subsequent development of mesial temporal sclerosis and temporal lobe epilepsy, and this remains a controversial issue. While the typical febrile seizure is generalized, it is plausible that temporal-lobe localizing features such as altered consciousness or behavior arrest may go unnoticed. Another argument for this possible relationship is that the limbic system is the region of the brain most susceptible to seizures. One hospital-based study found that none of the 289 children with febrile seizures had developed hippocampal sclerosis after 12-year follow-up. Six cases of later epilepsy were identified but all were found to be idiopathic generalized forms, arguing for a genetic mechanism for the development of epilepsy, rather than the epilepsy being a result of a structural change induced by the febrile seizure itself [7]. While prior prospective studies have failed to show a significant epileptogenic potential in patients with prolonged febrile seizures, some retrospective studies have linked a prior history of complex febrile seizures (in particular prolonged events) with temporal lobe epilepsy [26]. The FEBSTAT study is an ongoing prospective study designed to look at just this relationship. The study group reported that the majority of children presenting in febrile status epilepticus were experiencing their initial febrile seizure event, and the group has now established a long-term cohort to examine the possible relationship with mesial temporal sclerosis and temporal lobe epilepsy [27] (Figure 19.1). Interestingly, a neuroimaging study found evidence on magnetic resonance imaging (MRI) that there was subtle evidence of pre-existing hippocampal malformation in those with subsequent development of familial febrile seizures and mesial temporal sclerosis, again arguing for

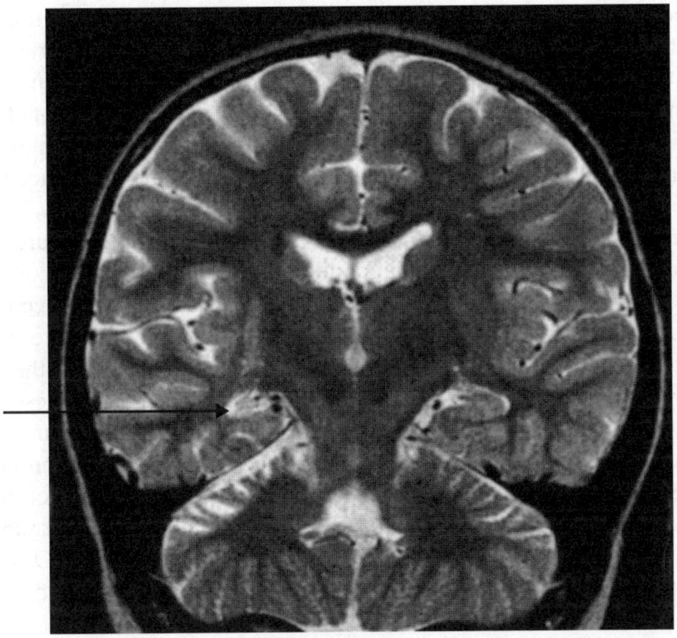

Figure 19.1 Coronal T2-weighted brain magnetic resonance imaging (MRI) scan in a young adult showing typical changes of right-sided mesial temporal sclerosis (the right side of the brain is on the left side of the figure). The hippocampus is atrophic and bright with distorted internal architecture (arrow).

a significant genetic etiological contribution and underscoring the multifactorial nature of seizures [28]. Thus it appears that febrile seizures may represent both a manifestation of epilepsy and a potential cause of said epilepsy syndrome.

19.8 Management in practice

According to data gained from widespread surveys, practice management has changed somewhat over the decades. In the mid-1980s, in a survey that included an estimated 5000 participants including pediatricians, neurologists, child neurologists, general practitioners, and family practitioners, approximately one-third or less of physicians prescribed anticonvulsive medications limited to the time of febrile illness, while most patients with features of complex febrile seizures (i.e., prolonged duration, focal features) were prescribed maintenance antiepileptic drugs or at minimum referred to a child neurologist for further evaluation. In the following decade a survey of Illinois pediatricians revealed that 90% prescribed phenobarbital for regular prophylaxis in the treatment of complex febrile seizures (mean duration of 2 years) and that more than 50% used EEGs to help decide whether or not to prescribe phenobarbital for prophylaxis. A questionnaire given to members of the Child Neurology Society in North America at a similar time showed that prolonged courses of phenobarbital were prescribed for prophylaxis of febrile seizures in 89% of children with complex febrile seizures and in 43% of children with simple febrile seizures. Since more recent practice parameters and guidelines have been published, there has been a decrease in the prophylactic use of antiepileptic drugs following simple febrile seizure, but this does not necessarily carry over to complex febrile seizures as there is a relative paucity of guidelines for complex rather than simple febrile seizures. Furthermore, formal consensus guidelines are needed for those patients with a history of afebrile seizures and neurologically abnormal children presenting with a seizure in the context of fever [25].

In 2006, a retrospective review was conducted to examine the adherence to AAP guidelines among community emergency department physicians. In this review, lumbar puncture was not commonly performed in the majority of patients with febrile seizures (8.4% in children less than 18 months old and 3.3% in children more than 18 months old in the studied population of 1029 patients aged between 6 months and 6 years and meeting the criteria for febrile seizures). Furthermore, the vast majority of those patients were sent home, with an overall rate of admission/transfer of 12%. However, in contrast to the AAP practice parameters, the study identified relatively frequent use of head CT in these patients (11% of the total). A subcohort limited to patients with first-time febrile seizures and non-focal neurological examination ($n = 457$) was matched and compared with previous historical emergency department (ED) cohorts. In this group, rates of lumbar puncture and hospital admission declined slightly in comparison to the historical group, the rate of urine and blood culture was unchanged, and the use of head CT increased [29]. Of note, the study design consisted of a chart review, and a distinction between simple and complex febrile seizures was not made.

19.9 Genetics

Febrile seizures as a group appear to be the consequence of a sophisticated interplay between genetics and environment in which a genetic predisposition for developing febrile seizures at a particular age is inherited, while environmental factors (i.e., fever, infection) influence this inheritance [24]. Advances in genetics have helped elucidate some of the potential familial linkages seen in epilepsy syndromes. To date, more than five genetic mutations have been found to be associated with channelopathies resulting in manifestation of febrile seizures. For instance, the gamma-2 subunit gene of the $GABA_A$ receptor has been implicated in genetic predisposition to febrile seizures by way of mediating synaptic inhibitions [30]. Multiple modes of inheritance in the genetic predisposition to febrile seizures have been implicated and include a suspected polygenic/multifactorial mode of inheritance. The genetic loci differ among families and ethnic backgrounds (Table 19.1). Mutations associated with febrile seizures in Caucasians include *FEB1* on chromosome 8, *FEB2* on chromosome 19, *FEB3* on chromosome 2, *FEB4* on chromosome 5, *FEB5* on chromosome 6, *FEB6* on chromosome 18, *FEB7* on chromosome 21, *FEB8* on chromosome 5, and *FEB9* on chromosome 3. Mutations associated with febrile seizures in Japanese children include *FEB4* and *FEB6*.

There are also specific febrile seizure syndromes for which genetic links have been identified. Generalized epilepsy with febrile seizures (GEFS+) is one such syndrome, which refers to patients with febrile seizures who later go on to develop afebrile seizures. At least five gene mutations have been identified at the time of this writing, including *SCN1A*, *SCN2A*, and *SCN1B*, which encode subunits of the sodium channel, as well as *GABRG2* and *GABRD*, which encode subunits of the $GABA_A$ receptor. Another associated locus has been reported on chromosome 2p24; however, the specific gene has yet to be identified. Severe myoclonic epilepsy of infancy (SMEI), or Dravet syndrome, is an epileptic encephalopathy that first manifests as febrile seizures around 6 months of age, and later develops into a

Table 19.1 Genetic mutations associated with febrile seizures and febrile seizure syndromes.

Chromosomal region	Gene/locus	Population
Febrile seizures		
8q13-q21	*FEB1*	Australia
19p13.3	*FEB2*	United States, China
2q23-q24	*FEB3*	United States, Italy
5q14-q15	*FEB4*	Japan
6q22-q24	*FEB5*	France
18p11	*FEB6*	Japan
21q22	*FEB7*	United States
5q31.1-q33.1	*FEB8*	Belgium
3p24.2-p23	*FEB9*	France
GEFS+		
2q21-q33	*SCN1A*	France
2q24	*SCN2A*	Japan
19q13.1	*SCN1B*	Australia
5q31.1-q33.1	*GABRG2*	France, Australia
1p36.3	*GABRD*	Australia
2p24	Unknown	Belgium

GEFS+, generalized epilepsy with febrile seizures plus.
Reprinted from Brain & Development 31 (2009), Nakayama, Progress in searching for the febrile seizure susceptibility genes, 359–365, © 2009, with permission from Elsevier.

relatively medically refractory epilepsy with multiple afebrile seizures and developmental delay. Some association has been made with *SCN1A* and *GABRG2* mutations, although not in all cases of SMEI [31].

19.10 Parent counseling

As one can imagine, there is significant parental fear and anxiety associated with children who experience febrile seizures, manifest as preoccupation with their child having another seizure or developing epilepsy as well as excessive concern about future fevers. These emotional reactions may lead to negative influences on parental behavior, daily life in the family, and future parent–child relationships due to the parents' perceived "vulnerability" of the child. Parents may also manifest physical reactions as a consequence of their child suffering a febrile seizure. Some commonly reported symptoms include sleep disruption, loss of appetite, and dyspepsia [10]. In general, it may help to provide educational resources in addition to emotional support to the parents of affected patients. Reassurance regarding the generally benign nature of febrile seizures may be of great comfort to parents. Some authors even suggest that in those families who remain quite anxious, intermittent secondary prophylaxis with benzodiazepine such as rectal diazepam may be offered "as a practical therapeutic option" [32]. It is alright for parents to monitor temperatures in children with frequent febrile illnesses, but as previously discussed, there is no evidence that early treatment of increased temperature will actually prevent febrile seizures. In addition, while it is appropriate for parents to consider using antipyretics to treat fevers, febrile seizures frequently occur in the initial stages of illness before signs of illness are apparent; thus parents should be counseled that it is most often not possible to prevent a febrile seizure from occurring [33]. Parents should be counseled on general seizure precautions including recommendations to remain calm during the seizure, to avoid trying to hold the child or stop seizure activity, as well as to not force anything into the child's mouth. Furthermore, reassuring parents that no children have died during a febrile seizure may aid in allaying their fears. As a general rule, parents should be encouraged to bring the child in for evaluation in the case of an initial febrile seizure, and the emergency services should be called if the seizure lasts more than a few minutes in those with recurrent febrile events. Other indications for seeking further medical attention include nausea, vomiting, rash, tremors, abnormal movements, coordination difficulties, altered mentation, drowsiness, irritability, and confusion, occurring either before or after the seizure.

19.11 Conclusion

In summary, febrile seizures are common in the pediatric population. While risk factors including genetic influences should be considered when discussing prognosis, they generally do not portend a lifetime of epilepsy for affected children. There is a relatively high recurrence rate of febrile seizures but otherwise as a group they are considered to follow a benign course. Limited neurodiagnostic workup for simple febrile seizures is recommended according to published practice guidelines, while further studies and recommendations are needed in the evaluation of complex febrile seizures. In general antiepileptic drugs are not recommended for prophylaxis, while antipyretics may be given to make the child more comfortable, though these have no clear role in preventing the recurrence of febrile seizures. As with all clinical decision-making, each child's specific circumstance should be considered. Appropriate education, emotional support, and reassurance are key when discussing febrile seizures with the parents of affected children.

References

[1] Nelson KB, Ellenberg JH. Predictors of epilepsy in children who have experienced febrile seizures. *N Engl J Med* 1976;**295**:1029–1033.
[2] ILAE. Guidelines for epidemiologic studies on epilepsy. *Epilepsia* 1993;**34**:592–596.
[3] Baumann RJ. Technical report: treatment of the child with simple febrile seizures. *Pediatrics* 1999;**103**:e86.
[4] Berg AT, Shinnar S. Complex febrile seizures. *Epilepsia* 1996;**37**:126–133.
[5] Shinnar S, O'Dell C. Profiles in seizure management. In: Leppik IE (ed.), *Managing Febrile Seizures in Young Children and Epilepsy in the Elderly*. Princeton Media Associates, 2003; pp. 3–15.
[6] Waruiru C, Appleton R. Febrile seizures: an update. *Arch Dis Child* 2004;**89**:751–756.
[7] Knudsen F. Febrile seizures: treatment and prognosis. *Epilepsia* 2000;**41**:2–9.
[8] Shanhope JM, Brody JA, Brink E, Morris CE. Convulsions among the Cahmorro people of Guam, Mariana Islands. II. Febrile convulsions. *Am J Epidemiol* 1972;**95**:299–304.
[9] Applegate MS, Lo W. Febrile seizures: current concepts concerning prognosis and clinical management. *J Fam Pract* 1989;**29**:422–428.
[10] Jones T, Jacobsen S. Childhood febrile seizures: overview and implications. *Int J Med Sci* 2007;**4**:110–114.

[11] Shibasaki K, Suzuki M, Mizuno A, Tominaga M. Effects of body temperature on neural activity in the hippocampus: regulation of resting membrane potentials by transient receptor potential vanilloid 4. *J Neurosci* 2007;**27**:1566–1575.

[12] Gatti S, Vezzani A, Bartfai T. Mechanisms of fever and febrile seizures: putative role of interleukin-1 system. In: Baram TZ, Shinnar S (eds), *Febrile Seizures*. San Diego: Academic Press, 2002; pp. 169–188.

[13] Vezzani A, Granata T. Brain inflammation in epilepsy: experimental and clinical evidence. *Epilepsia* 2005;**46**:1724–1743.

[14] Schuchmann S, Schmitz D, Rivera C, *et al.* Experimental febrile seizures are precipitated by a hyperthermia-induced respiratory alkalosis. *Nat Med* 2006;**12**:817–823.

[15] Nelson KB, Ellenberg JH. (1978) Prognosis in children with febrile seizures. *Pediatrics* **61**:720–727.

[16] van Stuijvenberg M, Derksen-Lubsen G, Steyerberg EW, *et al.* Randomized, controlled trial of ibuprofen syrup administered during febrile illness to prevent febrile seizure recurrences. *Pediatrics* 1998;**102**:E51.

[17] Lowenstein DH, Alldredge BK. Status epilepticus. *N Engl J Med* 1998;**338**:970–976.

[18] Warden C, Zibulewsky J, Mace S, Gold C, Gausche-Hill M. Evaluation and management of febrile seizures in the out-of-hospital and emergency department settings. *Ann Emerg Med* 2003;**41**:215–222.

[19] American Academy of Pediatrics. Practice Parameter: The neurodiagnostic evaluation of the child with a first simple febrile seizure. *Pediatrics* 1996;**97**:769–772.

[20] Kimia A, Ben-Joseph EP, Rudloe T, *et al.* Yield of lumbar puncture among children who present with their first complex febrile seizure. *Pediatrics* 2010;**126**:62–69.

[21] Baumann R, Duffner P. Treatment of children with simple febrile seizures: the AAP practice parameter. *Pediatr Neurol* 2000;**23**:11–17.

[22] Farwell JR, Lee JY, Hirtz DG, Sulzbacher SI, Ellenberg JH, Nelson KB. Phenobarbital for febrile seizures: effects on intelligence and seizure recurrence. *N Engl J Med* 1990;**322**:364–369.

[23] American Academy of Pediatrics. Practice Parameter: Febrile seizures: clinical practice guideline for the long-term management of the child with simple febrile seizures. *Pediatrics* 2008;**121**:1281–1286.

[24] Verity CM, Golding J. Risk of epilepsy after febrile convulsions: a national cohort study. *Brit Med J* 1991;**303**:1373–1376.

[25] Annegers JF, Hauser WA, Shirts SB, Kurland LT. Factors prognostic of unprovoked seizures after febrile convulsions. *N Engl J Med* 1987;**316**:493–498.

[26] Dube C, Brewster A, Baram T. Febrile seizures: mechanisms and relationship to epilepsy. *Brain Dev* 2009;**31**:366–371.

[27] Shinnar S, Hesdorffer DC, Nordli DR, *et al.* The FEBSTAT study team. Phenomenology of prolonged febrile seizures: results of the FEBSTAT study. *Neurology* 2008;**71**:170–176.

[28] Fernandez G, Effenberger O, Vinz B, *et al.* Hippocampal malformation as a cause of familial febrile convulsions and subsequent hippocampal sclerosis. *Neurology* 1998;**50**:909–917.

[29] Hampers L, Thompson D, Bajaj L, Tseng B, Rudolph J. Febrile seizure: measuring adherence to AAP guidelines among community ED physicians. *Pediatr Emerg Care* 2006;**22**:465–469.

[30] Kang JQ, Shen W, Macdonald RL. Why does fever trigger febrile seizures? $GABA_A$ receptor gamma2 subunit mutations associated with idiopathic generalized epilepsies have temperature-dependent trafficking deficiencies. *J Neurosci* 2006;**26**:2590–2597.

[31] Nakayama J. Progress in searching for the febrile seizure susceptibility genes. *Brain Dev* 2009;**31**:359–365.

[32] Lux A. Treatment of febrile seizures: historical perspective, current opinions, and potential future directions. *Brain Dev* 2010;**32**:42–50.

[33] Brown L. Febrile seizures. *Curr Treat Option Neurol* 2000;**2**:553–557.

20 Status epilepticus in childhood

Yu-Tze Ng[1] and Rama Maganti[2]

[1]*University of Oklahoma Health Sciences Center and The Children's Hospital, Pediatric Neurology, Oklahoma City, OK, USA*
[2]*Department of Neurology, Barrow Neurological Institute, St Joseph's Hospital and Medical Center, Phoenix, AZ, USA*

Status epilepticus (SE) is the commonest neurological emergency in childhood [1]. Many different types of seizures (including non-convulsive seizures) may present in protracted, refractory fashion even though convulsive status epilepticus is the most common and easily recognizable form. Certainly, it remains a potential life-threatening emergency although the concept of a subset of patients presenting with refractory status epilepticus is probably not well known. Numerous therapies, including medical and non-medical treatments both old and new, continue to be used with efficacy although with suboptimal results at times.

20.1 Definition

The traditional definition is a seizure that persists for a sufficient length of time or is repeated frequently enough that recovery between attacks does not occur [2]. Several authors have defined this duration as seizures that persist for more than 20 to 30 minutes. However, more recent operational definitions advocate a much shorter duration: either continuous seizures lasting at least 5 minutes or two or more discrete seizures between which there is incomplete recovery of consciousness [3,4]. These definitions are somewhat arbitrary;

Epilepsy in Children and Adolescents, First Edition. Edited by James W. Wheless.

however, the definition using the shorter duration is favorable as the earlier that treatment is initiated, the more effective it usually is. The incomplete recovery of consciousness between consecutive seizures typically is due to a postictal state; however, a persistent, ictal, non-convulsive state may not be evident without electroencephalography (EEG). The only completed class I randomized, double-blind study for the treatment of status epilepticus (in adult patients) involved EEG confirmation of cessation of seizures in patients who had stopped convulsing but remained comatose [4].

Refractory status epilepticus is the severe end of the spectrum. The definition of this form of status epilepticus involves a duration of greater than 60 minutes and resistance to therapies [3,5,6]. The seizures persist despite an appropriate treatment, which includes a benzodiazepine, fosphenytoin, or phenobarbital. There are several variant forms of status epilepticus, as described below.

Absence status epilepticus

This form of status epilepticus may be seen in patients with absence epilepsy or other types of idiopathic generalized epilepsy. It may occur *de novo* and has a characteristic EEG pattern [7–9]. The patients although not at baseline are typically not in a comatose state but are in an encephalopathic state with varying degrees of confusion and levels of consciousness and alertness. Minor motor findings such as rhythmic eye blinking and subtle clonic twitching that fluctuates may be present [9]. These symptoms may persist for minutes up to a few days and diagnosis can usually only be made by an EEG during such an episode. The EEG should show a generalized spike or polyspike-and-slow-wave pattern, which may wax and wane.

Complex partial status epilepticus

Complex partial status epilepticus is characterized by confusion and clouding of consciousness of variable degree, and can be associated with automatisms; it is probably relatively more common amongst adult patients [9]. Complex partial status epilepticus can also occur with primarily motor manifestations (tonic, clonic, myoclonic seizures), which are focal and involve loss of awareness.

Epilepsia partialis continua

Epilepsia partialis continua, or Kojewnikoff syndrome, was first described in 1895 [10,11]. The definition does vary between papers, although epilepsia partialis continua refers to clonic muscular twitching repeated at fairly regular short intervals in one part of the body for a prolonged period of time (up to days or even weeks) [11]. This is a form of simple partial seizure status epilepticus and hence by definition, the patient does not experience any loss of awareness. There is no secondary spread of the seizure activity although it may be associated with partial seizures or follow a bout of focal or generalized seizures [11].

Aura continua

This refers to prolonged episodes of sensory symptoms lasting hours to days and is also from the older German literature [12,13]. The term is an appropriate clinical description for this rare subtype of simple partial seizure status epilepticus [13]. As with most simple partial seizure forms, there is often no ictal pattern on scalp EEG monitoring.

Subtle status epilepticus

Initially described by Treiman [14], subtle status epilepticus essentially refers to the phase between convulsive and non-convulsive status epilepticus. Usually it occurs as a progression of untreated or insufficiently treated episodes of convulsive status epilepticus where some (to most) of the motor phenomena are exhausted, but not necessarily all. Minor motor findings may be apparent such as rhythmical twitching of facial or ocular muscles or distal extremities in comatose or at least unresponsive patients.

Status gelasticus

This term refers to a patient with a prolonged cluster of gelastic seizures (i.e., for 20–30 min, a duration similar to that for status epilepticus) [15]. Nearly always this is associated with a congenital lesion, a hypothalamic hamartoma, but not always [16,17].

Non-convulsive status epilepticus

This is a confusing and somewhat more broadly encompassing term. In most patients, untreated convulsive status epilepticus may progress to non-convulsive status epilepticus [9]. Any of the above-mentioned "other forms of status epilepticus" in patients who are either comatose or not, who are not having overt convulsive activity (i.e., excluding epilepsia partialis continua) may be classified under this more encompassing umbrella term. The term "non-convulsive" has been used interchangeably with "subclinical" [18].

Status myoclonicus

Generalized status myoclonicus has been defined as a fixed and enduring state lasting at least 30 minutes and characterized by continuous, generalized, and at times asynchronous rhythmic myoclonic jerks incessantly repeated at a frequency of 1–5 seconds [19]. The critical feature was the presence of rhythmic myoclonic jerks affecting the entire body, lasting at least 30 minutes and occurring in patients with an acute encephalopathy. This definition does not distinguish whether or not the myoclonic activity is epileptic in origin but nevertheless carries a grave prognosis [19].

Psychogenic non-epileptic status or pseudostatus epilepticus

This term is included here for completeness. It applies to patients who have prolonged convulsive movements of psychogenic origin. The first cases were probably reported in 1979 as "status epilepticus: an uncommon hysterical conversion syndrome," a case series of three young adults [20]. Markedly prolonged non-epileptic psychogenic events (non-epileptic psychogenic status) have been reported to occur in 27–78% of those patients with psychogenic non-epileptic seizures [21]. Presumably, the condition "pseudononconvulsive status epilepticus" exists!

20.2 Epidemiology

The incidence rates of convulsive and non-convulsive status epilepticus in children are difficult to ascertain. While most reports come from tertiary care institutions, minimal incidence rates range from 10 to 38/100 000 population [1,22–25]. Studies also showed a bimodal distribution with incidence being highest in children (age 0–4 years) and in the elderly [26]. In a population-based study, SE most commonly occurred in children less than 1 year of age and progressively decreased into the teenage years, both in a community hospital setting and a university hospital setting [27]. Chin *et al.* also found that the incidence of convulsive status epilepticus in childhood is highest among children less than 1 year of age (51/100 000/year) compared to those aged 1–4 (29/100 000/year), 5–9 (9/100 000/year), and 10–15 years (2/100 000/year) [22]. Socioeconomic factors may also play a role as prevalence is found to be higher in children of poor socioeconomic status in developed countries [28]. Similarly, the incidence in developing countries is also reported to be much higher. In one study from Kenya, incidence rates as high as 238/100 000 were reported [29].

Episodes of status epilepticus may be higher in children with pre-existing epilepsy, seen in about 10–20% [30,31]. SE may be the first manifestation of seizures in children who develop epilepsy, seen in up to 30% of cases [22,32,33]. Among children less than 2 years of age, febrile status epilepticus accounts for most cases whereas cryptogenic and remote symptomatic etiologies account for most cases in older children [22,32]. Febrile status epilepticus occurs in up to 5% of all cases of febrile seizures [34].

Incidence and prevalence rates of non-convulsive status epilepticus (NCSE) are difficult to ascertain in children. In one study, mostly consisting of adults, up to 25% of cases with SE were NCSE [8]. Among the critically ill, prevalence is higher in children less than 18 years of age compared to adults [35]. Even among children, NCSE is highest among those who are less than 1 year of age, constituting over 35% of cases [36,37]. Among those who are critically ill and utilizing continuous EEG monitoring, NCSE is detected in up to 33% of children [37]. The prevalence of NCSE is also high among children with prior epilepsy, accounting for up to 70% of cases [38,39].

20.3 Pathophysiology

Status epilepticus may be associated with neuronal loss as well as cognitive/behavioral consequences. Based on the currently available literature, there are several unresolved issues:

1. It is difficult to assess exactly the full spectrum of consequences associated with status epilepticus in humans.
2. It is difficult to extrapolate data from animal studies to humans.
3. It is unclear if the neuronal changes associated with SE are similar in animals and humans with prior epilepsy compared with those who have *de novo* SE.

Evidence of neuronal damage associated with SE comes mostly from animal studies. The earliest studies examined the effects of SE in baboons with generalized convulsive SE [40], which showed neuronal loss both in hippocampi and in neocortical regions. Pathological changes reported in animal models of complex partial SE include neuronal loss in the hippocampus, extrahippocampal structures, and mossy fibers sprouting similar to those seen in human temporal lobe epilepsy [41]. A number of mechanisms have been proposed including activation of glutamate receptors (NMDA type) [42], influx of calcium ions [43], mitochondrial dysfunction, reactive oxygen and nitrogen species, and activation of intracellular proteases and lipases [44], all of which indicate excitotoxicity. Similar changes have been reported in immature brains as well [45]. In contrast, absence status is felt to be a more benign entity with no neuronal loss demonstrated in animal models [46]. The thalamocortical discharges in absence status are dependent on GABAergic mechanisms, whereas limbic epilepsies are dependent on glutaminergic mechanisms, which may explain the fundamental differences in pathophysiology between the two syndromes.

Although the data on animals are robust, evidence of pathological changes associated with convulsive and non-convulsive status epilepticus in humans is largely indirect and anecdotal. In autopsy studies, reduced hippocampal neuronal density was reported among patients who had partial complex SE [47]. Similar observations have been noted in children [48]. Other indirect evidence comes from increased levels of neuron-specific enolase, a marker of neuronal injury, in cerebrospinal fluid of patients who had non-convulsive status epilepticus [49,50]. Moreover, radiological studies demonstrated evidence of neuronal loss on magnetic resonance spectroscopy following SE [51].

20.4 Etiology

The North London Convulsive Status Epilepticus in Childhood Surveillance Study (NL-STEPSS) was the first modern-era prospective study to focus specifically on childhood convulsive status epilepticus [22]. Unlike adult patients, the commonest presentation for a child with status epilepticus is a new-onset seizure [22]. Prolonged febrile seizures were the most common cause, accounting for 32% of total first-ever convulsive status epilepticus episodes in this population of children. Within this group of patients, with febrile status epilepticus, acute bacterial and viral central nervous system infections accounted for 19%, although only one-fifth of this group of patients had acute bacterial meningitis [52]. Subsequent extrapolation of these data by the same group of authors, however, concluded that amongst the group of patients with febrile status epilepticus, the incidence of bacterial meningitis is 15–18%, not surprisingly much higher than the incidence amongst patients with self-limited febrile seizures [53]. There were 176 first-ever episodes out of a total of 304 episodes. Other causes in decreasing order of frequency were: acute symptomatic in 17%, and remote symptomatic in 16%. Twelve percent of patients had previously diagnosed epilepsy (10% idiopathic epilepsy and 2% cryptogenic epilepsy) and finally 7% were of unknown cause [52].

A recent US study of 144 pediatric patients (average age 3.4 years) with new-onset seizures presenting as status epilepticus had similar findings [54]. Thirty-two percent of patients had true febrile status epilepticus, excluding central nervous system infections. Fever was present in a few other patients. Twenty-four percent of patients had acute symptomatic etiologies, which within this group included: a majority with primary central nervous system infection, followed by vascular, electrolyte imbalance, trauma, and toxins. Nearly 18% of patients had symptomatic etiologies, with cerebral dysgenesis and inborn errors of metabolism being the most common, followed by remote vascular and mesiotemporal sclerosis, remote infection, and chromosomal abnormalities [54]. The remaining patients were classified as cryptogenic (29%) or idiopathic (i.e., genetic cause) in 4.2%. Compared to the distribution of seizure type in adult patients' studies, primarily (idiopathic) generalized seizures occurred more often in children, whereas simple partial and secondarily generalized seizures occurred more often in adults [54]. This study had similar rates of prolonged febrile convulsions and acute symptomatic seizures but fewer cases due to remote and idiopathic etiologies and more cases of cryptogenic etiology [22,54].

A practice parameter from the American Academy of Neurology concerning the child with status epilepticus classified the different etiologies as (with the percentages in parentheses): acute symptomatic (26%), remote symptomatic (33%), remote symptomatic with an acute precipitant (1%), progressive encephalopathy (3%), febrile (22%), and cryptogenic (15%) [55].

20.5 Diagnosis and investigations

The AAN practice parameter stated that there are insufficient data to support or refute whether blood cultures or lumbar punctures should be performed routinely in children presenting with status epilepticus [55]. Other tests include blood tests predominantly for electrolytes. Certainly, alcoholism and secondary thiamine deficiency are extremely unlikely causes of status epilepticus in children; however, disturbances of glucose, predominantly hypoglycemia, and other electrolytes are rare but known causes and hence should be investigated. Antiepileptic drug (AED) levels should be considered when a child with epilepsy on AED prophylaxis develops status epilepticus [26]. When electrolytes and other "routine" blood tests are drawn, AED levels should be drawn to potentially confirm partial adherence as a major cause of status epilepticus in this group of patients. Toxicology testing may be considered in children with status epilepticus when no apparent etiology is immediately identified, as the frequency of ingestion of toxic substances as a diagnosis was at least 3.6% [26]. Similar consideration should be given for studies of inborn errors of metabolism, genetic testing, and even EEG [26].

It has been suggested that EEG should be performed in at least two situations. One is when generalized status epilepticus needs to be distinguished from a focal presentation predominantly for prognostic and therapeutic implications. The other is to exclude pseudostatus epilepticus [56]. Pseudoseizures are not as common as in adults and can often be distinguished clinically by someone with significant clinical experience – for more challenging cases video-EEG monitoring may be necessary. We believe the main reason for an EEG is when a patient is no longer convulsing but has yet to rouse significantly, that is, when he or she may be in subtle or non-convulsive status epilepticus. The only class I study ever performed in patients with status epilepticus included a protocol where EEGs were performed on every patient [4].

Finally, neuroimaging should be considered for the evaluation of the child with status epilepticus if there are clinical indications or if the etiology is unknown [55]. Neuroimaging – either computed tomography (CT) or magnetic resonance imaging (MRI) – helped make the diagnosis in 30% and altered the acute management in 24% of patients [54]. CT scans remain more readily available and obtainable and may be performed more quickly without sedation as compared to MRI scans despite the risk of exposing children to radiation and their decreased resolution and sensitivity [57]. Therefore, although CT scans may be and often are used in the emergency setting, MRI is preferred when available [58]. Consideration should be given to performing the MRI study with contrast and diffusion-weighted imaging (DWI) to highlight any focal lesions or infective or inflammatory process, and "DWI positive" lesions may signify specific focal areas of ictal activity.

We would suggest, however, that if the child with epilepsy is presenting with "routine" breakthrough seizuresonly , he or she does not inappropriately receive some form of neuroimaging (usually a CT scan) each time in the emergency room.

20.6 EEG patterns in status epilepticus

The diagnosis of SE is obvious in those with convulsive manifestations but may be difficult in patients with non-convulsive status epilepticus where there are no overt signs of any seizure activity. As there are no clinical or radiographic findings specific to non-convulsive status epilepticus, diagnosis may often rely on EEG findings in these patients. Thus, the EEG remains the gold standard for making this diagnosis among those with non-convulsive status epilepticus. Even among patients with convulsive status epilepticus, as non-convulsive status epilepticus often follows it, EEG is essential in further establishing the diagnosis and monitoring the progression/resolution. In cases of convulsive status epilepticus, EEG can provide prognostic information, and evidence that status epilepticus has ended. In critically ill patients, there may be no clinical manifestations of seizure activity at all, and a high degree of suspicion is required to detect non-convulsive status epilepticus. Moreover, a standard bedside EEG may not detect non-convulsive status epilepticus and continuous EEG monitoring may be required. Studies of continuous EEG monitoring in patients in neurological intensive care units (ICUs) have shown that electrographic seizures occur in 27–34% of patients with encephalopathy/coma [59]. Furthermore, prolonged monitoring is required to make the diagnosis in most cases of unexplained encephalopathy. Pandian *et al.* reported twice as many electrographic seizures captured with continuous EEG monitoring as compared with a routine diagnostic EEG, in a cohort of 105 patients [60].

In ambulatory patients, the most common EEG patterns associated with non-convulsive status epilepticus are generalized spike-and-wave or generalized polyspike-and-wave discharges (in the case of absence status epilepticus), or rhythmic focal discharges (in the case of complex partial status epilepticus) [61]. In contrast, in obtunded or comatose patients, the EEG patterns are more complex and controversial with rhythmic or periodic patterns that do not clearly fall into the "ictal" or "non-ictal" category predominating. These patterns include rhythmic delta activity, generalized triphasic waves, periodic lateralizing epileptiform discharges (PLEDs), generalized periodic epileptiform discharges (GPEDs), bilaterally independent periodic lateralizing epileptiform discharges (BIPLEDs), and stimulus-induced, rhythmic, periodic, or ictal discharges (SIRPIDs) [61,62]. PLEDs have been further divided by some authors into 'PLEDs-proper" and "PLEDs-plus;" and GPEDs have been divided into periodic short-interval diffuse discharges and periodic long-interval diffuse discharges [63,64]. To date, EEG patterns have been better defined in adult patients.

Periodic lateralizing epileptiform discharges (PLEDs)

PLEDs have been the most commonly studied periodic pattern. Chatrian *et al.* first described PLEDs as an EEG finding associated with an acute unilateral forebrain lesion [65]. Initially, it was thought that PLEDs required disconnection between cortical and subcortical structures, but studies have shown that PLEDs can be associated with lesions of the cortical

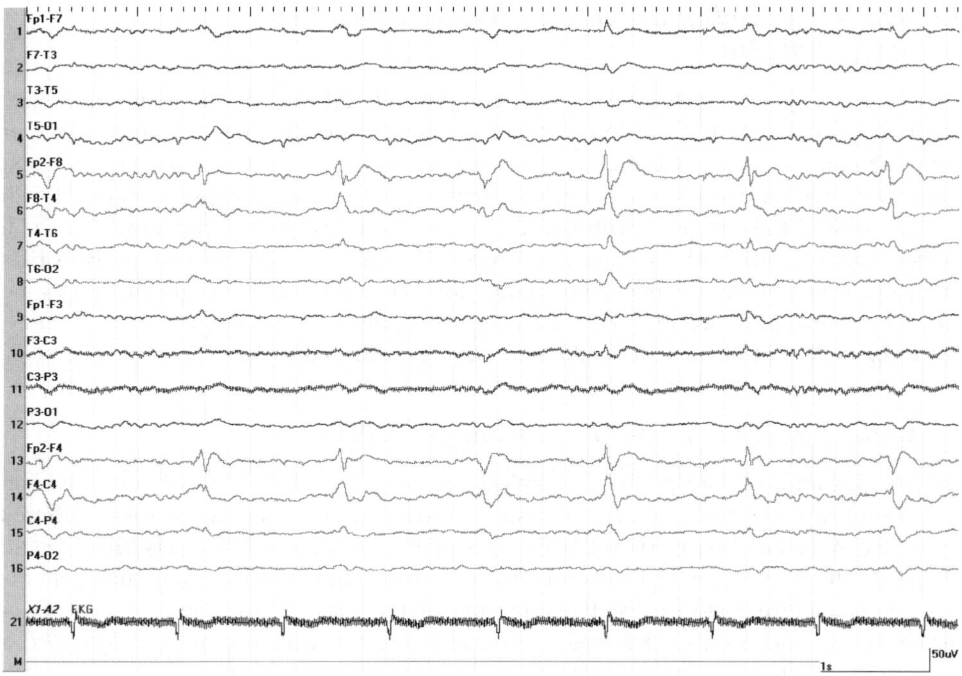

Figure 20.1 Example of periodic lateralized epileptiform discharges in a 14-year-old comatose patient with glioma.

gray matter, subcortical white matter, subcortical gray matter, or a combination of these [66]. In addition, PLEDs have been reported in patients with no focal lesion at all [67] or with chronic brain lesions such as a tumor, infarct, or encephalitis, with or without a superimposed metabolic disturbance [59]. Alcohol withdrawal has been emphasized as an associated factor [68]. Although herpes simplex encephalitis is classically associated with PLEDs, they have been reported with other CNS infections, theophylline toxicity, and with metabolic problems such as non-ketotic hyperglycemia [69]. PLEDs consist of periodic spike-and-slow-wave or sharp-and-slow-wave complexes, typically with a frequency of 1–2 Hz (Figure 20.1). The complexes can be reflected synchronously in the contralateral hemisphere [61]. The incidence of clinical seizures in the acute setting of PLEDs ranges from 58% to 100%; most commonly these are focal motor seizures or epilepsia partialis continua [70]. Whether PLEDs represent a definitively ictal pattern is debated in the literature. PLEDs have been reported to be "time-locked" with focal motor movements; they have also been reported to be associated with a reversible confusional state [59]. Focal changes in blood flow and glucose metabolism have been documented using single-photon emission computed tomography (SPECT) and positron emission tomography (PET), respectively [71,72]. These findings suggest that PLEDs can sometimes be ictal. However, longstanding PLEDs in ambulatory patients without apparent sequelae have been reported [73], so that they can sometimes not be ictal. Although more work is needed in clearly delineating whether PLEDs represent an ictal pattern or an ictal/interictal continuum, we believe that treatment should be individualized among patients depending on the clinical scenario.

Bilaterally independent periodic lateralizing epileptiform discharges (BiPLEDs)

BiPLEDs are, by definition, asynchronous and typically differ in morphology, amplitude, and frequency [61]. There are fewer studies addressing the etiology and significance of BiPLEDs compared with PLEDs. De la Paz and Brenner [74] reported that the most frequent causes were anoxic encephalopathy, CNS infection, and chronic epilepsy. Compared with patients with PLEDs, patients with BiPLEDs were more likely to be comatose and had a higher mortality rate [74]. Fushimi *et al.* reported a case of "benign" chronic BiPLEDs in a patient with bilateral hippocampal infarctions, with mild memory impairment as the only clinical manifestation [75]. BiPLEDs are also highly associated with clinical seizures, occurring in 78% of the patients in the series by de la Paz and Brenner [74].

Generalized periodic epileptiform discharges (GPEDs)

GPEDs (Figure 20.2) are periodic complexes that are bilaterally synchronous, and can have a variety of morphologies. Again, limited data are available, and studies have differed somewhat in their inclusion criteria. In their series of 25 patients with GPEDs, Husain *et al.* included "sharp, slow, and triphasic-like waves," but excluded suppression-burst patterns and continuous triphasic waves. Forty percent of the patients had anoxia and a toxic-metabolic encephalopathy, 28% had a toxic-metabolic encephalopathy, and 32% had a primary neurological process (predominantly seizures and stroke) [76]. Thirty-two percent of patients met criteria for status epilepticus, defined as electrographic seizure activity, tonic-clonic movements, or a positive response to antiepileptic drug treatment either clinically or electrographically. In this group, GPED amplitude, duration, and inter-GPED amplitude were significantly elevated. These patients also had a lower mortality (50%) compared with patients not in status epilepticus (71%). Yemisci *et al.* reported 37 cases of GPEDs; 89.2% of

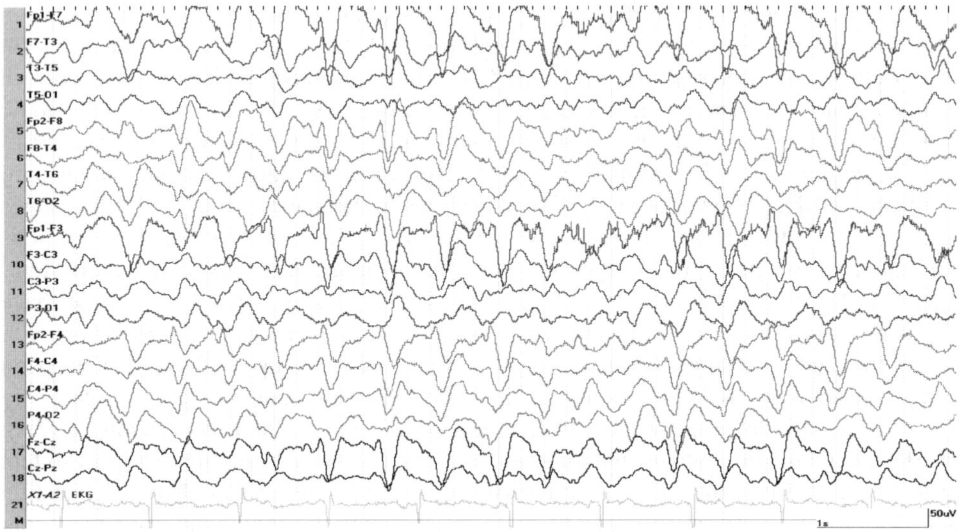

Figure 20.2 Example of generalized periodic epileptiform discharges (GPEDs) in patient with status epilepticus following a craniotomy for brain tumor.

patients had clinical seizures within 48 hours of GPED detection by EEG [77]. Four patients had suppression-burst patterns, 15 had periodic long-interval diffuse discharges (PLIDDs) (interdischarge interval in the range 4–30 s), and 15 had periodic short-interval diffuse discharges (PSIDDs) (interdischarge interval in the range 0.5–4 s). The most common etiology was metabolic and/or infectious disease (59.5%), followed by subacute sclerosing panencephalitis (SSPE) (29.7%) and Creutzfeldt–Jakob disease (10.8%). Three patients had hypoxic encephalopathy after cardiac arrest. SSPE was more commonly seen in patients with PLIDDs, whereas metabolic/infectious disease and Creutzfeldt–Jakob disease were more common in patients with PSIDDs. One-month mortality was 53.3% for PSIDDs, 20% for PLIDDs, and 100% for suppression-burst patterns. Classically, three conditions are recognized as being associated with GPEDs: SSPE, Creutzfeldt–Jakob disease, and anoxia [66]. SSPE is typically associated with PLIDDs, whereas Creutzfeldt–Jakob disease is typically associated with PSIDDs (although not in cases of new-variant disease). In the setting of anoxic injury, GPEDs are universally associated with a poor prognosis [76,77].

Stimulus-induced rhythmic, periodic, or ictal discharges (SIRPIDs)

SIRPIDs are the most recently described periodic EEG pattern [62]. They are defined as "periodic, rhythmic or ictal-appearing discharges . . . consistently induced by alerting stimuli." Of 150 consecutive, critically ill patients undergoing continuous EEG monitoring, 22% were found to have SIRPIDs. The stimulus-induced pattern was PEDs (including GPEDs, PLEDs, BIPLEDs, and triphasic waves) in 64%; 54% of patients showed evolving patterns that met criteria for "ictal discharges." Frontal rhythmic delta activity was present in 42%. Fifty-two percent of patients exhibited more than one pattern. Seventy-three percent of patients had an acute brain injury. Fifty-two percent had either clinical or subclinical seizures at some time during their illness, in addition to SIRPIDs. Clinical status epilepticus (but not isolated clinical seizure activity) was more frequent in patients with focal or ictal-appearing SIRPIDs compared with patients without SIRPIDs. The authors concluded that "further research is necessary to determine the pathophysiologic, prognostic, and therapeutic significance of SIRPIDs."

Triphasic waves (TWs)

Generalized triphasic waves (TWs) consist of an initial small negative phase, a larger positive phase (usually with the largest amplitude of the three), followed by a final negative phase. The waveforms typically have a duration of 0.25–0.5 s. A phase lag, either anterior to posterior or posterior to anterior, can be seen in the longitudinal bipolar montage. TWs can appear in a periodic or quasiperiodic pattern at 0.5- to 1-second intervals [78]. "Typical" TWs have been distinguished as bilaterally synchronous, symmetric, medium- to high-voltage TWs occurring in rhythmical trains at 1.5–2.5 Hz [79]. However, other authors consider this an unimportant distinction. Although "TWs" is the term usually used to imply a pattern of metabolic encephalopathy, this pattern can be indistinguishable from electrographic NCSE, and both NCSE and triphasic waves have been shown to clear with intravenous benzodiazepines [61,66]. It is not clear from the literature when TWs should be considered epileptiform as they may sometimes be indistinguishable from GPEDs. Some authors consider blunted peaks, anteroposterior amplitude gradient, and a time lag as features consistent with TWs, and use these criteria to make the distinction [80].

Others report that focal or bilaterally asymmetric TWs are more likely to be epileptiform [78,81]. A recent series reported improvement in mental status and resolution of TWs with antiepileptic treatment in 11 of 15 patients with focal or bilaterally asymmetric TWs [81]. Boulanger *et al.* reported that TWs associated with metabolic encephalopathies (as opposed to epileptiform discharges in non-convulsive status epilepticus) tend to have a lower frequency, a dominant phase 2 wave, an anterior–posterior lag, and associated diffuse background slowing. Interestingly, they also reported that TWs were seen in response to stimulation in 51% of patients; this puts them in the category of SIRPIDs (see above) [82]. However, this was a retrospective study comparing patients who had been diagnosed with non-convulsive status epilepticus among patients with metabolic encephalopathy. Half of the patients diagnosed with non-convulsive status epilepticus had anoxic injury, which typically produces EEG patterns that are quite distinct from TWs. This may have biased the findings. In summary, to quote Chong and Hirsch, "electroencephalographers should avoid being dogmatic when trying to distinguish metabolic periodic discharges from seizure-related periodic discharges because this distinction is often not possible with EEG alone" [66].

In conclusion, there are a number of EEG patterns that are seen in patients with encephalopathy. Some patterns clearly represent non-convulsive status epilepticus, whereas others are ambiguous. Moreover, different patterns may be seen within the same patient at different times. Thus, further work is needed to clearly define which patterns represent non-convulsive status epilepticus and which patterns do not.

20.7 Treatment

We will discuss the treatment of status epilepticus "sequentially" without specifically separating the treatments for refractory status epilepticus; that is, typically one would begin with more "first-line" conventional treatments before necessarily medically inducing a coma. Treatment should be done in a timely manner, as it is known that the earlier seizures are treated, the better response to the treatment [4,83].

There are a few approved out-of-hospital treatments available that may be administered by family members. Rectal diazepam (Diastat®) at a dose of 0.2–0.5 mg/kg (age dependent) (maximum 20 mg) is one of the most widely available commercial products and arguably best-known treatments. Midazolam administered via buccal and nasal routes has been described and appears safe and effective but is not available as a commercial formulation in the United States [84]. Clonazepam oral disintegrating tablets (Klonopin®=ODT) may be useful for treating seizure clusters and is less costly than rectal diazepam [85]. The dosing regimen for clonazapem is based on the child's size and height – 0.25 mg for a baby, 0.5 mg for a toddler, 1 mg for a child who is as tall as an adult's waist, and 2 mg for one who comes up to an adult's shoulder [85].

The only randomized, double-blind prospective study on the hospital treatment of status epilepticus was performed in adult patients [4]. This study found essentially similar results from four randomized intravenous (i.v.) treatment arms: (i) lorazepam, (ii) phenobarbital, (iii) diazepam and phenytoin, and (iv) phenytoin alone (with the *exception* that lorazepam was more effective than phenytoin alone) (64.9% as compared to 43.6%) [28].

A suggested treatment algorithm is given in Box 20.1 [6,86,87]. The dosing and administration of two of the agents most traditionally used, namely phenobarbital and fosphenytoin,

Box 20.1 Status epilepticus (SE) management algorithm

Out of hospital or no intravenous (i.v.) access available

- Rectal **diazepam (0.3–0.5 mg/kg – age dependent)** or
- Buccal or intranasal **midazolam (0.2 mg/kg)**

Emergency room/hospital treatment

- Check ABCs (airway, breathing, circulation), give oxygen
- Obtain i.v. access – check bedside glucose
- Begin EEG monitoring, avoid hyperthermia, hypo- or hyperglycemia
- Testing (individualize): bedside glucose, electrolytes, magnesium, phosphate, hematology, liver function tests, toxicology, cultures, antiepileptic drug levels, head CT (if <2 years, consider vitamin B6 100 mg i.v.)
- **Lorazepam 0.1 mg/kg** (max. 6 mg) over 2–3 min (allow 5 min to see if seizure stops). If seizure continues:
  - **Fosphenytoin 25–30 mg phenytoin equivalent (PE)/kg** at maximum rate of 3 mg/kg/min (max. 150 mg PE/min). (If unavailable, phenytoin 25–30 mg/kg at 1 mg/kg/min (max. 50 mg/min)).

If seizure continues 10 minutes after fosphenytoin (phenytoin) infusion then prepare to begin anesthetic agents (pharmacological coma initiation).

Admit to pediatric intensive care unit (PICU)

- Prepare to secure airway, mechanically ventilate, obtain central venous access and continuous hemodynamic monitoring (arterial line)
- EEG monitoring to assess response
- **Midazolam 0.2 mg/kg** bolus (max. 10 mg) over 2 min then infuse 0.1 mg/kg/h. (May repeat bolus × 2 if needed, titrate midazolam to max. infusion dose of 2–3 mg/kg/h (or as tolerated)
- If seizures continue:
  - **Pentobarbital 3–5 mg/kg** bolus, then infuse 0.3–3 mg/kg/h (max. dose 10 mg/kg/h)
  - (Consider addition of valproic acid, levetiracetam, lacosamide, or topiramate)
- Continue anesthetic agents for 24–48 h after last seizure, EEG goal of burst-suppression
- Check medicine levels

are extremely straightforward. The loading and administered doses of both medications correspond to the desired serum levels approximately. Hence a loading dose of 20 mg/kg of fosphenytoin and 20–30 mg/kg of phenobarbital should result in levels of around 20 mg/dL and 20–30 mg/dL, respectively. Furthermore, if a child has a serum level of 10 mg/dL of either of these drugs and you wish to obtain a desired level of 20 mg/dL, a further 10 mg/dL should be administered. Two newer non-anesthetic intravenous agents are valproic acid and levetiracetam. Anecdotal studies on the use of valproic acid in children with status epilepticus have reported efficacy of between 70 and 100% with loading doses of 20 to 40 mg/kg. We favor reserving the use of this agent for spike-wave stupor status epilepticus, non-convulsive (absence) status epilepticus, and in the treatment of status migranosus. A prospective study involving 30 children between the ages of 6 months and 14 years demonstrated the safety of an intravenous levetiracetam loading dose of 50 mg/kg (maximum 2500 mg) over 20 minutes [87]. These results are supported by another larger prospective intravenous levetiracetam safety study in children and adults [88].

Refractory status epilepticus

Anesthetic agents are the next line of treatment, if necessary. These involve sedation and medically induced coma requiring intubation, mechanical ventilation, and at times inotropic support in the intensive care. At this stage of treatment, continuous EEG monitoring is necessary. Traditionally a burst-suppression pattern is targeted without a specified ratio of burst to suppression. Intravenous midazolam may be used to induce coma, and a meta-analysis of 111 children indicated that midazolam was effective with low mortality [89]. Dosing has been suggested with an initial bolus of 0.1–0.5 mg/kg followed by an infusion of 1–2 μg/kg/min up to a maximum of 30 μg/kg/min [90]. Pentobarbital is an intravenous anesthetic barbiturate that is also commonly used in this setting. Studies suggest that pentobarbital is effective and induces a suppression pattern on EEG quickly but has complications of hypotension. The initial bolus is 5 mg/kg followed by an infusion rate of 1 mg/kg/h (maximum 3 mg/kg/h) [90].

Propofol is used relatively commonly in adult patients but rarely in children because of safety concerns. A Dutch study looked retrospectively at results from 33 patients with refractory status epilepticus [91]. These patients with status epilepticus all failed to respond to phenytoin and midazolam and had been seizing for more than 60 minutes. Propofol at a loading dose of 1–2 mg/kg then 1–2 mg/kg/h (up to 5 mg/kg/h) in 22 episodes was compared to thiopental dosed to a level of 20 mg/mL. Seizure control occurred in 14/22 (64%) of the propofol-treated group as compared to 11/20 (55%) in the thiopental group. Although there were no deaths attributed to propofol and two deaths were felt to be related to thiopental (eight children in total did die from this group of children with refractory status epilepticus), four patients discontinued propofol therapy – due to rhabdomyolysis in one and increased triglycerides in three. These complications completely resolved following the discontinuation. The authors' conclusion was that propofol is fast acting, has reversible complications, and is probably safe if used at a dose of less than 5 mg/kg/h [91]. The propofol infusion syndrome is a rare, fatal syndrome resulting in cardiac failure, rhabdomyolysis, renal failure, and severe metabolic acidosis. In a series of 21 pediatric and 14 adult cases, there were five deaths in children aged between 4 weeks and 6 years [92]. Propofol impairs free fatty acid utilization and mitochondrial activity, leading to cardiac and peripheral muscle necrosis [93,94]. However, propofol is a seemingly effective therapy that may be an appropriate option if used with caution (particularly if used for more than 48 hours) and at a dose of greater than 5 mg/kg/h with daily testing of muscle enzymes and triglycerides.

Other less conventional treatments include the inhaled anesthetic isoflurane, ketamine, pyridoxine, immunomodulating therapies including corticosteroids, hypothermia, the ketogenic diet, and even electroconvulsive therapy which have guarded results and safety concerns [39].

Neurosurgery has a very limited role as a treatment for refractory status epilepticus [95,96]. Lesional cases are clearly relatively more straightforward; non-lesional surgery may be performed, but usually requires invasive monitoring or other initial testing. Nevertheless surgical options, even other than resection – e.g. multiple subpial transections (MSTs) for eloquent cortex – should be considered, and not necessarily only as a last resort. Prolonged medical management is associated with other complications, such as hypotension, myocardial and respiratory depression, and increased risks of infection and poikilothermia. Delaying surgery may be an option for patients whose status epilepticus is controlled with medication. Surgical intervention should be considered earlier in the course of refractory status epilepticus. There has been a recent gradual overall increase in the awareness and consideration for this form of therapy but it is probably still underutilized [97].

20.8 Prognosis

Outcomes have improved over the last three decades. Whereas earlier studies had shown a mortality rate of 11% in children younger than 15 years, more recent studies report rates of only 5% and 2% in patients less than 1 year and 1 to 19 years of age, respectively [98]. Case fatality for first-time episodes of convulsive status epilepticus was 3% in a north London study [22]. In a systematic review of available outcome studies, short-term mortality after convulsive status epilepticus was as low as 2.7%, but with intensive care unit children only mortality was between 5% and 8% [99], confirming that cases of refractory status epilepticus are different. Long-term complications other than death include secondary epilepsy, cognitive and behavioral problems, and focal neurological deficits, which may affect 15–50% of children [98].

References

[1] Chin RF, Verhulst L, Neville BG, *et al.* Inappropriate emergency management of status epilepticus in children contributes to need for intensive care. *J Neurol Neurosurg Psychiatry* 2004;**75**:1584–1588.
[2] Proposal for revised clinical and electroencephalographic classification of epileptic seizures. From the Commission on Classification and Terminology of the International League Against Epilepsy. *Epilepsia* 1981;**22**:489–501.
[3] Lowenstein DH, Alldredge BK. Status epilepticus. *N Engl J Med* 1998;**338**:970–976.
[4] Treiman DM, Meyers PD, Walton NY, *et al.* A comparison of four treatments for generalized convulsive status epilepticus. Veterans Affairs Status Epilepticus Cooperative Study Group. *N Engl J Med* 1998;**339**:792–798.
[5] Sahin M, Menache CC, Holmes GL, *et al.* Prolonged treatment for acute symptomatic refractory status epilepticus: outcome in children. *Neurology* 2003;**61**:398–401.
[6] Riviello JJ Jr, Holmes GL. The treatment of status epilepticus. *Semin Pediatr Neurol* 2004;**11**:129–138 [review].
[7] Thomas P, Beaumanoir A, Genton P, *et al.* 'De novo' absence status of late onset: report of 11 cases. *Neurology* 1992;**42**:104–110.
[8] Dunne JW, Summers QA, Stewart-Wynne EG. Non-convulsive status epilepticus: a prospective study in an adult general hospital. *Q J Med* 1987;**62**:117–126.
[9] Maganti R, Gerber P, Drees C, *et al.* Nonconvulsive status epilepticus. *Epilepsy Behav* 2008;**12**:572–586 [review].

[10] Koshewnikow AY. Eine besondere Form von corticler Epilepsie. *Neurol Centralbl* 1895;**14**:1895.
[11] Juul-Jensen P, Denny-Brown D. Epilepsia partialis continua. *Arch Neurol* 1996;**15**:563–578.
[12] Wieser HG. Simple partial status epilepticus. In: Engel J, Pedley T (eds), *Epilepsy: a Comprehensive Textbook*. Philadelphia: Lippincott-Raven Press, 1997; pp. 709–723.
[13] Yager JY, Seshia SS. Sublingual lorazepam in childhood serial seizures. *Am J Dis Child* 1993;**142**:931–932.
[14] Treiman DM. Generalized convulsive status epilepticus in the adult. *Epilepsia* 1993;**34**(Suppl. 1):S2–11.
[15] Ng YT, Rekate HL. Coining of a new term, "Status Gelasticus". *Epilepsia* 2006;**47**:661–662.
[16] Kerrigan JF, Ng YT, Chung S, *et al.* The hypothalamic hamartoma: a model of subcortical epileptogenesis and encephalopathy. *Sem Pediatr Neurol* 2005;**12**:119–131 [review].
[17] Pustorino G, Spano M, Sgro DL, *et al.* Status gelasticus associated with levetiracetam as add-on treatment. *Epileptic Disord* 2007;**9**:186–189.
[18] Bauer G, Trinka E. Nonconvulsive status epilepticus and coma. *Epilepsia* 2010;**51**:177–190.
[19] Celesia GG, Grigg MM, Ross E. Generalized status myoclonicus in acute anoxic and toxic-metabolic encephalopathies. *Arch Neurol* 1998;**45**:781–784.
[20] Toone BK, Roberts J. Status epilepticus. An uncommon hysterical conversion syndrome *J Nerv Ment Dis* 1979;**167**:548–552.
[21] Reuber M, Pukrop R, Mitchell AJ, *et al.* Clinical significance of recurrent psychogenic nonepileptic seizure status. *J Neurol* 2003;**250**:1355–1362.
[22] Chin RF, Neville BG, Peckham C, *et al.* Incidence, cause, and short-term outcome of convulsive status epilepticus in childhood: prospective population-based study. *Lancet* 2006;**368**:222–229.
[23] Coeytaux A, Jallon P, Galobardes B, *et al.* The incidence of status epilepticus in French speaking Switzerland. *Neurology* 2000;**55**:693–697.
[24] Hesdorffer DC, Logroscino G, Cascino G, *et al.* Incidence of status epilepticus in Rochester, Minnesota, 1965–1984. *Neurology* 1998;**50**:735–741.
[25] Knake S, Rosenow F, Vescovi M, *et al.*, Status Epilepticus Study Group Hessen (SESGH). Incidence of status epilepticus in adults in Germany: a prospective, population-based study. *Epilepsia* 2001;**42**:714–718.
[26] Govoni V, Fallica E, Monetti VC, *et al.* Incidence of status epilepticus in southern Europe: a population study in the health district of Ferrara, Italy. *Eur Neurol* 2008;**59**:120–126.
[27] DeLorenzo RJ, Kirmani B, Deshpande LS, *et al.* Comparisons of the mortality and clinical presentations of status epilepticus in private practice community and university hospital settings in Richmond, Virginia. *Seizure* 2009;**18**:405–411.
[28] DeLorenzo RJ, Hauser WA, Towne AR, *et al.* A prospective, population-based epidemiologic study of status epilepticus in Richmond, Virginia. *Neurology* 1996;**46**:1029–1035.
[29] Sadarangani M, Seaton C, Scott JA, *et al.* Incidence and outcome of convulsive status epilepticus in Kenyan children: a cohort study. *Lancet Neurol* 2008;**7**:145–150.
[30] Sillanpää M, Shinnar S. Status epilepticus in a population-based cohort with childhood-onset epilepsy in Finland. *Ann Neurol* 2002;**52**:303–310.
[31] Berg AT, Shinnar S, Testa FM, *et al.* Status epilepticus after the initial diagnosis of epilepsy in children. *Neurology* 2004;**63**:1027–1034.
[32] Shinnar S, Pellock JM, Moshé SL, *et al.* In whom does status epilepticus occur: age-related differences in children. *Epilepsia* 1997;**38**:907–914.
[33] Berg AT, Levy SR, Novotny EJ, *et al.* Predictors of intractable epilepsy in children: A case-control study. *Epilepsia* 1996;**37**:24–30.
[34] Ahmad S, Marsh ED. Febrile status epilepticus: current state of clinical and basic research. *Semin Pediatr Neurol* 2010;**17**:150–154.
[35] Claassen J, Mayer SA, Kowalski RG, *et al.* Detection of electrographic seizures with continuous EEG monitoring in critically ill patients. *Neurology* 2004;**62**:1743–1748 [review].

[36] Hosain SA, Solomon GE, Kobylarz EJ. Electroencephalographic patterns in unresponsive pediatric patients. *Pediatr Neurol* 2005;**32**:162–165.
[37] Tay SK, Hirsch LJ, Leary L, *et al.* Nonconvulsive status epilepticus in children: clinical and EEG characteristics. *Epilepsia* 2006;**47**:1504–1509.
[38] Jette N, Claassen J, Emerson RG, *et al.* Frequency and predictors of nonconvulsive seizures during continuous electroencephalographic monitoring in critically ill children. *Arch Neurol* 2008;**63**:1750–1755.
[39] Abend NS, Dlugos DJ. Treatment of refractory status epilepticus: literature review and a proposed protocol. *Pediatr Neurol* 2008;**38**:377–390 [review].
[40] Meldrum BS, Brierley JB. Neuronal loss and gliosis in the hippocampus following repetitive epileptic seizures induced in adolescent baboons by allylglycine. *Brain Res* 1972;**48**:361–365.
[41] Hosford DA. Animal models of nonconvulsive status epilepticus. *J Clin Neurophysiol* 1999;**16**:306–313.
[42] Fountain NB, Lothman EW. Pathophysiology of status epilepticus. *J Clin Neurophysiol* 1995;**12**:326–342.
[43] Pal S, Sombati S, Limbrick DD, *et al.* In vitro status epilepticus causes sustained elevation of intracellular calcium levels in hippocampal neurons. *Brain Res* 1999;**851**:20–31.
[44] Jope RS, Johnson GV, Baird MS. Seizure-induced protein tyrosine phosphorylation in rat brain regions. *Epilepsia* 1991;**32**:755–760.
[45] Sankar R, Shin DH, Liu H, *et al.* Patterns of status epilepticus-induced neuronal injury during development and long-term consequences. *J Neurosci* 1998;**18**:8382–8393.
[46] Nehlig A, de Vasconcelos AP. The model of pentylenetetrazol-induced status epilepticus in the immature rat: short- and long-term effects. *Epilepsy Res* 1996;**26**:93–103.
[47] DeGiorgio CM, Gott PS, Rabinowicz AL, *et al.* Neuron-specific enolase, a marker of acute neuronal injury, is increased in complex partial status epilepticus. *Epilepsia* 1996;**37**:606–609.
[48] Tsuchida TN, Barkovich AJ, Bollen AW, *et al.* Childhood status epilepticus and excitotoxic neuronal injury. *Pediatr Neurol* 2007;**36**:253–257.
[49] Rabinowicz AL, Correale JD, Bracht KA, *et al.* Neuron-specific enolase is increased after nonconvulsive status epilepticus. *Epilepsia* 1995;**36**:475–479.
[50] O'Regan ME, Brown JK. Serum neuron specific enolase: a marker for neuronal dysfunction in children with continuous EEG epileptiform activity. *Eur J Paediatr Neurol* 1998;**2**:193–197.
[51] Lazeyras F, Blanke O, Zimine I, *et al.* MRI, 1H-MRS, and functional MRI during and after prolonged nonconvulsive seizure activity. *Neurology* 2000;**55**:1677–1682.
[52] Neville BG, Chin RF, Scott RC. Childhood convulsive status epilepticus: epidemiology, management and outcome. *Acta Neurol Scand Suppl* 2007;**186**:21–24 [review].
[53] Chin RF, Neville BG, Scott RC. Meningitis is a common cause of convulsive status epilepticus with fever. *Arch Dis Child* 2005;**90**:66–69.
[54] Singh RK, Stephens S, Berl MM, *et al.* Prospective study of new-onset seizures presenting as status epilepticus in childhood. *Neurology* 2010;**74**:636–642.
[55] Riviello JJ Jr, Ashwal S, Hirtz D, *et al.*, American Academy of Neurology Subcommittee, Practice Committee of the Child Neurology Society. Practice parameter: diagnostic assessment of the child with status epilepticus (an evidence-based review): report of the Quality Standards Subcommittee of the American Academy of Neurology and the Practice Committee of the Child Neurology Society. *Neurology* 2006;**67**:1542–1550 [review].
[56] Scott RC, Kirkham FJ. Clinical update: childhood convulsive status epilepticus. *Lancet* 2007;**370**:724–726 [review].
[57] Gaillard WD, Chiron C, Cross JH, *et al.*, ILAE, Committee for Neuroimaging, Subcommittee for Pediatric. Guidelines for imaging infants and children with recent-onset epilepsy. *Epilepsia* 2009;**50**:2147–2153.
[58] Freilich ER, Zelleke T, Gaillard WD. Identification and evaluation of the child in status epilepticus. *Semin Pediatr Neurol* 2010;**17**:144–149 [review].

[59] Jirsch J, Hirsch LJ. Nonconvulsive seizures: developing a rational approach to the diagnosis and management in the critically ill population. *Clin Neurophysiol* 2007;**118**:1660–1670.

[60] Pandian JD, Cascino GD, So EL, *et al.* Digital video-electroencephalographic monitoring in the neurological-neurosurgical intensive care unit: clinical features and outcome. *Arch Neurol* 2004;**61**:1090–1094.

[61] Brenner RP. EEG in convulsive and nonconvulsive status epilepticus. *J Clin Neurophysiol* 2004;**21**:319–331.

[62] Hirsch LJ, Claassen J, Mayer SA, *et al.* Stimulus-induced rhythmic, periodic, or ictal discharges (SIRPIDs): a common EEG phenomenon in the critically ill. *Epilepsia* 2004;**45**:109–123.

[63] Brenner RP, Schaul N. Periodic EEG patterns: classification, clinical correlation, and pathophysiology. *J Clin Neurophysiol* 1990;**7**:249–267.

[64] Reiher J, Rivest J, Grand'Maison F, *et al.* Periodic lateralized epileptiform discharges with transitional rhythmic discharges: association with seizures. *Electroencephalogr Clin Neurophysiol* 1991;**78**:12–17.

[65] Chatrian G-E, Shaw CM, Leffman H. The significance of periodic lateralized epileptiform discharges in EEG: an electrographic, clinical and pathological study. *Electroencephalogr Clin Neurophysiol* 1964;**17**:177–193.

[66] Chong DJ, Hirsch LJ. Which EEG patterns warrant treatment in the critically ill? Reviewing the evidence for treatment of periodic epileptiform discharges and related patterns. *J Clin Neurophysiol* 2005;**22**:79–91.

[67] Garcia-Morales I, Teresa Garcia M, Galan-Davila L, *et al.* Periodic lateralized epileptiform discharges: etiology, clinical aspects, seizures, and evolution in 130 patients. *J Clin Neurophysiol* 2002;**19**:172–177.

[68] Westmoreland BF, Klass DW, Sharbrough FW. Chronic periodic lateralized epileptiform discharges. *Arch Neurol* 1986;**43**:494–496.

[69] Chu NS. Periodic lateralized epileptiform discharges with preexisting focal brain lesions: role of alcohol withdrawal and anoxic encephalopathy. *Arch Neurol* 1980;**37**:551–554.

[70] Yoshikawa H, Abe T. Periodic lateralized epileptiform discharges in children. *J Child Neurol* 2003;**18**:803–805.

[71] Pohlmann-Eden B, Hoch DB, Cochuis JL, *et al.* Periodic lateralized epileptiform discharges: a critical review. *J Clin Neurophysiol* 1996;**13**:519–530.

[72] Handforth A, Cheng JT, Mandelkern MA, *et al.* Markedly increased mesiotemporal lobe metabolism in a case with PLEDs: further evidence that PLEDs are a manifestation of partial status epilepticus. *Epilepsia* 1994;**35**:876–881.

[73] Assal F, Papazyan JP, Slosman DO, *et al.* SPECT in periodic lateralized epileptiform discharges (PLEDs): a form of partial status epilepticus? *Seizure* 2001;**10**:260–264.

[74] De la Paz D, Brenner RP. Bilateral periodic lateralized epileptiform discharges: clinical significance. *Arch Neurol* 1981;**38**:713–715.

[75] Fushimi M, Matsubuchi N, Sekine A, *et al.* Benign bilateral independent periodic lateralized epileptiform discharges. *Acta Neurol Scand* 2003;**108**:55–59.

[76] Husain AM, Mebust KA, Radtke RA. Generalized periodic epileptiform discharges: etiologies, relationship to status epilepticus, and prognosis. *J Clin Neurophysiol* 1999;**16**:51–58.

[77] Yemisci M, Gurer G, Saygi S, *et al.* Generalised periodic epileptiform discharges: clinical features, neuroradiological evaluation and prognosis in 37 adult patients. *Seizure* 2003;**12**:465–472.

[78] Fisch BJ. Electrographic seizure patterns, pseudoperiodic patterns, and pseudoepileptiform patterns. In: Fisch BJ, Spehlmann R (eds), *EEG Primer: Basic Principles of Digital and Analog EEG*. Amsterdam: Elsevier, 1999; pp. 307–348.

[79] Bauer G. Coma and brain death. In: Niedermayer E, Da Silva FL (eds), *Electroencephalography: Basic Principles, Clinical Applications and Related Fields*. Baltimore: Lippincott Williams & Wilkins, 2005; pp. 471–487.

[80] Kaplan PW, Birbeck G. Lithium-induced confusional states: nonconvulsive status epilepticus or triphasic encephalopathy? *Epilepsia* 2006;**47**:2071–2074.

[81] Kaya D, Bingol CA. Significance of atypical triphasic waves for diagnosing nonconvulsive status epilepticus. *Epilepsy Behav* 2007;**11**:567–577.

[82] Boulanger JM, Deacon C, Lécuyer D, *et al.* Triphasic waves versus nonconvulsive status epilepticus: EEG distinction. *Can J Neurol Sci* 2006;**33**:175–180.

[83] Shinnar S, Berg AT, Moshe SL, *et al.* How long do new-onset seizures in children last? *Ann Neurol* 2001;**49**:659–664.

[84] Scott RC, Besag FM, Neville BG. Buccal midazolam and rectal diazepam for treatment of prolonged seizures in childhood and adolescence: a randomised trial. *Lancet* 1999;**353**:623–626.

[85] Troester MM, Hastriter EV, Ng YT. Dissolving oral clonazepam wafers in the acute treatment of prolonged seizures. *J Child Neurol* 2010;**25**:1468–1472.

[86] Venkataraman V, Wheless JW. Safety of rapid intravenous infusion of valproate loading doses in epilepsy patients. *Epilepsy Res* 1999;**35**:147–153.

[87] Ng YT, Hastriter EV, Cardenas JF, *et al.* Intravenous levetiracetam in children with seizures: a prospective safety study. *J Child Neurol* 2010;**25**:551–555.

[88] Wheless JW, Clarke D, Hovinga CA, *et al.* Rapid infusion of a loading dose of intravenous levetiracetam with minimal dilution: a safety study. *J Child Neurol* 2009;**24**:946–951.

[89] Gilbert DL, Gartside PS, Glauser TA. Efficacy and mortality in treatment of refractory generalized convulsive status epilepticus in children: a meta-analysis. *J Child Neurol* 1999;**14**:602–609.

[90] Abend NS, Gutierrez-Colina AM, Dlugos DJ. Medical treatment of pediatric status epilepticus. *Semin Pediatr Neurol* 2010;**17**:169–175 [review].

[91] van Gestel JP, Blussé van Oud-Alblas HJ, Malingré M, *et al.* Propofol and thiopental for refractory status epilepticus in children. *Neurology* 2005;**65**:591–592.

[92] Vasile B, Rasulo F, Candiani A, *et al.* The pathophysiology of propofol infusion syndrome: a simple name for a complex syndrome. *Intensive Care Med* 2003;**29**:1417–1425.

[93] Parke TJ, Stevens JE, Rice AS, *et al.* Metabolic acidosis and fatal myocardial failure after propofol infusion in children: five case reports. *Brit Med J* 1992;**305**:613–616.

[94] Hanna JP, Ramundo ML. Rhabdomyolysis and hypoxia associated with prolonged propofol infusion in children. *Neurology* 1998;**50**:301–303.

[95] Ng YT, Kerrigan JF, Rekate HL. Neurosurgical treatment of status epilepticus. *J Neurosurg (Pediatrics)* 2006;**105**:378–381.

[96] Ng YT, Bristol RE, Schrader DW, *et al.* The role of neurosurgery in status epilepticus. *Neurocrit Care* 2007;**7**:86–91.

[97] Vendrame M, Loddenkemper T. Surgical treatment of refractory status epilepticus in children: candidate selection and outcome. *Semin Pediatr Neurol* 2010;**17**:182–189 [review].

[98] Arzimanoglou A. Outcome of status epilepticus in children. *Epilepsia* 2007;**48**(Suppl. 8):91–93 [review].

[99] Raspall-Chaure M, Chin RF, Neville BG, *et al.* Outcome of paediatric convulsive status epilepticus: a systematic review. *Lancet Neurol* 2006;**5**:769–779.

Index

Epilepsy in Children and Adolescents, First Edition. Edited by James W. Wheless.